The OMAHA SYSTEM

A Key to Practice, Documentation, and Information Management

CONTENTS

The OMAHA SYSTEM

A Key to Practice, Documentation, and Information Management

KAREN S. MARTIN, RN, MSN, FAAN
Health Care Consultant
Omaha, Nebraska

REPRINTED SECOND EDITION

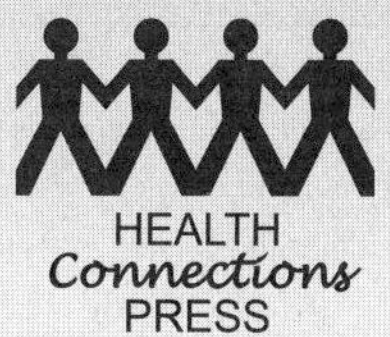

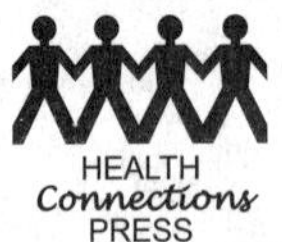

www.healthconnectionspress.com

THE OMAHA SYSTEM: A KEY TO PRACTICE, DOCUMENTATION, AND INFORMATION MANAGEMENT, REPRINTED SECOND EDITION

ISBN: 978-0-9825727-1-9
LCCN: 2009943955

Health Connections Press reprinted and reissued this book after Elsevier, Inc. transferred the copyright to Karen S. Martin in 2009. The content and page numbers are identical to the book initially published by Elsevier, Inc. in 2005; the covers have been revised and include the new publisher's name and logo. To reference this book, use: Martin KS. (2005). *The Omaha System: A Key to Practice, Documentation, and Information Management* (Reprinted 2nd ed.). Omaha, NE: Health Connections Press.

Out of Print Titles

- *The Omaha System: Applications for Community Health Nursing,* 1992, Saunders, ISBN 0-7216-6126-2
- *The Omaha System: A Pocket Guide for Community Health Nursing,* 1992, Saunders, ISBN 0-7216-6123-8
- *The Omaha System: A Key to Practice, Documentation, and Information Management,* 2005, Elsevier ISBN 0-7216-0130-4

Printed in the USA
10 9 8 7 6 5 4

CONTRIBUTORS and REVIEWERS

CONTRIBUTORS

Kathryn H. Bowles, RN, PhD
Associate Professor
School of Nursing
University of Pennsylvania
Philadelphia, Pennsylvania
Chapter 5 *Use of the Omaha System in Research*

Victoria L. Elfrink, RNBC, PhD
Senior Associate, iTelehealth, Inc.
Frederick, Maryland
Adjunct Professor, UNITEC Polytechnic Institute
Auckland, New Zealand
Chapter 4 *Use of the Omaha System in Education*

Karen A. Monsen, RN, MS
Program Manager
Washington County Department of Public Health and Environment
Stillwater, Minnesota
Chapter 3 *Use of the Omaha System in Practice*

REVIEWERS

Jean R. Christensen, RN, RHV, BSc (Hons)
Project Manager, National Service Framework for Children
Young People and Maternity Services
Welsh Assembly Government, Cathays Park
Cardiff, Wales, United Kingdom

Debra J. Konicek, RN, MSN, BC
Terminology Manager, Nursing, SNOMED® International
College of American Pathologists
Northfield, Illinois

David L. Rosebaugh, BS, MURP
Chief Executive Officer, CHAMP Software, Inc.
Mankato, Minnesota

FOREWORD

More than three decades ago, there was a dream at the Visiting Nurse Association of Omaha, a dream that it was possible to develop a better way to describe the care that patients needed and nurses provided. Although nurses understood the dimensions of care, they did not have a verbal or written method to describe those dimensions. The diagnoses captured by the International Classification of Diseases and the treatments captured by the Current Procedural Terminology, as well as the various definitions of skilled nursing care, were not sufficient, especially since home visits and community practice were involved.

A group of nurses who were managing and delivering daily care began to devise a classification that could more adequately describe care. This classification would become standardized so that care could be quantified to support clinical decision-making, clinical management, financial management, quality improvement, and research. Although it was unusual to have such leadership originate from a health care service organization, the Visiting Nurse Association of Omaha began the process of building a system that would change the way care was provided and documented. Suggestions were elicited from administrators, and practitioners employed by many agencies throughout the United States. The Visiting Nurse Association of Omaha wrote proposals for development and testing that were funded by the Division of Nursing, U.S. Department of Health and Human Services. I had the opportunity to serve on the national advisory committee for this project, a most exciting appointment. Dr. Avedis Donabedian, the guru of quality assurance, and others were members of this advisory committee. The thrill of being a small part of the "Omaha System" development remains with me as I observe the current expansion and use of the Omaha System around the world.

Twice during my tenure as a dean, I supported the selection of the Omaha System as the basis for a clinical information system. First, under the leadership of Dr. Sally Lundeen, the University of Wisconsin-Milwaukee College of Nursing implemented an extensive information system for clients in a community-based nurse managed center. That center and its information system continue to thrive and expand. The center's practitioners, students, and programs are described in this book. Data generated by the information system contributed to the nursing center's ability to secure federal research funds, and to conduct research that investigated the delivery of care. Later, while dean at the University of Pennsylvania School of Nursing, one of the school-owned practices sought a computerized information system for the care of frail elders. Dr. Lois Evans and other key leaders selected the Omaha System as the terminology to be incorporated in the information system. In addition, several nurse researchers recognized that the Omaha System provided a way to classify and quantify problems, interventions, and outcomes of care from extensive narrative patient records. A number of their research projects were funded.

The uniqueness of the Omaha System is that it combines problems, actions, and outcomes in a set of terms that is manageable in size and can be easily understood and used by various health care professionals. This new edition provides relevant examples and descriptions of the national and international application of the Omaha System in ever-expanding settings. The goal for the next decade should be to increase the use of the terminology with clinical and administrative practice, decision support, financial reimbursement, quality improvement, and health care policy. This book is a major contribution to that goal.

Norma M. Lang, RN, PhD, FRCN, FAAN
Lillian S. Brunner Professor of Nursing
School of Nursing, University of Pennsylvania
Philadelphia, Pennsylvania

Florence Nightingale once wrote, "If you find it helps you to note down such things on a bit of paper with a pencil, by all means do so" (Nightingale, 1860, p. 112). Nightingale was right to recognise that nurses needed to document their observations, but more than a century later, the "bit of paper with a pencil" is not enough. Computers are everywhere. Although computers are less flexible, they can store, aggregate, and manipulate vast quantities of data, making data available in different formats and for multiple purposes.

Whether documentation is computerised or paper-based, it must be carefully structured to be useful, and, if it is to be meaningful to other readers, it must be expressed in a standardised language. Without a language to describe what nurses observe, diagnose, plan, and do, nursing remains largely invisible to the rest of the world. Nursing's contribution to care goes unrecorded, unrecognised, and therefore is under-valued. Too often, nurses must use a documentation system to meet today's legal and administrative requirements. However, if nurses also capture the clinical decisions that are the core of their professional practice, their documentation ceases to be just an "end of shift chore." It becomes a valuable resource for communicating and sharing care with other health professionals; providing data for service planning, quality improvement, and resource management; guiding educational curricula; providing data for research; and articulating the knowledge base of nursing which Benner (1984, p. 36) described as "embedded in clinical practice."

I first heard about the Omaha System in 1992 when I was working on the International Council of Nurses' project to develop an International Classification for Nursing Practice. One of our early tasks was to identify and review the existing terminologies. The Omaha System was among those already recognised by the American Nurses Association. It struck me that this System had advantages over the others. In particular, the Omaha System's problem-oriented structure enabled interventions to be linked directly to problems and, by measuring change, enabled the identification and measurement of outcomes.

Later, when I was seeking a system to help community health nurses in the United Kingdom document their practice and identify their outcomes, we chose the Omaha

System, and *The Omaha System: Applications for Community Health Nursing* (1992) became our bible. We selected the Omaha System because it was simple and logical and reflected our way of thinking. Moreover it represented the reality of community nursing practice in a way that most other terminologies, developed primarily for use in acute care hospitals, did not. Most important, because it links diagnoses, interventions, and outcomes, it enables practising nurses to review the care they provide while enabling service managers to use the aggregated data for resource management and program planning.

In the United Kingdom, documentation requirements are less stringent than in the United States. Community nurses still have limited access to computers, but the world of information technology is moving quickly; soon computerised records will be universal. As the world changes, so does health care. It is a pleasure and privilege to write a Foreword to this expanded book. It provides more information about computerisation than the first edition but continues to support those who are not automated.

The Omaha System was tried and tested over many years, and it is used in places as far apart as the United States, United Kingdom, and Japan. Although the community health nursing practice of these countries differs in detail, the core principles are common. Similarly, the requirements for documenting practice vary and become ever more complex, but the core principles remain the same. Our ability to capture what we do, using standardised language in structured documentation, whether computerised or paper-based, enables us to compare our practice and share our knowledge.

REFERENCES

Benner, P. (1984) *From Novice to Expert: Excellence and Power in Clinical Nursing Practice.* Menlo Park, California, Addison-Wesley.

Nightingale, F. (1859) *Notes on Nursing: What it is, and What it is not.* London, Harrison.

Dame June Clark, RN, PhD, RHV, FRCN

Professor of Community Nursing
School of Health Science, University of Wales
Swansea, Wales, United Kingdom

PREFACE

This book is dedicated to Omaha System supporters everywhere. May your creativity and perseverance result in quality care and improved information today and in the future.

Health and health care are global issues that are causing practitioners, providers, politicians, and the public to ask difficult questions. What services can be provided effectively? Who, when, where, and how can those services be provided and at what cost? Where are data to describe the outcomes of those services? Although the Omaha System does not answer all of those difficult questions, it provides a strategy to address critical practice, documentation, and information management issues. It helps organize and standardize qualitative and quantitative clinical data. It encourages consideration of both "the forest and the trees." Some practitioners focus on the individual, family, or community at the moment and fail to consider the trends and aggregate data in the bigger picture (forest). Some managers, auditors, or providers focus on the bigger picture and fail to consider unique patterns of specific clients (trees).

ORGANIZATION OF THE BOOK

This book is intended to be useful. The tabs help to find specific sections; the spiral spine helps to you use the book while documenting care in automated or manual records. The tabs can assist you to find a specific section. Box 2-1 and Figures 2-3, 2-4, 2-5, and 2-6 in Chapter 2, and Appendixes A, B, and F are in the public domain and may be reproduced for educational and clinical purposes.

Section I includes six chapters. Chapter 1 is an overview of the Omaha System, and Chapter 2 suggests how to use the System consistently and accurately. Chapters 3 through 5 describe the implementation experiences of individuals, groups, and organizations in diverse practice, education, and research settings. Chapter 6 offers suggestions for those considering or implementing software and examples of software screens. Boxes that summarize diverse authors' experiences are scattered throughout the six chapters. Section II consists of the User's Guide, integrating the structure, terms, and definitions of the entire Omaha System with examples for frequent use.

The Appendix has six sections. The complete Omaha System with its revised terms and definitions appears in Appendix A; the structure, terms, and definitions exist in the public domain. The 18 diverse case studies in Appendix B were designed to provide practice opportunities. Appendix C illustrates the relationship between client problems, selected conditions, medical diagnoses, and treatments. The process used to revise the Omaha System is described in Appendix D. Appendix E consists of codes so users, especially programmers and system analysts, can update their software. Appendix F is a survey for readers to complete. Please familiarize yourself with the Glossary before you begin to read the book.

ACKNOWLEDGEMENTS

So many people have contributed to the continuing growth and development of the Omaha System and the publication of this new edition. DeLanne Simmons, Nancy Scheet, and staff members of the Visiting Nurse Association of Omaha were acknowledged in previous publications. More individuals are identified in this book, including the chapter, box, and case study authors; reviewers; and members of the Omaha System Board.

Three additional groups provided invaluable assistance. The first group consists of Pamela Correll, Bangor, Maine; Ruth Pieken, Omaha, Nebraska; Judith Riemer, Riverside, California; and Shelly Whitwer, Beatrice, Nebraska. The second group is the Minnesota Omaha System Users Group, with members from Bethel College, CareFacts Information Systems, Carver County, Central Minnesota Nurse Managed Center, CHAMP Software, Chisago County, Crow Wing County, Dakota County, Douglas County, Hennepin County, Le Sueur County, McLeod County, Minnesota Department of Health, Olmsted County, Scott County, St. Paul/Ramsey County, and Washington County. The third group was led by managing editor Linda Thomas and her team at Elsevier.

Although I planned a short-term commitment when I began working with the Omaha System in 1978, it evolved into a satisfying career. I want to thank my family for their patience and good humor to make that possible. I also want to thank each person who participated in Omaha System research, used the System in service or academic settings, mentored others, developed software, gave speeches, displayed posters, wrote for publication, sent messages to the listserv, helped with the Web site, and provided other support, even if his or her name has not been published. You are fantastic gardeners!

Karen S. Martin

HOW TO GROW A GARDEN OF RELIABLE DATA: PLANTING INSTRUCTIONS

1. Prepare soil *(the infrastructure for documentation)* using education in the Omaha System and agency policies and procedures. This will provide bulbs with a solid "grounding" in the Omaha System.
2. Place healthy bulbs (*practitioners*) and nutrient rich soil *(infrastructure)* in pot *(client situation)*.
3. Add fertilizer *(Omaha System updates, record review, and case studies)* often and on a regular basis.
4. Water *(consult with Omaha System specialists)* liberally to share expertise and increase uptake of nutrients.
5. Use tools *(computers and software)* consistently to tend the garden.
6. Provide plenty of warm sunlight *(support and leadership)* to stimulate growth.
7. Watch beautiful flowers *(reliable data)* blossom!

Courtesy Emily A. Robb, RN, BA, SANE, and the Family Health Public Health Nurses, Washington County Department of Public Health and Environment, Stillwater, Minnesota.

CONTENTS

SECTION

I

Using the Omaha System

1

THE PAST, PRESENT, AND FUTURE OF THE OMAHA SYSTEM

Karen S. Martin

Early in the 1970s, Visiting Nurse Association (VNA) of Omaha practitioners, managers, and administrators began to predict future health care changes and the critical need for practice, documentation, and information management systems that would address those changes. They anticipated the importance of naming and quantifying professional health care practice as later articulated by Lang (Clark & Lang, 1992). Under the leadership of DeLanne Simmons, these early pioneers developed an action plan. The combined efforts of the VNA, test agencies, and others resulted in the research-based Omaha System.

Five attributes were associated with the VNA, a large home care and public health agency, and with present and future health care practitioners who are passionately committed to the concepts of continuity, quality improvement, and the provision of the best possible client care (Martin & Scheet, 1992a):

- Vision: identification of the best long-term interests for the public and the profession based on knowledge and clinical expertise.
- Inspiration: loyalty, communication skills, and the commitment to work well with others within and outside the organization.
- Flexibility: willingness to take risks, reconsider action plans, and change as needed.
- Critical thinking: willingness to thoughtfully collect valid and reliable quantitative and qualitative data, use those data, and arrive at accurate conclusions, the essential foundation for evidence-based practice.
- Mobilization: implementation of innovative and creative strategies that involve practitioners, administrators, skills, materials, and programs.

OMAHA SYSTEM DEVELOPMENT

Between 1975 and 1986, the Division of Nursing of the U.S. Department of Health and Human Services funded three research projects. The purpose of the research was to develop and refine the structure and content of the Omaha System components, the *Problem Classification Scheme*, the *Intervention Scheme*, and the *Problem Rating Scale for Outcomes.* A National Institute of Nursing Research, National Institutes of Health RO-1 grant (1989-1993) funded a fourth research project designed to address reliability, validity, and usability of the entire Omaha System. Research project team members developed inductive methods and procedures and data collection instruments that were used throughout the four research projects. Expert, practicing public health and home care nurses employed by the VNA of Omaha and seven diverse test sites located throughout the United States collected individual and family data and submitted those data for inclusion in the Omaha System. Numerous multidisciplinary health care and nonhealth care experts participated in the research as advisory members and consultants. Relevant research and literature were reviewed extensively and referenced in the previous book (Martin & Scheet, 1992a). Table 1-1 summarizes the research purposes, participants, sample and design, and findings. Details about the first three studies are available in

Table 1-1 Omaha System Research, 1975-1993

Study Funding	Setting	Purpose	Sample, Design, and Procedure	Findings
1975-1976 Funded by Division of Nursing USDHHS	VNA of Omaha	Develop and conduct preliminary test of the Problem Classification Scheme	Descriptive, prospective; inductive approach. 61 RNs collected collected initial data from 338 records; 16 RNs used 99 records during test and revision.	1341 client problems sorted and collapsed to 49 unique problems for initial Problem Classification Scheme and signs/symptoms
1977-1980 Funded by Division of Nursing US DHHS	4 agencies: Texas (home care), Delaware (public health), Iowa (both), and Nebraska (both)	Field test the Problem Classification Scheme and develop the Expected Outcome-Outcome Criteria Scheme	Descriptive, prospective; inductive approach. For Problem Classification Scheme, about 75 RNs oriented and participated in initial test with 270 records from Texas, Delaware, and Iowa; retest with 125 records from 4 agencies. For Expected Outcome-Outcome Criteria Scheme, RNs oriented and participated with about 400 records during a 6-stage process.	36 problems for the Problem Classification Scheme; problem-specific Expected Outcome-Outcome Criteria Scheme drafted

Table 1-1 Omaha System Research, 1975-1993—cont'd

Study Funding	Setting	Purpose	Sample, Design, and Procedure	Findings
1984-1986 Funded by Division of Nursing, USDHHS	4 agencies: Indiana (home care), Delaware (public health), Iowa (both), and Nebraska (both)	Develop and test the Intervention Scheme and Problem Rating Scale for Outcomes; test and retest, and evaluate reliability, validity, and usefulness of the Problem Classification Scheme	Descriptive, prospective; inductive approach. About 50 RNs oriented and participated in a 4-stage process: more than 200 records from 4 sites, interviews taped with all supervisors and at least 50% of RNs, testing, and retesting.	40 problems for Problem Classification Scheme; categories and targets for Intervention Scheme; replaced Expected Outcome-Outcome Criteria Scheme with Problem Rating Scale for Outcomes
1989-1993 Funded by National Institute of Nursing Research, NIH	4 home care agencies: Nebraska (small, rural, hospital based), Wisconsin (small, rural, county), New Jersey (large, urban, free-standing), and Nebraska (large, urban, free-standing)	Evaluate reliability, validity, and usefulness of the entire Omaha System	Descriptive, prospective; inductive approach. 80 RNs oriented with a pre-post test format and participated during 18 months of data collection: 2403 records from 4 sites; 1 research assistant made shared visits for interrater reliability with RNs and families at each agency every 3 months; content validity evaluated with 10 randomly selected problems and panel of experts.	Revised Omaha System based on 9107 problems and 96,000+ interventions and at least 0.52 improvement in *Knowledge, Behavior,* and *Status* ratings noted between admission and dismissal; median age 68.6 years; circulation and neoplasms most frequent medical diagnoses

Compiled from Martin, K.S., Norris, J., & Leak, G.K. (1999, January/March). Psychometric analysis of the Problem Rating Scale for Outcomes. *Outcomes Management for Nursing Practice*, *3*(1):20-25; Martin, K.S. & Scheet, N.J. (1992a). *The Omaha System: Applications for Community Health Nursing.* Philadelphia, Saunders; and Martin, K.S., Scheet, N.J., & Stegman, M.R. (1993, December). Home health clients: Characteristics, outcomes of care, and nursing interventions. *American Journal of Public Health, 83*(12):1730-1734.

Chapter 4 of Martin and Scheet (1992a), and details about the fourth study are in other articles (Martin, Scheet, & Stegman, 1993; Martin, Norris, & Leak, 1999).

The resulting Omaha System is a research-based, comprehensive classification designed to generate meaningful data following documentation of client care. The Omaha System is intended to have characteristics of a sound terminology (Cimino, 1998; Zielstorff, 1998). While it is impossible for one classification or terminology to capture or meet every data need for all health care professionals, the Omaha System is designed to meet many needs for a variety of health care disciplines and has proven successful in doing so. In addition, ongoing efforts are intended to continually evaluate, update, and improve the Omaha System.

The Omaha System consists of three interrelated, reliable, and valid components: the *Problem Classification Scheme*, the *Intervention Scheme*, and the *Problem Rating Scale for Outcomes*. These components provide a structure to document client needs and strengths, describe practitioner interventions, and measure client outcomes in a simple yet comprehensive manner. When the three components are used together, the Omaha System offers a way to link clinical data to demographic, financial, administrative, and staffing data. This linkage is similar to arranging diverse pieces and completing a puzzle. The Omaha System offers a tool for making accurate decisions and can produce a vivid portrait of client needs, the health care services provided, and the outcomes of the services.

Because the Omaha System follows taxonomic or classification principles, it consists of terms arranged from general to specific. Terms within each level of the classification are stated at the same degree of abstraction. Definitions of each level determine the placement of terms. Terms selected for inclusion are simple, clear, concise, and easily understood by health care professionals and the general public. The Omaha System is logically consistent by virtue of development and organization, and has criteria for classes and subclasses that are relatively exhaustive and mutually exclusive (Aydelotte & Peterson, 1987; Levine, 1987; Martin & Scheet, 1992a; Zielstorff, 1998). Terms are intended to be appropriate for individuals, families, and communities, and for clients of all ages, medical diagnoses, socioeconomic status, education, spiritual beliefs, ethnicity, and cultural values.

From the onset, the entire Omaha System was intended to be as comprehensive and yet as brief and flexible as possible, and to be useful to nurses as well as to members of various disciplines in multiple settings. VNA administrators, managers, practitioners, research project staff, and the test sites shared the philosophy that "more is not necessarily better." While every addition, deletion, and revision was carefully considered and field-tested, the decision was made to err on the side of simple and brief structure, terms, and definitions, rather than extra verbiage. This philosophy and its result have been strengths of the Omaha System.

Since the initial research, the Omaha System's structure, terms, definitions, and codes were not copyrighted so that they are equally accessible to all potential users. They do not represent new knowledge, but a systematic organization of what compassionate health care professionals need to know, do, and communicate. Appendixes A and E include the structure, terms, and definitions of the newly revised (2005) version of the Omaha System; definitions are organized by topic in the Glossary. As publisher, Saunders, a division of Elsevier, has copyrighted the remainder of this book. Box 2-1, Figures 2-3 through 2-5, and Appendixes B and F are copyrighted but may be reproduced without permission for educational or clinical use. More details about copyright and suggestions for use are included in Chapter 2. Applications of the Omaha System are described in Chapters 3 through 5 and are illustrated in the case studies in Appendix B.

OMAHA SYSTEM MODEL

The Omaha System model incorporates the circular, dynamic, epidemiological, interactive nature of the problem solving process, the practitioner-client relationship, and concepts of critical thinking, clinical decision making, quality improvement, and novice-to-expert stages (Figure 1-1). It attempts to depict the complex blend of art and science that characterizes excellent evidence-based health care practice, and the ever-increasing emphasis on the "knowledge work" of health care professionals. The model was originally developed by the research team and the participants of the second research study.

Initial and current assumptions of the model include the following (Martin & Scheet, 1992a):

1. Most practitioners have the skills necessary to identify client problems, use interventions, measure client progress, and document accurately and consistently.
2. Mutuality of concern and effort between health care professionals and clients is essential to identify, use, and record realistic client problems, interventions, and outcomes.
3. Complex forces influence the health status of clients; practitioners recognize, but may not be able to control, these forces.
4. Most individuals, families, and communities are interested in increasing their competence, enhancing control over their lives, and promoting their functioning at the highest possible level. When clients are not able or willing to do so, practitioners need to identify problems and provide interventions in clients' best interests and maximize clients' safely.
5. The problem-oriented system and record is adaptable to and provides for an effective approach to the delivery of health care and social services. Most health care

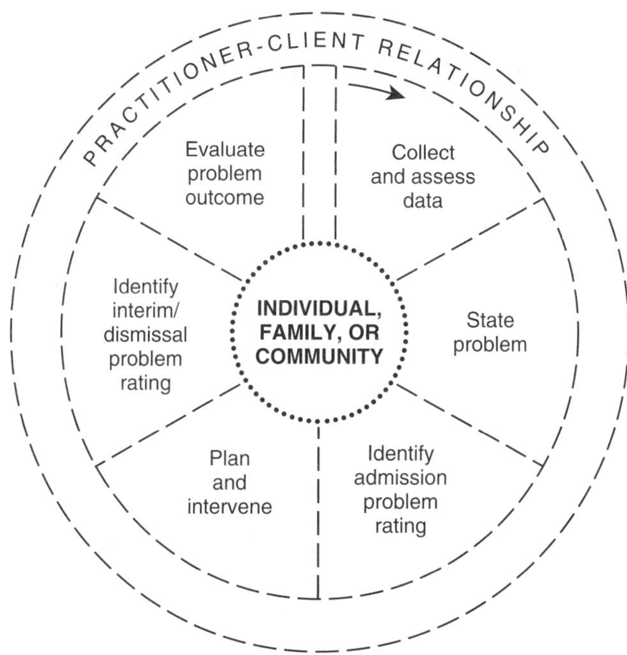

Figure 1-1 Omaha System model of the problem solving process.

professionals recognize the need to identify and document strengths and assets as well as problems; this approach is incorporated into the Omaha System.

6. Most practitioners have the expertise to use a valid and reliable organized system of practice, documentation, and information management.
7. Health care professionals, managers, and administrators can implement the Omaha System in diverse settings, and identify benefits to users, clients, external personnel, and the public.

The importance of the client is emphasized by placement at the center of the Omaha System model (see Figure 1-1). The client is defined as an individual, family, or community. Although health care professionals have traditionally provided services to individuals and families, the advent of community services is more recent. Details about community services are included in Chapter 2. The outer circle of the model notes the significance of a positive, caring, and appropriate client-practitioner relationship. This relationship is essential for access to and collection of accurate client data and maximizing client outcomes. When health care professionals have access to data, they must use their senses of sight, hearing, smell, and touch to collect and interpret data accurately.

The steps of the problem solving process provide practitioners with a relatively simple system of feedback loops, as noted by the arrow and open lines in the Omaha System model. The six wedges provide a method for health care professionals in diverse settings to operationalize the problem solving and critical thinking processes, and track the delivery of care from admission through discharge. *Data collection* and *assessment* begin the process and are followed by *problem identification* or *nursing diagnosis*. These steps are equivalent to the Problem Classification Scheme. Accurately identifying the client problem is critical to the success of care. *Plans* and *interventions*, equivalent to the Intervention Scheme, reflect the art and science of health care delivery. Interventions should be based on research evidence. The practitioner's skill in selecting and implementing optimal interventions is crucial to achieving the best possible outcomes. The final phase, *evaluation*, is equivalent to the Problem Rating Scale for Outcomes. Often, evaluation and outcomes measurement receive too little attention in practice settings. Without examining the results of care during and at the end of service, accurate conclusions about the efficiency and effectiveness of care are not possible.

THE CONTEXT OF THE OMAHA SYSTEM

It is important to recognize that the Omaha System with its history, purpose, model, concepts, and terms exists within a larger context. Although certain aspects of the Omaha System are unique, it is closely related to global concepts, models, theories, standards, and developments of health care practice, documentation, and information management.

Problem-Solving Approach

In the early 1970s, VNA of Omaha public health and home care personnel adopted Weed's problem-oriented approach and began revising their client records as the first step to developing a uniform documentation system (Weed, 1968; Martin & Scheet, 1992a). The problem-solving approach had many advantages: the concepts were familiar and relatively easy to operationalize; the approach was applicable to all clients and multidisciplinary practitioners; the combination of problems, interventions, and outcomes spanned the process of care from admission to discharge; the approach enabled practitioners to think holistically, focus care, and document clients' needs and preferences; care and outcomes could be quantified; and the approach could be automated. The problem-solving approach complements the "strength-based approach," which focuses on building developmental assets and increasing the health of youth and communities. See the following Web site for more information about developmental assets: http://www.search-institute.org/assets/.

The long-term vision was to develop a documentation system that would become the basis of an automated clinical information system for the VNA, and for other health care employers interested in implementing automated documentation systems. Since the initial VNA efforts, this vision has become reality, thanks to advances in information technology including the Internet and commercially available information systems, emphasis on outcomes measurement, development and dissemination of standardized terminologies, concern about high quality and safe health care, and public demands (Koch, 1998; Institute of Medicine, 1991; Carty, 2000; Institute of Medicine, 2000; Institute of Medicine, 2001; Coenen et al., 2001b; Elfrink et al., 2001; Frank-Stromborg, Christensen, & Elmhurst, 2001a and 2001b; Englebardt & Nelson, 2002; Landro, 2002; Monsen & Martin, 2002a and 2002b; Androwich et al., 2003; Institute of Medicine, 2003; Landro, 2003; American Nurses Association, 2004; Institute of Medicine, 2004).

Data Models

The pyramid in Figure 1-2 illustrates the initial vision and the transformation of clinical data to information that is necessary for evidence-based practice, even though it was not developed until the Omaha System was completed (Monsen & Martin, 2002a). Data flow upward from the base through the five levels to the top and reverse the flow from the top back to the base:

1. *Client records:* the base or foundation of the pyramid. In most community-based agencies in the United States, a record is initiated after a referral is received for home, clinic, school, or parish services and initial care is provided. Practitioners document diverse data that often include assessment, interventions, and evaluation details. These data are very granular and specific. Many practitioners and health care organizations use a similar approach to documentation nationally and globally, although the focus, style, and length of client records vary dramatically.
2. *Client information system:* the second level of the pyramid. The client information system is the repository of the clinical data collected and documented when nurses, other health care professionals, and paraprofessionals provide care. The client information system is maintained by a single provider agency or organization or by multiple providers in a health care system.
3. *Agency information system:* the third level of the pyramid. The agency information system is the repository where clinical data are merged with statistical, financial, staffing, supply, and other data. The agency information system is maintained by a single provider agency or organization or by multiple providers in a health care system.
4. *Develop reports:* the fourth level of the pyramid. Clinical and nonclinical data are abstracted, summarized, aggregated, and analyzed at this level. Although some clinical reports have been generated for more than 100 years by practitioners, it is only recently that automation offered technology to easily obtain timely and useful reports that are based on clinical data.
5. *Use reports:* the fifth and final level of the pyramid. Because of automation, many providers now have an abundance or even an excess of reports. However, few providers are able to interpret and apply clinical reports, develop essential feedback loops, and use their reports to influence best practices and provider operations.

Others have published similar graphic conceptualizations or models to depict the flow and use of data. Very specific (atomic level or granular) data obtained from individual clients

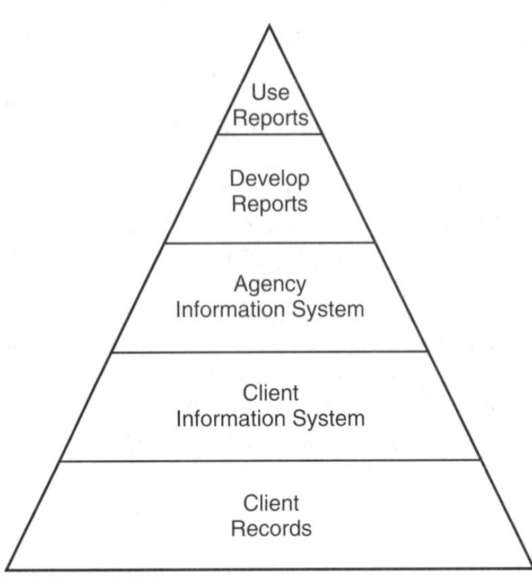

Figure 1-2 Pyramid model depicting the transformation of clinical data to information.
(Adapted from Monsen, K.A. & Martin, K.S. [2002a, April/June]. Developing an outcomes management program in a public health department. Outcomes Management, 6(2):62-66.)

evolve to information at the worldwide level according to Zielstorff, Hudgings, & Grobe (1993). Figure 6-1 is a more complex illustration of the relationships among data, information, knowledge, and clinical information systems (Androwich et al., 2003). During the development of the International Classification for Nursing Practice, a model was developed to depict the spirals from nursing practice to the minimum data set and nursing information systems (International Council of Nurses, 1996). Goossen, Epping, & Dassen (1997) developed a nursing information reference model with four layers that illustrate the progression of data from decisions at the clinical, management, and policy levels. Tidd (1998) illustrated the relationship of data and information to performance improvement.

In 1986 Blum described data, information, and knowledge as the hierarchy of health care computing applications. Data are pertinent specifics such as a person's name, age, weight, or blood pressure. Information is a collection of related data that has been processed. Knowledge results when data and information are organized, analyzed, and synthesized and the relationships are formalized. In 1989 Graves and Corcoran used data, information, and knowledge to explain nursing informatics. During the same year, Nelson and Joos (1989) defined data as naming, collecting, and organizing; information as organizing and interpreting; knowledge as interpreting, integrating, and understanding; and added wisdom as understanding that is applied with sound judgment. Tidd (1998) linked data, information, and performance improvement, while Turley (2000) emphasized the communication aspects of knowledge and encouraged the shift of informatics farther from the technological to the professional perspective.

Theory Building

The Omaha System both contributes to and is influenced by theory building. The Omaha System is a first level or middle-range theory that complements other theories (Englebardt & Nelson, 2002; Androwich et al., 2003). The System supports Donabedian's structure, process, and outcome approach (1966), the Neuman Systems Model (Neuman, 1995; Lowry & Martin, 2004), and other theories. Similarly, it supports critical thinking (Oermann, 1998; Carty, 2000; Finkelman, 2001; Englebardt & Nelson, 2002; Lunney, 2003; Profetto-McGrath et al., 2003) and the Dreyfus model of Skill Building (Dreyfus, 1979) that Benner synthesized from her qualitative descriptive research, in which she developed a novice-to-expert skill acquisition model for nurses (Benner, 1984, Benner, Tanner, & Chesla, 1996; Larrabee, 1999).

Other disciplines that require logical, scientific thinking and systematic nomenclature also employ a problem solving approach (Table 1-2). The problem solving process includes generalized information gathering, problem identification, and analysis, as well as critical thinking based on fact, intuition, and experiences. Physicians employ a medical diagnostic process that is similar to the nursing process and the problem-solving approach.

Terminologies and Standards

The value of using classification and taxonomic principles to organize and manage complex and often extensive data has been promoted for centuries, although opponents usually argue that classification leads to reductionism and linear thinking. Polanyi (1967) is an example of the authors who described the ability to understand the whole by first understanding the sum of the parts. Although the medical diagnoses of the International Classification of Diseases have existed for years, many physicians assign responsibility for their use to fellow employees, primarily for billing purposes. Few other practitioners or providers have been interested in developing terminologies, which often include data sets, classification schemes, models, and standards (Zielstorff et al., 1993; Ozbolt, 1996; Henry & Mead, 1997; Healthcare Information and Management Systems Society, 2003).

As use of the Omaha System increased, practitioners and providers recognized the opportunity and need to establish practice and documentation standards. The value of such standards and the relationship to accurate and consistent client data are described in the Benefits section of this chapter and Chapters 2 and 3.

Various national and global organizations have established professional and technical standards that relate to the Omaha System. Many of these organizations are promoting the development of information and terminology models. The models have the potential for increasing the comparability and compatibility of coded clinical data (interoperability) within and among health care settings when classifications such as the Omaha System

Table 1-2 Relationship of Nursing Process to Problem Solving and Medical Diagnostic Processes

Nursing Process	Problem-Solving Process	Medical Diagnostic Process
Data collection	Information gathering	History and physical examination
Nursing diagnosis	Problem	Diagnosis
Plan	Plan	Plan
Intervention	Action	Treatment
Evaluation	Evaluation	Evaluation

From Lowry, L.W. & Martin, K.S. (2004). Organizing Frameworks Applied to Community-Oriented Nursing. In Stanhope, M., & Lancaster, J., (Eds.) *Community and Public Health Nursing*, ed. 6 (p. 208). St. Louis, Mosby.

are used at the "point-of-care." The Omaha System and similar terminologies are referred to as "front end" or interface terminologies, in contrast to reference terminologies that function behind the scenes and link data from various sources successfully (Hardiker, Hoy, & Casey, 2000; Harris et al., 2000; Ozbolt, 2000). Complex technical standards related to automation are summarized in Chapter 6. Omaha System representatives submitted reports and applications to diverse technical standard organizations, and testified at meetings. The result is acknowledgment, recognition, inclusion, and partnerships. Specifically, the Omaha System is congruent with the reference terminology model for the International Organization for Standardization (ISO), is registered (recognized) by Health Level Seven (HL7), and is integrated into Logical Observation Identifiers, Names, and Codes (LOINC).

The evolution of professional standards has had a challenging history (Hardiker, Hoy, & Casey, 2000; Harris et al., 2000; Ozbolt, 2000; Evers, 2001). A significant milestone occurred in 1985 when the Nursing Minimum Data Set Conference was held in Milwaukee, Wisconsin, and co-chaired by Drs. Harriet Werley and Norma Lang (Werley & Lang, 1988; Lang, 1995). The 1985 conference recognized and celebrated nurses and their work with standardized terminologies and automation; another purpose was to improve the communication and data sharing among practice, education, and research. Papers focused on NANDA-International, the Omaha System, other terminology projects, the need to describe and quantify nursing practice, and projected information technology developments.

The conference stimulated increased activities by the American Nurses Association. A committee was formed to establish criteria for terminology recognition. Criteria included completing reliability tests conducted on terms and validating usefulness of the terms for clinical purposes (Coenen et al., 2001a and 2001b). In 1992, the American Nurses Association recognized NANDA-International, the Omaha System, Nursing Interventions Classification, and the Home Health Care Classification as terminologies to be considered by nurses to describe clinical data and to improve and standardize their practice. The Committee also stated that the goal for the nursing profession was to be multilingual and to promote unified, not uniform, data and information, as well as professional standards (Lang, 1995). Currently, 13 terminologies that support nursing practice have been recognized and disseminated by the American Nurses Association. Some terminologies are designed for use by nurses only while others such as the Omaha System are designed for multidisciplinary use (American Nurses Association, 2004).

The terminologies are also part of the Nursing Information and Data Set Evaluation Center (NIDSEC) standards and scoring guidelines, which merge professional and technical components (American Nurses Association, 2004). The initial standards were published in 1997 and revised in 2003; they are designed to encourage vendors to add standardized terminologies that support nursing practice to their software applications. The new standards address four areas:

- Standardized terminologies: the thirteen terminologies recognized by the American Nurses Association
- Clinical content associations: the choices displayed on data entry screens to record assessments, diagnoses, interventions, and outcomes
- Clinical data repositories: the physical or logical compendia of longitudinally-stored client health data
- Decision support, administrative, clinical, and support requirements: the hardware/software system requirements for supporting repository use, linkage to management/administrative data, and point-of-care decision support

These events stimulated increased global interest in the Omaha System and more partnerships involving professional standards. For example, the Omaha System is integrated into the National Library of Medicine's Metathesaurus, CINAHL, Alternative Link and SNOMED Clinical Terms (SNOMED CT®), which includes the Read Codes. The System can be used collaboratively with Medicare's Outcome and Assessment Information Set (OASIS) and the International Classification of Diseases. It contributes to successful surveys and audits conducted by professional and payer groups. The Omaha System has been linked to the International Classification of Nursing Practice, NANDA-International, Nursing Interventions Classification, Nursing Outcomes Classification, and other terminologies.

BENEFITS OF USING THE OMAHA SYSTEM

Practitioners in all health care settings must have health education, technology, case management, critical thinking, and communication skills. Those skills are increasingly important because of the complexity of practice and the need to articulate and measure the outcomes of that practice, mergers and the shift in health delivery from inpatient acute care to community settings, the philosophy of seamless health care delivery, reimbursement changes, and decreased length of stay. Practitioners need to develop skills to function and communicate across multiple settings. They need competencies that include client assessment and diagnosis, targeted interventions, outcomes measurement, documentation using automated record systems, and the ability to transform clinical data to information and to communicate that information to others.

When implemented in practice, education, and research settings, the Omaha System can facilitate evidence-based practice, documentation, and information management. The System can be used to introduce novice multidisciplinary health care and social service professionals and students to professional practice through a standardized, easily understood system of client problems, practitioner interventions, and client outcomes. For all practitioners, the Omaha System offers a series of cues or feedback loops that remind users about possible client problems and interventions and ways to evaluate the effect of the care provided, creating a bridge to the identification of best practices. When novices use the Omaha System to reflect on their client data, they will progress along the novice-to-expert practice continuum, as well as the documentation continuum.

Regardless if health care providers are in the novice, advanced beginner, competent, proficient, or expert stage of their clinical practice, they will face a definite learning curve when they are introduced to the Omaha System. Those who are more expert practitioners may find the learning curve more stressful than their novice peers. Although the schedule may differ, it is not unlike the learning curve experienced by practitioners when they learn to use clinical information software (see Box 6-3) (Benner, 1984; Larrabee, 1999; Mallard, 2000). The accuracy and speed at which professionals arrive at their conclusions is related to their attitudes and to multiple educational, employment, and life experiences, and to the resources and support they receive during orientation.

Fortunately, heightened interest in health care quality and outcomes measurement is occurring globally. Driving forces include the desire to quantify outcomes, new accreditation and national regulations, legislation, escalating health care costs, and increasingly vocal consumers. Many people are asking for, or demanding, comparable data (Landro, 2002; Landro, 2003; Institute of Medicine, 2004; *Nursing Outlook,* 2004). Examples of important federal initiatives in the United States involving data and information are the original Health Insurance and Portability Act of 1996 (Pub. L. 104-191), and the revisions to this act referred to as the Health Insurance Portability and Accountability Act (HIPAA). The relationships between quality and reimbursement concerns for functional status data are now being publicized (Centers for Medicare and Medicaid Services, 2003a). Beginning in 1999, Medicare-certified home care agencies have been required to use the Outcome and Assessment Information Set (OASIS) as part of the conditions of participation (Centers for Medicare and Medicaid Services, 2003b). During 2003, federal pressure and proposed legislation in support of electronic health records increased dramatically and appeared to establish the beginning of a new era (Johnson, 2003; U.S. Department of Health and Human Services, 2003).

Data generated by using the Omaha System can provide essential information. Clinical data can be aggregated and converted into compellingly illustrated trends and graphics (Monsen & Martin, 2002a and 2002b; Monsen & Kerr, 2004). The information can be used to improve practice, facilitate communication with employees, enhance communication with board members and the general public, complete reports for third party payers, meet accreditation requirements, plan new agency programs, and integrate with other, nonclinical information within the provider's management information system. The increasing portion of health care services in community settings in the United States that are reimbursed by third party payers such as managed care companies illustrates the new challenges. Managed care companies want their enrollees to improve their health, prevent illness, and limit the amount of expensive sickness care they require. Therefore, managed care is changing the type of programs that agencies offer, their need for valid and reliable outcomes data, and the types of clients they serve (Martin & Martin, 1997; Monsen & Martin, 2002a and 2002b).

NATIONAL AND INTERNATIONAL USERS

Initial adopters of the Omaha System included home care, public health, and school health practice settings, as well as some educators in the United States. A survey was developed for collecting data about Omaha System users (similar to the survey in Appendix F). When the results of the first survey were published in 1992, more than 200 settings were identified as users and were located in the United States, three Canadian provinces, the United Kingdom, Denmark, and the Netherlands (Martin & Scheet, 1992a). Although some agencies and groups developed automated systems for their own use, most used manual record systems. Approximately 100 users responded to the survey, including:

- More than 70 agencies that offered home health and preventive services and employed almost 4000 nurses.
- Almost 20 schools and colleges of nursing.
- Ten others who were primarily consultants.

During the early years, information about the Omaha System was disseminated through workshops and conference presentations. Both continue to be popular methods to share information. The first article was published by VNA of Omaha staff in 1981, followed by more articles, chapters, and books. Since then, other practitioners, managers, administrators, researchers, educators, and students have completed numerous publications. Many are listed in this book and on the Omaha System Web site (www.omahasystem.org). Dissemination also increased because of American Nurses Association recognition and inclusion in the National Library of Medicine's Metathesaurus, which made the terminologies available to those who conduct electronic searches.

Since the 1980s, different groups have organized Omaha System conferences. Beginning in 2001, the first biennial Omaha System International Conference was held at Bethel College in St. Paul, Minnesota (Plowfield & Raymond, 2001). The second conference was held at the University of Wisconsin-Milwaukee in 2003. Information about conferences is available on the Omaha System Web site (2004) (www.omahasystem.org).

In addition, the Web site includes a summary of the Omaha System, an extensive list of references, news, hot links, directions for joining the Omaha System listserv, and a users' survey.

The Omaha System was translated into Danish about 1985. Since then, translations include Dutch, Japanese, Chinese, Swedish, Korean, Slovene, Spanish, Turkish, German, Estonian, and Thai. The International Council of Nurses International Classification for Nursing Practice project introduced the Omaha System to nurses in many countries and stimulated interest in adoption. The Omaha System pocket guide was translated into Japanese in 1997 (Martin & Scheet, 1992b; Martin & Scheet, 1997b).

Since the 1990s, both the number and type of users have expanded dramatically to include nurse-managed center staff, hospital-based and managed care case managers, educators, parish nurses, occupational health nurses, acute and long-term care staff, researchers, members of various disciplines, software vendors, and the international community. The increase in the use of the Omaha System is due in part to the global desire for outcomes measurement, the increasing elder population, the shift of health care delivery from institutions to community settings, and advances in technology including listservs and the Internet. The availability of computerized information systems based on the Omaha System and designed for use in clinical and educational settings is a very important reason for the increase, as described in other chapters in this book and in other publications (Martin, 1999; Monsen & Martin, 2002b). An organization, a school, or a group must invest time, energy, and money in hardware and software required for automation. This investment tends to increase the commitment to the Omaha System as well as the likelihood that it will be used consistently and accurately.

A survey was conducted between 2001 and 2003 to identify the number and type of Omaha System adopters and trends in the depth and range of its use. As mentioned, the Omaha System is not copyrighted and has been disseminated through workshops, publications, and various Internet publications including the Omaha System Web site. For these reasons, Table 1-3 underrepresents the total user population and provides an estimate of the number and type of practitioners, educators, and students who have implemented the Omaha System. The table identifies 169 user organizations and their 8000 employees. As in the survey, a user is defined as one individual, agency, group, organization, center, school, or college that uses the Omaha System. Many user organizations provide health care services, whereas others are software vendors and consultants. The definition of use is equally flexible: adopters implemented part or all of the Omaha System, and have automated or manual records.

Practice, education, and research users in 14 countries returned 169 surveys, suggesting that the type and location of users has expanded. The countries represented are Andorra, Canada, Estonia, Ireland, Japan, Korea, New Zealand, Slovenia, Sweden, Taiwan, Thailand, Turkey, the United Kingdom, and the United States. The predominant users are nurses employed by community organizations in 26 states in the United States, although the number and location of nonnurses, schools and universities, noncommunity organizations, and global users is increasing. The number of practitioners in the 103 user organizations ranges from one to 869 for a total of 2401 (see Table 1-3, Types of Settings 1-5). The users in 54 schools and universities, with 239 educators and 2974 students, total 3213. Note that the School and University category includes the range of educators and programs described in Chapter 4. A program may have several educators who include the Omaha System in their course work, or the curriculum may be based on the Omaha System. Nurses, clinical specialists, nurse practitioners, and other health care professionals use the Omaha System to document services in nurse-managed health centers.

Table 1-3 Omaha System Users: Analysis of 169 organizations that responded to the 2001-2003 Omaha System survey

Type of Setting	Number of Organizations and Description	Total Number of Employees	Number and Type of Employees	Number and Percent Automated
Home Care	21: provide intermittent, hospice, and/or long-term care services	358	329 RNs, 15 SWs, 7 PTs, 3 OTs, 2 RDs, 2 SLPs	19 (90%)
Public Health	44: provide high risk parent-child, high risk elder, communicable disease, parish, and/or community services	687	672 RNs, 12 SWs, 3 RDs	25 (57%)
Home Care and Public Health	33: provide combined home care and public health services	465	447 RNs, 6 SW, 8 PTs, 3 OTs, 1 SLPs	29 (88%)
Residential Long-term Care	1: provides assisted living, long-term care, and/or chronic illness hospital services	869	700 RNs, 40 SWs, 30 PTs, 20 OTs, 15 RDs, 12 SLPs, 40 RTs, 10 psychologists, 2 pastoral care workers	In process
Other Service Providers	4: provide care/case management and/or clinic services	16	12 RNs, 4 outreach workers	1 (25%)
Schools and Universities	54: schools of nursing, other health education programs, and/or nurse managed centers	3213	239 educators, 2974 students	*
Others	12: organizations who do not provide client services	12 groups	Software vendors/ programmers, consultants	N/A

*Some schools use automation with a specific clinical group and/or nurse managed center, but data cannot be analyzed accurately.
OT, Occupational therapist; *PT*, physical therapist; *RD*, registered dietician/nutritionist; *RN*, registered nurse; *RT*, recreational therapist; *SLP*, speech and language pathologist; *SW*, social worker.

When the survey data published in 1992 and in 2005 are compared, the most dramatic change involves automation. Previously, only a few users entered any clinical data electronically, and no user had a completely automated clinical information system. Now, those users who have computerized client records predominate, especially in the United States. Approximately 75% of home care and public health organizations reported using Omaha System software. Minnesota has the highest number of automated users. Of the 87 counties in Minnesota, 74, or 85%, have one or more automated Omaha System providers who serve their residents (Monsen & Martin, 2002b).

If you are a new Omaha System user and have not completed a survey, please complete the form in Appendix F and return it.

PREDICTIONS FOR FUTURE USE OF THE OMAHA SYSTEM

The rate of change is accelerating. Although the basic premises of client-practitioner relationships, professional skill development, and quality improvement continue, many aspects of health care practice, education, and research are changing rapidly. The changes, summarized in this chapter and described more completely in the following chapters, are causing the momentum associated with the Omaha System to escalate. Therefore, it is likely that the following will increase:

- Interest in and use of evidence-based practice, outcomes measurement, and information technology.
- Dissemination of Omaha System information.
- Number and type of national and global Omaha System users and software applications.

When the Omaha System research began in the 1970s, the vision included comparing evidence-based client data to describe trends and improve the outcomes of practice, and having automated information systems. Until recently, most users focused their energy on learning and applying the Omaha System. Now the trends to embrace information technology, automate, actually convert data to information, and use those data to influence best practices are evident through diverse publications, site visits, the Omaha System listserv, international conferences, and informal conversation. Practitioners and students need encouragement, commitment, and resources to question practice patterns and obtain the necessary accurate and consistent quantitative data to identify best practice patterns (Masson, 2003; Gorski, 2004; Martin, 2004). Educators need to become better informed about global trends and convey that information to students (Carty, 2000; Englebardt & Nelson, 2002; Pesut, 2002). Likewise, employers require a change in attitude or external pressures to address group practice and documentation on a monthly basis, schedule an annual record audit and quality improvement day, send new practitioners to an introductory Omaha System workshop, release managers to participate in an Omaha System users' group, purchase an automated clinical information system, or participate in quality indicator, benchmarking, or report card activities (Jennings, 1999; Monsen & Martin, 2002a and 2002b; Sawyer et al., 2002; Editorial, 2003; Halamandaris, 2003; Whitman, 2003; Monsen & Kerr, 2004; *Nursing Outlook,* 2004; Rosebaugh, 2004; Sienkiewicz, 2004). To publicly release such data and information is an important milestone. Providers are participating because of voluntary, competitive, regulatory, accreditation, and legislative initiatives.

Requests for national and global Omaha System site visits and presentations are increasing, as is communication with global professional and technical organizations such as the Association for Common European Nursing Diagnoses, Interventions, and Outcomes (ACENDIO) and others listed earlier in this chapter (Martin & Scheet, 1997a; Martin,

Bessho, & Saito, 1999; Elfrink et al., 2001; Martin, 2002; Monsen & Martin, 2002b). More international practitioners, managers, administrators, educators, students, and researchers are beginning to use the Omaha System in automated and manual versions and to write for publication (Jonkergouw, 1991; Huang, 1994; Martin, Bessho, & Saito, 1999; Park, Kim, & Cho, 2000; Clark et al., 2001; Clark, 2003; Wilson & Roy, 2003). Translations of this book into various languages are being negotiated. Global communication on the Omaha System listserv is thriving.

Additional formal activities are occurring in response to predictions and trends. A users' group was established in Minnesota in 2001. Representatives of state and county public health agencies, home care agencies, educators, and software vendors meet bimonthly to share ideas about Omaha System use in these diverse settings. They provide mutual support and work together to learn from each other and solve problems (Monsen & Martin, 2002b). Because of this opportunity to share information and ideas, agencies have improved accurate and consistent use of the Omaha System in their own settings, begun to analyze aggregate data, and encouraged each other to speak, present posters, and publish.

Also in 2001, a 12-member Omaha System Advisory Board was formed, which is comprised of representatives from diverse service and educational settings nationally and globally (see Appendix D). Board members participate in diverse Omaha System activities. They plan and participate in conferences including a biennial international conference, write for publication, help manage the website and listserv, and participate in terminology review and revision as validation experts. Omaha System review and revision is necessary for ongoing improvement, and to ensure that the terms and definitions address practice changes and meet other requirements. For example, the criteria for terminology recognition initially established by the American Nurses Association will be revised periodically, and the Omaha System will need to be resubmitted for review. The Advisory Board members will participate in that process.

SUMMARY

The Omaha System consists of the Problem Classification Scheme, Intervention Scheme, and Problem Rating Scale for Outcomes, and is designed to facilitate health care practice, documentation, and information management. The Omaha System was developed and revised during four federally-funded research projects that were conducted from 1975 to 1993. Use continues to expand nationally and internationally in practice, education, and research contexts. Technological steps such as automation and the Internet have contributed to expansion. It is important for developments and experiences to be published, presented, indexed, and shared with the nursing and health care communities. A process is in place for systematic and deliberate Omaha System revisions and ongoing development. Therefore, it is equally important for the Omaha System to be revised periodically and disseminated in publications such as this book. With this exciting past, present, and future, the Omaha System can continue contributing to the art and science of health care.

REFERENCES

American Nurses Association. (2004). *Recognized Languages for Nursing.* Retrieved March 8, 2004 from the Internet: http://www.nursingworld.org/nidsec/classlst.htm.

Androwich, I.M., Bickford, C.J., Button, P.S., Hunter, K.M., Murphy, J., & Sensmeier, J. (2003). *Clinical Information Systems: A Framework for Reaching the Vision.* Washington, DC, American Nurses Publishing.

Aydelotte, M. & Peterson, K. (1987). Keynote address: Nursing taxonomies—state of the art. In McLane, A. (Ed.), *Classification of Nursing Diagnoses: Proceedings of the Seventh Conference* (pp. 1-16). St. Louis, Mosby.

Benner, P. (1984). *From Novice to Expert: Excellence and Power in Clinical Nursing Practice.* Menlo Park, California, Addison-Wesley.

Benner, P.A., Tanner, C.A., & Chesla, C.A. (Eds.). (1996). *Expertise in Nursing Practice: Caring, Clinical Judgment, and Ethics.* New York, Springer.

Blum, B.I. (1986). *Clinical Information Systems.* New York, Springer.

Carty, B. (Ed.). (2000). *Nursing Informatics: Education for Practice.* New York, Springer.

Centers for Medicare and Medicaid Services. (Spring, 2003a). *Health Care Financing Review, 24*(3). Pub. Number 03448. Baltimore, MD: USDHHS.

Centers for Medicare and Medicaid Services. (2003b). *Conditions of Participation: Home health agencies.* Retrieved September 1, 2003 from the Internet: http://www/cms.hhs.gov/medicare.

Cimino, J.J. (1998, November). Desiderata for controlled medical vocabularies in the twenty-first century. *Methods of Information in Medicine, 37*(4-5):394-403.

Clark, J. (2003). *Naming Nursing: Proceedings of the First ACENDIO Ireland/UK Conference.* Bern, Switzerland, Hans Huber.

Clark, J., Christensen, J., Mooney, G., Davies, P., Edwards, J., Fitchett, L., Spowart, B., & Thomas, P. (2001, March). New methods of documenting health visiting practice. *Community Practitioner, 74*(3):108-112.

Clark, J. & Lang, N.M. (1992, July-August). Nursing's next advance: An international classification for nursing practice. *International Nursing Review, 39*(4):109-111, 128.

Coenen, A., Marin, H.F., Park, H-A., & Bakken, S. (2001a, May/June). Collaborative efforts for representing nursing concepts in computer-based systems: International perspectives. *Journal of the American Medical Informatics Association, 8*(3):202-211.

Coenen, A., McNeil, B., Bakken, S., Bickford, C., & Warren, J.J. (2001b, November/December). Toward comparable nursing data: American Nurses Association criteria for data sets, classification systems, and nomenclatures. *Computers in Nursing, 19*(6):240-246.

Donabedian, A. (1966, July). Evaluating the quality of medical care. *Milbank Memorial Fund Quarterly, 44*(2):166-206.

Dreyfus, H.L. (1979). *What Computers Can't Do: The Limits of Artificial Intelligence.* New York, Harper & Row.

Editorial. (2003, April). Home health quality goes public. *Caring, XXII*(4):18-20.

Elfrink, V., Bakken, S., Coenen, A., McNeil, B., & Bickford, C. (2001, February). Standardized nursing vocabularies: A foundation for quality care. Seminars in Oncology Nursing, 17(1):18-23.

Englebardt, S.P. & Nelson, R. (Eds.). (2002). *Health Care Informatics: An Interdisciplinary Approach.* St. Louis, Mosby.

Evers, G.C.M. (2001). Naming nursing—Evidence based nursing. In Oud, N. (Ed.), *ACENDIO 2001: Proceedings of the 3rd European Conference of the Association of Common European Nursing Diagnoses, Interventions, and Outcomes in Berlin* (pp. 55-60). Bern, Switzerland, Hans Huber.

Finkelman, A.W. (2001, December). Problem-solving, decision-making, and critical thinking: How do they mix and why bother? *Home Care Provider, 6*(6):194-197.

Frank-Stromborg, M., Christensen, A., & Elmhurst, D. (2001a, May). Nurse documentation: Not done or worse, done the wrong way—Part I. *Oncology Nursing Forum, 28*(4):697-702.

Frank-Stromborg, M., Christensen, A., & Elmhurst, D. (2001b, June). Nurse documentation: Not done or worse, done the wrong way–Part II. *Oncology Nursing Forum, 28*(5):841-846.

Goossen, W.T.E., Epping, P.J.M.M., & Dassen, T.W.N. (1997, November/December). Criteria for nursing information systems as a component of the electronic patient record: An international Delphi study. *Computers in Nursing, 15*(6):307-315.

Gorski, L.A. (2004, April). Making a commitment to clinical data. *Home Health Care Management and Practice, 16*(3):206-211.

Graves, J.R. & Corcoran, S. (1989, Winter). The study of nursing informatics. *Image: The Journal of Nursing Scholarship, 21*(4):227-230.

Halamandaris, V.U. (2003, March). Government report cards on health care quality: Blessing or curse? *Caring, XXII*(3):47-48.

Harris, M.R., Graves, J.R., Solbrig, H.R., Elkin, P.L., & Chute, C.G. (2000, November/December). Embedded structures and representation of nursing knowledge. *Journal of the American Medical Informatics Association, 7*(6):539-549.

Hardiker, N.R., Hoy, D., & Casey, A. (2000, November/December). Standards for nursing terminology. *Journal of the American Medical Informatics Association*, *7*(6):523-528.

Healthcare Information and Management Systems Society. (2003, July). *An analysis of health information standards development initiatives.* Retrieved September 8, 2003 from the Internet: http://himss.org/content/files

Henry, S.B. & Mead, C.N. (1997, May/June). Nursing classification systems: Necessary but not sufficient for representing "What nurses do" for inclusion in computer-based patient record systems. *Journal of the American Medical Informatics Association*, *4*(3):222-232.

Huang, L.H. (1994, September). The Omaha System application in home health nursing. *Journal of Nursing of the Republic of China*, *41*(3):14-17.

Institute of Medicine. (1991). *The Computer-based Patient Record: An Essential Technology for Change.* Dick, R., & Steen, E. (Eds.). Washington, DC, National Academies Press.

Institute of Medicine. (2000). *To Err is Human: Building a Safer Health Care System.* Kohn, L.T., Corrrigan, J.M., & Donaldson, M.S. (Eds.). Washington, DC, National Academies Press.

Institute of Medicine. (2001). *Crossing the Quality Chasm.* Committee on Quality of Health Care in America. (Ed.). Washington, DC, National Academies Press.

Institute of Medicine. (2003). *Health Professions Education: A Bridge to Quality.* Greiner, A.C. & Knebel, E. (Eds.). Washington, DC, National Academies Press.

Institute of Medicine. (2004). *Keeping Patients Safe: Transforming the Work Environment of Nurses.* Page, A. (Ed.). Washington, DC, National Academies Press.

International Council of Nurses. (1996). *The International Classification of Nursing Practice: A Unifying Framework—the Alpha Version.* Geneva, Switzerland, ICN.

Jennings, B.M. (1999, October/December). Evaluating outcomes versus "McAnswers"—where are we going? *Outcomes Management for Nursing Practice*, *3*(4):144-146.

Johnson, N. (2003, July 24). *National Health Information Infrastructure Act of 2003.* Retrieved August 1, 2003 from the Internet: http://www.house.gov/nancyjohnson/pr_nhii.htm.

Jonkergouw, P.H. (1991). Computerisation of the nursing process. In Hovenga, E.J.S., Hannah, K.J., McCormick, K.A., & Ronald, J.S. (Eds.), *Nursing Informatics '91: Proceedings of the Fourth International Conference* (pp. 457-463). New York, Springer.

Koch, L.A. (1998, September). Eight essential steps for effective data collection and use. *Caring*, *XVII*(9):58-67.

Landro, L. (2002, August 15). Electronic medical records call for common language by doctors. *Wall Street Journal*, *CCXL*(33):D3.

Landro, L. (2003, July 1). Wired patients. *Wall Street Journal*, *CCXLII(1)*:A10.

Lang, N.M. (Ed.). (1995). *Nursing Data Systems: The Emerging Framework.* Washington, DC, American Nurses Publishing.

Larrabee, S.B. (1999, August). Benner's novice to expert nursing theory applied to the implementation of laptops in the home care setting. *Home Health Care Management and Practice, 11*(4):41-47.

Levine, M.E. (1987). Approaches to the development of a nursing diagnosis taxonomy. In McLane, A. (Ed.), *Classification of Nursing Diagnoses: Proceedings of the Seventh Conference* (pp. 45-52). St. Louis, Mosby.

Lowry, L.W. & Martin, K.S. (2004). Organizing frameworks applied to community-oriented nursing. In Stanhope, M. & Lancaster, J. (Eds.), *Community and Public Health Nursing* (6th ed.) (pp. 194-219). St. Louis, Mosby.

Lunney, M. (2003, September). Critical thinking and accuracy of nurses' diagnoses. *International Journal of Nursing Terminologies and Classifications, 14*(3):96-107.

Mallard, C.O. (2000). Nursing informatics in the home health care environment. In Carty, B. (Ed.), *Nursing Informatics: Education for Practice* (pp. 252-270). New York, Springer.

Martin, K.S. (1999, Winter). The Omaha System: Past, present, and future. *On-line Journal of Nursing Informatics*, *3*, 1-6. Retrieved March 8, 2004 from the Internet: http://www.eaa-knowledge.com/ojni/ni/dm/ojni.html.

Martin, K.S. (2002). The Omaha System. In Oud, N. (Ed.), *ACENDIO 2002: Proceedings of the Special Conference of the Association of Common European Nursing Diagnoses, Interventions, and Outcomes in Vienna* (pp. 91-100). Bern, Switzerland, Hans Huber.

Martin, K.S. (2004, April). Your mission. *Home Health Care Management and Practice, 16*(3):170.

Martin, K.S., Bessho, Y., & Saito, Y. (1999, April). The introduction to the Omaha System. *The Japanese Journal of Total Care*, *9*(4):64-72.

Martin, K.S. & Martin, D.L. (1997). How can the quality of nursing practice be measured? In McCloskey J.C. & Grace, H.K. (Eds.), *Current Issues in Nursing* (5th ed.) (pp. 315-321). St. Louis, Mosby.

Martin, K.S., Norris, J., & Leak, G.K. (1999, January/March). Psychometric analysis of the Problem Rating Scale for Outcomes. *Outcomes Management for Nursing Practice, 3*(1):20-25.

Martin, K.S. & Scheet, N.J. (1992a). *The Omaha System: Applications for Community Health Nursing.* Philadelphia, Saunders.

Martin, K.S. & Scheet, N.J. (1992b). *The Omaha System: A Pocket Guide for Community Health Nursing.* Philadelphia, Saunders.

Martin, K.S. & Scheet, N.J. (1997a). The Omaha System. In Kastermans, M. & Oud, N. (Eds.), *Handboek verpleegkundige diagnostiek, interventies en resultaten (Handbook of Nursing Diagnoses, Interventions, and Outcomes)* (A1900.1-A1900.24). The Netherlands, Bohn Stafleu Van Loghum, Houten.

Martin, K.S. & Scheet, N.J. (1997b). *The Omaha System: A Pocket Guide for Community Health Nursing.* Tokyo, Ishiyaku. (Reprinted).

Martin, K.S., Scheet, N.J., & Stegman, M.R. (1993, December). Home health clients: Characteristics, outcomes of care, and nursing interventions. *American Journal of Public Health, 83*(12):1730-1734.

Masson, V. (2003, May). Questioning current practice. *American Journal of Nursing, 103*(5):13.

Monsen, K.A. & Kerr, M.J. (2004, April). Mining quality documentation data for golden outcomes. *Home Health Care Management and Practice, 16*(3):192-199.

Monsen, K.A. & Martin, K.S. (2002a, April/June). Developing an outcomes management program in a public health department. *Outcomes Management, 6*(2):62-66.

Monsen, K.A. & Martin, K.S. (2002b, July/September). Using an outcomes management program in a public health department. *Outcomes Management, 6*(3):120-124.

Nelson, R. & Joos, I. (1989, Summer). On language in nursing: From data to wisdom. *Pennsylvania League for Nursing Visions, 1*(5):6.

Neuman, B. (1995). *The Neuman Systems Model,* 3rd ed. Stamford, CT, Appleton-Lange.

Nursing Outlook, 52(1). (2004, January/February). Entire issue.

Oermann, M.H. (1998, November/December). How to assess critical thinking in clinical practice. *Dimensions of Critical Care Nursing, 17*(6):322-327.

Omaha System Web site. (2004). Retrieved March 8, 2004 from the Internet: http://www.omahasystem.org.

Ozbolt, J.G. (1996, Spring). From minimum data to maximum impact: Using clinical data to strengthen patient care. *Advanced Practice Nursing Quarterly, 1*(4):62-69.

Ozbolt, J. (2000, November/December). Terminology standards for nursing. *Journal of the American Medical Informatics Association, 7*(6):517-522.

Park, H.A., Kim, J.E., & Cho, I. (2000). *Nursing Diagnoses, Interventions, and Outcomes Classification.* Seoul, Korea, Seoul National University Press.

Pesut, D.J. (2002, January-February). Nursing nomenclatures and eye-roll anxiety control. *Journal of Professional Nursing, 18*(1):3-4.

Plowfield, L.A. & Raymond, J.E. (2001, July 30). Capturing nursing interventions and patient outcomes. *Greater Philadelphia Advance for Nurses, 3*(15):21-22, 34.

Polanyi, M. (1967). *The Tacit Dimension.* London, Cox & Wyman.

Profetto-McGrath, J., Hesketh, K.L., Lang, S., & Estabrooks, C.A. (2003, April). A study of critical thinking and research utilization among nurses. *Western Journal of Nursing Research, 25*(3):322-337.

Rosebaugh, D.L. (2004, April). Getting ready for the software in your future. *Home Health Care Management and Practice 16*(3):228-234.

Sawyer, L.M., Berkowitz, B., Haber, J.E., Larrabee, J.H., Marino, B.L., Martin, K.S., Mason, K.P., Mastal, M.F., Nilsson, M.W., Waldridge, S.E., & Walker, M.K. (2002, April/June). Expanding American Nurses Association quality indicators to community-based practices. *Outcomes Management, 6*(2):53-61.

Sienkiewicz, J. (2004, June). The Quality Network Adverse-Event Benchmarking Project: A New Jersey perspective. *Home Health Care Management and Practice, 16*(4):280-285.

Tidd, C.W. (1998, February). From data to information: Management tools for home health care clinical directors. *Home Health Care Management and Practice, 10*(2):1-10.

Turley, J.P. (2000). Informatics and education: The start of a discussion. In Carty, B. (Ed.), *Introduction to Nursing Informatics: Education for Practice,* (pp. 271-293). New York, Springer.

U.S. Department of Health and Human Services. (2003, July 1). *HHS launches new efforts to promote paperless health care system.* Retrieved November 3, 2003 from the Internet: http://aspe.os.dhhs.gov/sp/nhii/News/NHIIJul1_03.htm.

Weed, L. (1968, March 14-21). Special article: Medical records that guide and teach. *New England Journal of Medicine, 278*(12):593-600, 652-657.

Werley, H.H. & Lang, N.M. (Eds.). (1988). *Identification of the Nursing Minimum Data Set.* New York, Springer.

Whitman, G.R. (2003, January/March). Making the grade. *Outcomes Management, 7*(1):4-7.

Wilson, S.K. & Roy, D. (2003). KIWIN: An automated documentation solution for nursing education. In Marin, H.D.F., Marques, E.P., Hovenga, E., & Goossen, W. (Eds.), *NI 2003: 8th International Conference in Nursing Informatics* (p. 707). Rio de Janeiro, Brazil, E-papers Servicos Editorials Ltd.

Zielstorff, R.D. (1998, September). Characteristics of a good nursing nomenclature from an informatics perspective. *Online Journal of Issues in Nursing,3*(2):1-10. Retrieved September 1, 2003 from the Internet: http://www.nursingworld.org/ojin/tpc7/tpc7_4.htm.

Zielstorff, R.D., Cimino, C., Barnett, G.O., Hassan, L., & Blewett, D.R. (1993). Representation of nursing terminology in the UMLS Metathesaurus: A pilot study. In Frisse, M.E. (Ed.), *Symposium on Computer Applications in Medical Care*, (pp. 392-396). New York, McGraw-Hill.

Zielstorff, R.D., Hudgings, C.I., & Grobe, S.J. (1993). *Next-generation Nursing Information Systems.* Washington, DC, American Nurses Association.

2

HOW TO USE THE OMAHA SYSTEM

Karen S. Martin

This chapter is an introduction for all who are interested in the Omaha System and are involved in health care practice, education, research, and information technology. It is designed for diverse learners regardless whether their educational experiences are self-directed or part of organized orientation. Those who have management, educational, or research responsibilities in any setting should also use this chapter for review and preparation prior to instructing others or conducting research.

When beginning to learn or teach the Omaha System, it is useful to consider Benner's novice, advanced beginner, competent, proficient, and expert continuum (Benner, 1984; Benner, Tanner, & Chesla, 1996). Based on a research methodology, Benner examined nurses' critical thinking skills and caregiving styles in work settings. Because novices had only context-free rules and lacked experience, they did not have discretionary judgment to guide their practice. Advanced beginners demonstrated marginally acceptable performance, because they had coped with enough real situations or had mentors who previously identified correct practice decisions. Typically, competent practitioners were nurses who had worked for 2 to 3 years and could relate their immediate actions to long-range goals or plans. Proficient practitioners perceived a situation as a whole and limited their number of reasonable options; case studies were a particularly effective teaching tool. Experts had an intuitive grasp of situations and zeroed in on accurate data, and were therefore able to provide care accurately and quickly; experts analyzed data without delay when novel situations occurred and events and behaviors did not respond as expected.

Omaha System skills can be evaluated and classified according to Benner's continuum. Learners should consider the novice-to-expert concepts to review their own skill performance and progress. They will be less frustrated if they recognize that it takes all Omaha System learners time and effort to gain critical thinking skills and progress through the five stages, especially if they are developing new software skills simultaneously (Larrabee, 1999). Teachers need to consider the novice-to-expert concepts to tailor educational strategies such as the teaching style, format, materials, and schedule (Oermann, 1998). If strategies match the learners' stages, the teaching and learning process will become more efficient and effective. In addition, Dreyfus (1979) identified and Benner (1984) elaborated on three general aspects of skill performance that must be incorporated into Omaha System teaching and learning strategies to develop and improve competence: reliance on past concrete experiences rather than abstract principles, synthesis of a situation into a whole, and conversion from a detached observer to an involved performer.

To help Omaha System learners recognize the context and anticipate what is expected of them, it is helpful to consider the "who, what, when, why, and how" phases of the educational process. Learners, regardless of their discipline, setting, desired outcome, or other variables, are referred to as "who." The first phase for most novices and advanced beginners involves knowing the "what" of the Omaha System structure: its origin, purpose, value, and the meaning of its terms. Knowing "when, why, and how" are the next phases. Learners must develop increasingly complex skills to recognize and select the correct terms of the Omaha System, apply them in their practice, document them in a timely manner, and evaluate how well they are using the terms. They must complete all the phases before they reach proficient or expert status and are able to obtain *accurate and consistent* data and information for aggregate data analysis. Even if some managers, administrators, educators, programmers, and software vendors do not provide client care, they can benefit from participation in interactive educational sessions and gain understanding about the Omaha System, especially if practitioners are focusing on "when, why, and how" case studies and related application activities.

This chapter describes the fundamentals of the Omaha System and serves as a general teaching and learning bridge to specific details and application examples in other chapters of the book. For example, "who" uses the Omaha System is only addressed briefly in this chapter. In contrast, Chapter 3 describes the importance of establishing a multidisciplinary project team in practice settings, its members' responsibilities, and implementation steps in detail, and Chapters 4 through 6 address "who" in relation to education, research, and information technology. Appendix C links client problem, medical diagnosis, and treatment information that is particularly useful to those who are not familiar with standardized terminologies. This chapter addresses the "what, when, why, and how" phases in the following way:

What:

- The first section of the chapter, Omaha System Components, describes the structure and terms of the Problem Classification Scheme, the Intervention Scheme, and the Problem Rating Scale for Outcomes.
- The second section, 2004 Omaha System Revision, summarizes the changes that have occurred since the 1992 books were published, and includes rationale for those changes.

How and *When:* The third section, Guidelines for Use, provides information needed to establish a strong knowledge base or foundation.

Why: The fourth section, Frequently Asked Questions, presents questions often posed by individuals and groups who are evaluating the Omaha System.

OMAHA SYSTEM COMPONENTS

The Omaha System is comprised of the Problem Classification Scheme, the Intervention Scheme, and the Problem Rating Scale for Outcomes. The three components were introduced in Chapter 1 and are summarized in this section. Before reading the rest of this chapter, review Figure 2-2, *B*; the structure, terms, and definitions that appear in Appendix A; and the Glossary. Suggestions and examples of application in practice, education, and research appear throughout the book. In these examples, terms that comprise the components are italicized consistently to facilitate recognition.

Problem Classification Scheme

The Scheme is a comprehensive, orderly, nonexhaustive, mutually exclusive classification designed to identify clients' health-related concerns (see Appendix A). It provides a structure, language, and system of cues and clues to help practitioners collect, sort, document, classify, analyze, retrieve, and communicate client needs and strengths. The Problem Classification Scheme enables practitioners to separate essential from nonessential data objectively and efficiently, organize the puzzle of data elements, and identify relationships and patterns among the data. Rather than expressing the values of practitioners, the Scheme is intended to summarize objective and subjective client data. It is a bridge between diagnosis and the delivery of care. Medical diagnoses, laboratory tests, and etiological or causation factors are not included in the Problem Classification Scheme, but need to be considered when using the Scheme. The Scheme does not replace other specialized terminologies. It is compatible with and complementary to medical diagnoses and other classifications (see Appendix C).

The Problem Classification Scheme is organized in the following way:

Level 1: Domains
- Level 2: Problems
  - Level 3: Modifiers
    - Level 4: Signs/symptoms

Terms that appear at the same level are not listed in hierarchical order; each is of equal importance. Each problem statement has multiple parts that flow from general to specific. The parts include a problem name, one modifier from the *Individual, Family,* and *Community* set, and one modifier from the *Health Promotion*, *Potential*, and *Actual* set. One or more signs/symptoms are identified for an *Actual* problem, as are risk factors for a *Potential* problem, and descriptive data for a *Health Promotion* problem.

Four domains appear at the first level and represent priority areas of practitioner and client health-related concerns. At the second level there are 42 terms referred to as client problems, foci, nursing diagnoses, areas of client needs, concerns, and strengths. Two sets of problem modifiers are at the third level. The modifiers are *Health Promotion, Potential,* or *Actual* as well as *Individual, Family,* or *Community.* At the fourth level, a cluster of signs and symptoms describes actual problems. In most automated and manual record systems, practitioners are encouraged to document a minimal amount of pertinent free text to describe client-specific details about the signs and symptoms for *Actual* problems. Likewise, they should document a minimal amount of free text when they identify risk factors for *Potential* problems and descriptive data for *Health Promotion* problems. During Problem Classification Scheme research, project staff recognized that the diversity and amount of risk factors and descriptive data were too great to organize formally.

The four domains are *Environmental, Psychosocial, Physiological,* and *Health-related Behaviors.* Examples of problems in each respective domain are *Income*, *Caretaking/parenting*, *Circulation,* and *Nutrition.* The first set of modifiers, *Health Promotion*, *Potential,* and *Actual,* is intended to depict a health-illness continuum. When the modifiers are compared, *Health Promotion* defines a positive state of client need and the absence of risk factors or signs and symptoms. Note that while anticipatory guidance and other wellness interventions are applicable, the modifier should not be interchanged with the intervention, health promotion, a term that is typically used in public health practice. The middle term, *Potential,* is used for clients who are at risk for developing a problem because of historic or current factors, but who do not currently exhibit any signs/symptoms. More aggressive educative and therapeutic interventions are required. *Actual* is the most negative of the three modifiers because one or more signs and symptoms are already present. Severity ranges from a relatively mild sign or symptom to several or many severe signs and symptoms. Interventions are designed to resolve or control the signs/symptoms. Based on data that have been available during client record audits at numerous locations, the frequency of modifier use varies. *Actual* is documented most often in all organizations, *Potential* is next and appears in more public health records, and *Health Promotion* is documented least often.

The second set of modifiers consists of *Individual, Family,* and *Community.* The modifiers comprise a continuum and suggest to whom the problem pertains. While acute and long-term care settings have traditionally had individual records, many community providers had family records. With the advent of automation, many community providers decided to maintain their family-centered approach to care, but stopped using family records. This approach usually yields more accurate and complete data for analysis. In addition, good software programs can produce family reports by aggregating data from individual members. The modifier *Community* is a new addition to the Omaha System; it facilitates documentation and analysis of population-focused interventions. Note that the definition is inclusive in order to accommodate a range of user activities. For example, nurse-managed centers use the modifier for their pregnant teen groups, and long-term care facilities for their exercise programs. Health departments select the modifier to capture program data for specific sites or for community-wide programs about tobacco use, communicable disease, housing, or other relevant topics. Appendix B includes examples of case studies that use this approach.

The last level of the Problem Classification Scheme, signs/symptoms, appears as a unique cluster for each problem. Examples of signs/symptoms for the problem *Income* include *uninsured medical expenses* and *difficulty buying necessities.*

The Problem Classification Scheme is comprehensive at the levels of domains, problems, and modifiers and nonexhaustive at the level of the signs/symptoms. The four domains, 42 problems, and two sets of modifiers represent the full spectrum of client issues, while the signs/symptoms offer an expandable, flexible coding structure with the term "other." The number and names of terms have been revised by adding, dividing, and combining since the initial version of the Scheme was developed in 1975. Each problem with its unique cluster of signs and symptoms is intended to represent a discrete area of concern narrow enough to be easily identified and differentiated from other problems and broad enough to represent a client-focused area addressed by practitioners. Signs/symptoms that meet the following criteria have been selected for inclusion: appeared most frequently in research findings, identified by test site practitioners as the most important, and offered a reasonable rather than cumbersome size to the total cluster. Use of the Problem Classification Scheme is based on five general assumptions:

1. Practitioners genuinely care about clients as individuals, families, and communities and develop interpersonal and interview skills sufficient to obtain valid and reliable client data. Clients are included across the age and health-illness spectrums and represent diverse social, cultural, spiritual, regional, political, and economic values.
2. The terms, problems, client needs, concerns, strengths, and nursing diagnoses are stated from the client's perspective. Clients, not practitioners, "own" problems. Ideally, a client acknowledges the problem and is willing to become involved in change. The practitioner's ability to identify problems and set priorities may be different from that of the client.
3. Health care professionals have the knowledge and skills to differentiate between *Health Promotion, Potential, Actual, Individual, Family,* and *Community* problems.
4. Identified problems are amenable to intervention. Problems are an essential component of the Omaha System model (see Figure 2-2, *B*). When practitioners identify prob-

lems as high priority, they develop care plans, identify ratings, and actively work with clients on those problems. In contrast, when practitioners identify problems as low priority, they may record details to leave a data trail for others, but not actively intervene. Health care professionals should be able to describe the rationale for these decisions, although such rationale may or may not be documented.

5. The Problem Classification Scheme is the holistic foundation of the Omaha System and is designed to consist of terms that are mutually exclusive and appear at comparable levels of abstraction (see Figure 2-2, *B*). Although revising the Scheme is possible (see Appendix D), transferring or repeating ideas from one problem to another problem or from a sign/symptom for one problem into a sign/symptom for another problem is not appropriate. If duplication between problems *or* signs and symptoms occurs, the Scheme is no longer a classification.

Intervention Scheme

The Scheme is a comprehensive, orderly, nonexhaustive, mutually exclusive classification used to describe practitioners' actions and activities (see Appendix A). The Scheme provides a structure, language, and system of cues and clues to help nurses and other practitioners classify, document, analyze, and communicate their client-focused actions, activities, or functions. It provides a quality improvement and legal data trail for practitioners' actions. The Intervention Scheme accommodates actions that are autonomous or independent, as well as collaborative or interdependent, and guides practitioners as they develop goal-directed care plans and document interventions. It is designed to be problem-specific, and to provide a bridge between diagnoses and outcomes measurement. Treatment code sets mandated by third party payers are not included in the Intervention Scheme. The Scheme does not replace other specialized terminologies, but is compatible with other treatment code sets.

The Intervention Scheme is organized in the following way:

Level 1: Categories
- Level 2: Targets
  - Level 3: Client-specific Information

Terms that appear at the same level are not listed in hierarchical order; each is of equal importance. Each intervention statement has multiple parts that flow from general to specific: a category name, one or more targets, and one or more client-specific information statements. Interventions are problem-specific when they appear in the care plan or progress notes. Most automated and manual records encourage health care professionals to document a few brief but pertinent words or phrases to describe the client-specific information statements. For example, when the category *Teaching, Guidance, and Counseling* is selected to describe an intervention that was provided, the practitioner should leave a data trail to describe the client's verbal and/or nonverbal responses.

Four broad categories of interventions appear at the first level of abstraction and represent priority areas of professional practice. An alphabetical list of 75 targets or objects of health care action and one "other" appears at the second level. Client-specific information generated by practitioners is at the third level.

The four categories are *Teaching, Guidance, and Counseling*; *Treatments and Procedures; Case Management;* and *Surveillance.* They are designed to address all 42 problems of the Problem Classification Scheme. Targets can be used with each of the four categories. For example, for the problem *Circulation* and the intervention category *Teaching, Guidance, and Counseling,* possible targets are *cardiac care* and *signs/symptoms-physical.* The target *signs/symptoms-physical* is also frequently used with the intervention category *Treatments and Procedures* and the category *Surveillance*. The third level of the Intervention Scheme is client-specific information. Examples for the problem *Caretaking/parenting* and the target *discipline* include methods, appropriateness, and consistency. During early Intervention Scheme research, project staff recognized that the diversity and amount of data referred to as client-specific information were too great to organize formally. Therefore practitioners at the Visiting Nurse Association (VNA) of Omaha developed care planning/intervention guides that were included in the previous Omaha System pocket guide (Martin and Scheet, 1992b). Many practitioners helped expand those guides for this book.

Some agencies and software vendors have integrated the Problem Classification and Intervention Schemes as a foundation for developing planning guides or pathways for problems that practitioners address frequently (see Chapter 3). When health care professionals use these guides appropriately, the guides provide an effective tool and reduce documentation time. When they do not use these guides appropriately, they are likely to ignore important problems and interventions, and address and document less important problems and interventions.

The Intervention Scheme is comprehensive at the level of categories and nonexhaustive at the levels of targets and client-specific information. The four categories represent the full spectrum of practitioner activities, while the targets and client-specific information offer an expandable, flexible coding structure with the term "other." As the Scheme evolved from 1984 to 1993, the number, names, and definitions of categories, targets, and client-specific information were revised. Each category was intended to represent a discrete area of action or activity narrow enough to be easily identified and differentiated from other categories and broad enough to represent an important intervention conducted by various health care disciplines. For example, as described previously, *Teaching, Guidance, and Counseling* was initially subdivided into several categories (Martin & Scheet, 1992a). However, research findings showed that the categories overlapped and did not provide users with mutually exclusive categories. Therefore, the categories were collapsed into one category. Also during the research, targets were organized in various ways, including domain-specific groupings. Practitioners who served as pilot and field testers decided that an alphabetic list was the most efficient and acceptable option.

Use of the Intervention Scheme is based on five general assumptions:

1. Expert health care professionals (a) select the best combination of interventions, (b) adapt them to meet clients' environmental, psychosocial, physiological, and health-related behavior needs and preferences, and (c) time the implementation and repetition of the interventions effectively. They provide evidence- or research-based interventions.
2. Practitioners can develop extensive professional judgment as a result of sound educational preparation, personal experience, and experience providing care to clients. Therefore, they recognize the benefits of practice, documentation, and information systems that offer flexibility as well as cues and clues; they tend to reject exhaustive standardized plans as burdensome.
3. In partnership with clients, practitioners identify strengths and set priorities among problems before developing plans and interventions. Priorities take into account factors such as the urgency of client needs, safety, dynamics, politics, and a comparison of costs and benefits. Likewise, client action is usually required to increase self-sufficiency and make progress.
4. Individuals, families, and communities have the right and responsibility to make their own decisions unless their safety or the safety of others is severely jeopardized. Decisions reflect their social and cultural systems and personal values.

5. The Intervention Scheme provides essential terms that describe practitioners' actions and activities in the Omaha System model (see Figure 2-2, *B*). Plans and interventions are based on categories, targets, and client-specific information, are closely linked, and are often developed or completed simultaneously.

Problem Rating Scale for Outcomes

The Scale is a comprehensive, systematic, recurring evaluation framework designed to measure client progress in relation to specific health-related problems (see Appendix A). It provides a bridge between client problems and the delivery of care, and serves as a guide to practice for practitioners. The Scale offers a quantitative method of documentation from admission through discharge. Because the design is simple, it is practical to implement and can be completed quickly by health care professionals. Although mortality, morbidity, cost, severity of illness, patient acuity, nursing intensity, Outcome and Assessment Information Set (OASIS), and other outcome indicators are not included in the Problem Rating Scale for Outcomes, they need to be considered when using the Scale. The Problem Rating Scale for Outcomes is compatible with and complementary to other outcome indicators and terminologies.

The Problem Rating Scale for Outcomes consists of three five-point scales or dimensions for measuring the entire range of severity for the concepts of *Knowledge*, *Behavior*, and *Status*. The Scale is based on the assumption that the interaction of a client and practitioner in relation to a specific problem affects what the client knows (*Knowledge*), what the client does (*Behavior*), and how the client is (*Status*). The purpose of the *Knowledge* subscale is to determine how well the client understands. The purpose of the *Behavior* subscale is to evaluate client practices, performances, and skills. The purpose of the *Status* subscale is to determine how the client's conditions or circumstances improve, remain stable, or deteriorate. Dr. Avedis Donabedian served as a consultant to develop a model that depicts the three concepts of *Knowledge*, *Behavior*, and *Status;* client-practitioner interactions relative to outcomes; and the problem solving process (Figure 2-1). The figure is closely related to Donabedian's (1966) structure, process, and outcome evaluation approach. The figure indicates that it is crucial for health care professionals to identify and maximize positive or driving forces and minimize negative or restraining forces to develop appropriate intervention strategies. Those interventions intersect with the three parallel subscales before changing direction and merging at the ultimate goals of client adaptation and coping.

Each of the three subscales is a continuum providing an evaluation framework for examining problem-specific client ratings at regular or predictable time intervals. Suggested times include admission, specific interim points, and dismissal. Users, preferably user organizations, need to determine a frequency or schedule of interim ratings and disseminate an organizational policy. For example, some educators require students to complete ratings as part of documentation for each client encounter. Students have relatively few opportunities to work with clients and need to practice the steps involved with ratings. In contrast, home care programs may establish a policy that ratings are evaluated when a significant client change occurs and/or when it is time to review and update assessment details and orders. Often, public health programs establish a 1- to 2-month review interval. It is likely that long-term care programs will establish a longer review interval and may expect practitioners to complete ratings every 3 or 6 months.

When establishing the initial ratings, practitioners create an independent data baseline to capture the condition and circumstances of clients before the delivery of service. Admission *Knowledge, Behavior,* and *Status* severity baselines are used to compare and

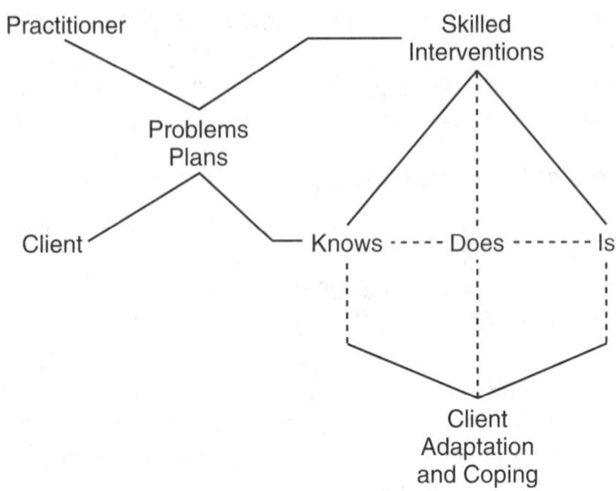

Figure 2-1 The outcome model depicts how practitioner-client interactions affect client adaptation and coping.

contrast clients' conditions and circumstances with the ratings completed at later intervals and at client dismissal. The comparison or change in ratings over time can be used to identify client progress in relation to the effectiveness of the plan of care and interventions for specific client problems.

The Problem Rating Scale for Outcomes is actually comprised of three summated or Likert-type ordinal scales (Martin, Norris, & Leak, 1999). Although the Scale has characteristics of both norm- and criterion-referenced instruments, it has more of the latter. The Scale was constructed for two primary purposes: to examine outcomes in relation to specific behavioral criteria and to determine how well clients have achieved specific knowledge, behavior, or status indicators.

The three scales are equal in importance, although they may not be equal when used with specific clients. For example, changes in the *Status* rating of a child who has been abused are of extreme concern to a nurse. The nurse, however, may be much less concerned about the *Knowledge* rating. In contrast, the *Knowledge* rating of an elder with a respiration problem may be of greater concern to a hospice nurse than the *Status* rating. Unlike some Likert-type scales, the Problem Rating Scale for Outcomes does not include a formal set of questions to be scored and summed and produce a final numeric rating. Instead, users need knowledge, experience, and guidance, and to refer to the examples in the User's Guide. The prototypical patterns are guidelines or anchors for rating each of the 42 problems.

Use of the Scale serves several purposes for practitioners. It encourages them to consider anticipated ratings or goals for client care. It helps them consider intervention alternatives relative to clients' circumstances or need for change or adaptation. By transforming abstract measurement concepts into ones that are concrete, it offers a feedback method to practitioners as they review and reflect on the patterns of the ratings.

Between 1978 and 1984, Omaha System research efforts produced a system of expected outcomes and outcome criteria that were intended to serve as an evaluation tool. During testing at four field sites, nurses reported extensive difficulties and dissatisfaction. The previous tool was discontinued and work began on the Problem Rating Scale for Outcomes, grounded on the principles of content validity. As the Scale evolved and was completed in 1986, three concepts were determined to be essential. The Scale has five categories or degrees for response to depict the most positive or desired to the most negative or severe client state in relation to a specific problem.

Prototypical patterns were included in the 1992 Omaha System pocket guide (Martin & Scheet, 1992b) and are in this book as examples, guidelines, or anchors. The prototypes illustrate the potential range of severity or intensity for each problem, but are not intended to be an exhaustive example for that problem. Thus, while practitioners should consider these anchors to rate each problem, they must still use their sound clinical judgment.

During the pilot and field tests, some nurses preferred selecting a numeric rating for the concepts of *Knowledge, Behavior,* and *Status;* others preferred using words. Therefore, the final Scale has both numbers and words. For example, when using the Scale for problems such as *Income* and *Circulation,* practitioners identify and document one baseline rating for each concept during the first home visit, hospital shift, or clinic encounter. One rating should again be identified for each of the three concepts at appropriate intervals and when the client is discharged from service.

Use of the Problem Rating Scale for Outcomes is based on five general assumptions:

1. Client change is inevitable and especially desirable when it involves movement in a positive direction. Most individuals, families, and communities value improvements that increase their competence, enhance control over their lives, and promote their functioning at the highest possible level.
2. Client change is influenced significantly by practitioners although cause-effect relationships can rarely be proven. Clients have their own unique problems and value systems and control some of the variables that affect change. In addition, some variables are beyond the control of clients, practitioners, or others in the health care and social service systems.
3. It is possible to implement measures of change in many ways, including practitioners using themselves as change agents. The more health care professionals understand and value outcomes measurement, the more likely they are to be successful change agents.
4. Most practitioners have the wisdom and skills to determine a specific rating from among the available choices. The best selection reflects clients' history and assessment, practice experience, disease pathology, and recent developments in treatments, pharmacology, and medical care. Practitioners also must recall *Knowledge, Behavior,* and *Status* patterns they observed with others in similar circumstances, whether those are family members, friends, or clients as individuals, families, or communities. Practitioners are expected to recognize that the continuum of each subscale represents the universe of clients, not just one community, the families in one practitioner's caseload, or the individuals who attend clinic during a specific week.
5. The Problem Rating Scale for Outcomes is an essential component of the Omaha System model (see Figure 2-2, *B*). *Knowledge, Behavior,* and *Status* ratings comprise the Scale and are a valid and reliable way to operationalize outcomes measurement.

2005 OMAHA SYSTEM REVISION

Research staff, practitioners, managers, and administrators at the VNA of Omaha recognized that it was critical to encourage accurate and consistent use of the Omaha System and maintain its integrity; they wanted to help it thrive and to guide it into the future. Those objectives were shared by the seven research field test sites located from 1975 through 1993 throughout the United States, and a relatively small number of additional practice, education, and research adopters and supporters.

The publication of this book with its revised version of the Omaha System (Appendix A) is an important milestone and describes how use and users have expanded since the initial VNA research. The revision is a result of a lengthy and comprehensive approach that included expert practice, education, and research users, and reflects changes and trends in practice and health care delivery that are occurring globally in the twenty-first century. The terms and definitions incorporate suggestions and research findings from a rapidly growing number of diverse global users, responses from the Omaha System surveys (Appendix F), a small communicable disease pilot test, an extensive field test, and an extensive review procedure (Appendix D). Information technology and reference terminology advances were also considered. Establishing a 12-member Advisory Board as a panel of experts was a critical milestone for the revision process. The Board will meet every 2 years to discuss the Omaha System and schedule a 5-year review process that begins with this 2005 revision. Details about the revision criteria, the Advisory Board, the field test and review process, and the retirement of terms and codes are in Appendix D.

The Omaha System revision is presented in four ways. First, terms that have been added, divided, combined, and retired are introduced with a brief rationale in this chapter. If a term was edited but not significantly, it is not listed. Second, the completed Omaha System with all revised terms and definitions is presented in Appendix A. Third, the revised Omaha System coding system appears in Appendix E. Codes were retired and cannot be reused for those terms that had significant changes in meaning. Likewise, new codes have been assigned to new terms. For these reasons, it was necessary to change the coding system extensively for this 2005 revision. Representatives from the Advisory Board, automated and manual System users, software vendors, and the National Library of Medicine evaluated alternatives. The final decisions are reflected in Appendixes A and E. While the order of terms and hierarchical structure of the Problem Classification and Intervention Schemes are essential and retained, the codes were removed for all point-of-care users of both automated and manual records (Appendix A). Simultaneously, all software and manual record developers are urged to adopt and use the new coding system consistently (Appendix E) so that data will be compared and analyzed across time and settings. Fourth, all terms, including new or revised definitions, are included in the Glossary.

Omaha System Model (Figure 2-2)

- Changed *Nurse-Client Relationship* to *Practitioner-Client Relationship* (outer circle).

Rationale: Change emphasizes multidisciplinary focus. The term, *Nurse-Client Relationship,* reflected federal funding for four research projects. While other disciplines were using the Omaha System in 1992 (Martin & Scheet, 1992a), the proportion is increasing rapidly.

- Changed *Individual or Family* to *Individual, Family, or Community* (inner circle).

Rationale: Change reflects expanded application. In the late 1980s and early 1990s, a group of community health graduate students selected certain problems and conducted successful community-wide assessments. This information was only briefly mentioned in the previous book. Now, various practice and education settings use the Omaha System to document population-based and community-level interventions for target groups, clinics, neighborhoods, census tracts, and other geographic areas and populations. The Minnesota Users Group, described in Chapter 1, contributed to the knowledge base for the *Community* modifier based on their practice experience with

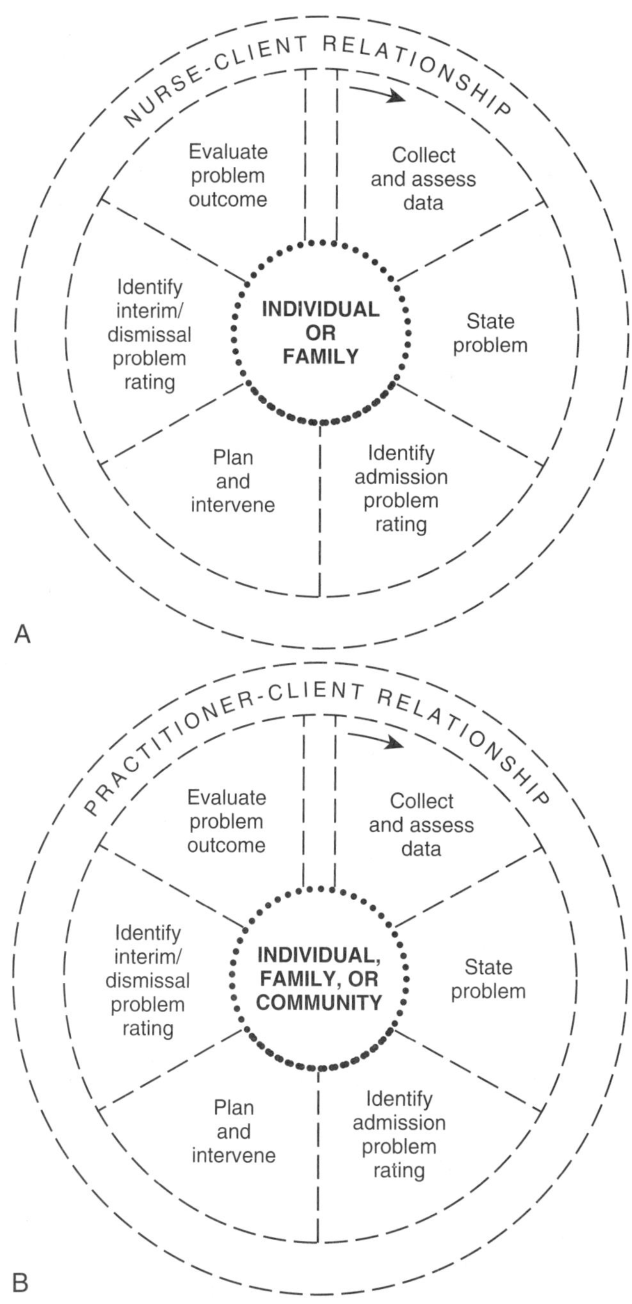

Figure 2-2 **A,** The original Omaha System Model. **B,** The revised Omaha System Model.

the Public Health Interventions Model. User Group members include developers and users of this Model, which defines the concepts of population-based individual, community, and systems-focused interventions (Keller et al., 1998; Keller et al., in press a and b). Practitioners and educators at the University of Wisconsin-Milwaukee nurse-managed center use the Omaha System with community groups. They incorporate before and after skills testing and demonstrations to increase the accuracy of data, including *Knowledge, Behavior,* and *Status* ratings. The definition and adoption of the *Community* modifier should be considered a work in progress; further research, use, and testing are needed and will be described in future publications.

- Changed *Conceptualization of the Family Nursing Process* to *Omaha System Model of the Problem Solving Process* (title).

Rationale: Change emphasizes multidisciplinary focus. While other disciplines were using the Omaha System in 1992 (Martin & Scheet, 1992a), their proportion is increasing rapidly.

Problem Classification Scheme

Additions, divisions, combinations, and retired terms are listed in the order that the problems appear in the four domains.

Modifiers:

- Changed the modifier options, *Deficit, Impairment,* or *Actual,* to *Actual.*

Rationale: Simplified use and documentation.

Environmental Domain:

- Added two signs/symptoms, *presence of mold and excessive pets*, for the problem, *Sanitation.*

Rationale: Offers needed options. The first new sign/symptom may be used to document community level interventions designed to prevent or decrease illness, especially after natural disasters such as floods and tornadoes.

- Added two signs/symptoms, *exposed wiring* and *structural barriers*, for the problem, *Residence.*

Rationale: Offers needed options.

- For the problem, *Neighborhood/workplace safety*, added five signs/symptoms, *inadequate space/resources to foster health, threats/reports of violence, vehicle/traffic hazards, chemical hazards,* and *radiological hazards.*

Rationale: The second new sign/symptom is useful with all three modifiers; the other four offer needed options, especially when documenting community resources, safety work such as alcohol-related traffic fatalities, and emergency preparedness.

Psychosocial Domain:

- Added five signs/symptoms for the problem, *Communication with community resources.* They are *cultural barrier, educational barrier, transportation barrier, limited access to care/services/goods,* and *unable to use/has inadequate communication devices/equipment.*

Rationale: Clarifies the intent and extent of the problem; incorporates the relevant instrumental activities of daily living.

- For the problem, *Role change*, combined the two signs/symptoms, *involuntary reversal of traditional male/female roles* and *involuntary reversal of dependent/independent roles*, to *involuntary role reversal.*

Rationale: Simplified for users and documentation.

- For the problem, *Interpersonal relationship,* added two signs/symptoms, *physically/emotionally abusive to partner,* and *difficulty problem solving without conflict.* Revised sign/symptom, *inappropriate suspicion/manipulation/compulsion/aggression,* to *inappropriate suspicion/manipulation/control.*

Rationale: Offers needed options. Through the revision process, *compulsion* and *aggression,* were moved to the problem, *Mental health.*

- Corrected the problem name, *Spiritual distress*, to *Spirituality.*

Rationale: Because of a typographical error, *Spirituality* was not printed in the 1992 books, but was included in other publications and software.

- Changed the problem name, *Emotional stability,* to *Mental health.* Divided the sign/symptom, *expresses wish to die/attempts suicide* to *expresses suicidal/homicidal thoughts* and *attempts suicide/homicide.* Added, combined, or revised nine signs/symptoms, *narrowed to scattered attention/focus, irritable/agitated/aggressive, purposeless/compulsive activity, difficulty managing anger, delusions, hallucinations/illusions*, *self-mutilation*, *mood swings*, and *flash-backs.*

Rationale: Simplified and clarified the problem name and expanded the signs/symptoms to coincide with data that clients are presenting.

- Changed the problem name, *Human sexuality,* to *Sexuality* and added three signs/symptoms, *unsafe sexual practices, sexual acting out/provocative behaviors/harassment,* and *sexual perpetration/assault.*

Rationale: Simplified; human is understood in the definition. Added needed sign/symptoms.

- Added the sign/symptom, *difficulty interpreting or responding to verbal/nonverbal communication*, for the problem, *Caretaking/parenting.*
- Changed the problem name, *Neglected child/adult,* to *Neglect.*

Rationale: Simplified; child or adult who is neglected is understood in definition.

- Changed the problem name, *Abused child/adult*, to *Abuse.*

Rationale: Simplified; child or adult who is abused is understood in definition.

Physiological Domain:

- Added two signs/symptoms, *difficulty hearing speech in large group settings,* and *difficulty hearing high-frequency sounds,* for the problem, *Hearing.*

Rationale: Offers needed options.

- Added the sign/symptoms, *floaters/flashes,* for the problem, *Vision.*

Rationale: Offers needed options.

- Changed the problem, *Dentition,* to *Oral health* and added three signs/symptoms, *caries, excess tartar,* and *sensitivity to hot or cold.* Revised *abnormalities of teeth* to *missing/broken/malformed teeth.*

Rationale: Expands problem and cluster of signs/symptoms.

- Added the sign/symptom, *wanders*, for the problem, *Cognition.*

Rationale: Adds an important option, especially for clients who have Alzheimer's disease.

- Changed the problem name, *Integument*, to *Skin* and added the sign/symptom, *delayed incisional healing.*

Rationale: New problem name preferred by global users; new sign/symptom can be used with surgical incisions and implanted devices.

- For the problem, *Neuro-musculo-skeletal function*, added three signs/symptoms: *difficulty transferring*, *fractures*, and *difficulty with thermoregulation.* Retired one sign/symptom, *difficulty managing activities of daily living.*

Rationale: Provides more specificity including data related to activities of daily living.

- Added the sign/symptom, *abnormal respiratory laboratory results,* for the problem, *Respiration.*

Rationale: Offers needed option.

- Added two signs/symptoms, *abnormal clotting,* and *abnormal cardiac laboratory results,* for the problem, *Circulation.*

Rationale: Offers needed option.

- Divided one problem, *Genito-urinary function,* into two problems, *Urinary function* and *Reproductive function.* The cluster of signs/symptoms for *Urinary function* is *burning/painful urination, incontinent of urine, urgency/frequency, difficulty initiating urination, difficulty emptying bladder, abnormal amount, hematuria/abnormal color, nocturia*, and *abnormal urinary laboratory results.* The cluster of signs/symptoms for *Reproductive function* is *abnormal discharge, abnormal menstrual pattern, difficulty managing menopause/andropause, abnormal lumps/swelling/tenderness of genital organs or breasts, pain during or after sexual intercourse, infertility*, and *impotency.*

Rationale: Each problem has a unique set of client concerns, risk factors, and signs/symptoms and corresponding interventions and ratings. Offers needed options for breast disease. Since the Scheme is not organized by physiological systems, this combination is possible.

- Divided one problem, *Antepartum/postpartum*, into two problems, *Pregnancy* and *Postpartum.* The cluster of signs/symptoms for *Pregnancy* is *difficulty bonding with unborn baby, difficulty coping with body changes, difficulty with prenatal exercise/rest/diet/behaviors, fears delivery procedure, prenatal complications/preterm labor,* and *inadequate social support.* The cluster of signs/symptoms for *Postpartum* is *difficulty breast-feeding, difficulty coping with postpartum changes, difficulty with postpartum exercise/rest/diet/behaviors, abnormal bleeding/vaginal discharge, postpartum complications,* and *abnormal depressed feelings.*

Rationale: Each problem has a unique set of client concerns, risk factors, and signs/symptoms and corresponding interventions and ratings. A primary reason that they were combined in previous versions was the burden of documentation using manual records. Information technology has decreased that burden.

- Added the problem, *Communicable/infectious condition*, with a cluster of signs/symptoms: *infection, infestation, fever, biological hazards, positive screening/culture/laboratory results, inadequate supplies/equipment/policies to prevent transmission, does not follow infection control regimen,* and *inadequate immunity.*

Rationale: A similar problem, Infection management: Communicable disease, was described previously (Martin & Scheet, 1992a); it was not added because the signs and symptoms duplicated those of other problems, reducing the discreteness of categories and interrater reliability. Since then, the incidence of tuberculosis and HIV/AIDS has increased globally, smallpox has become a threat, and diseases such as West Nile virus and Severe Acute Respiratory Syndrome (SARS) have been identified. Health care professionals provide diverse interventions, including those at the community level.

Health-related Behaviors Domain:

- For the problem, *Nutrition,* added one sign/symptom, *unable to obtain/prepare food.* Revised two signs/symptoms, *weighs 10% more than average,* to *overweight: adult BMI 25.0 or more; child BMI 95th percentile or more.* Revised sign/symptom, *weighs 10% percent less than average*, to *underweight: adult BMI 18.5 or less; child BMI 5th percentile or less.*

Rationale: Registered dieticians and other practitioners are using widely-accepted Body Mass Index charts for more precise calculation.

- Added two signs/symptoms, *sleep apnea* and *snoring,* for the problem, *Sleep and rest patterns.*

Rationale: Offers needed option.

- Changed the problem name, *Personal hygiene* to *Personal care.* Added four signs/symptoms, *difficulty with toileting activities, difficulty dressing lower body, difficulty dressing upper body,* and *unwilling/unable/forgets to complete personal care activities.*

Rationale: Expands problem and cluster of signs/symptoms including those related to activities of daily living.

- For the problem, *Substance use,* divided and revised the sign/symptom, *abuses over-the-counter/street drugs,* to *abuses over-the-counter/prescription medications* and *uses "street"-recreational drugs.* Added two signs/symptoms, *exposure to cigarette/cigar smoke* and *buys/sells illegal substances.*

Rationale: Offers needed options, Including those for community level interventions.

- For the problem, *Family planning,* added three signs/symptoms. They are *inappropriate/insufficient knowledge about preconceptual health practices, fears others' reactions regarding family planning choices,* and *difficulty obtaining family planning methods.*

Rationale: Offers needed options.

- For the problem, *Health care supervision,* added the sign/symptom, *inadequate source of health care,* and revised other signs/symptoms.

Rationale: Offers needed options. Five of the signs/symptoms needed editing to remain consistent with the problem's definition that now includes a range of practitioners in addition to physicians and dentists.

- Changed the problem name, *Prescribed mediation regimen,* to *Medication regimen,* and added two signs/symptoms, *inadequate medication regimen* and *unable to take medications without help.*

Rationale: Because the number and type of over-the-counter medications are increasingly rapidly, practitioners offer diverse services. Medications that are available only by prescription vary globally. The new sign/symptom reflects client needs.

- Retired the problem, *Technical procedure,* and its cluster of signs/symptoms.

Rationale: Simplified based on suggestions from field test and section review participants who indicated that the problem duplicated others. For example, use problems such as *Skin* (wound care), *Respiration* (tracheostomy care), *Urinary function* (catheter care), and *Medication regimen* (insulin, injections, intravenous fluids) instead.

Intervention Scheme

Categories:

- Changed *Health Teaching, Guidance, and Counseling* to *Teaching, Guidance, and Counseling.*

Rationale: Simplified; understood that all categories are related to health in a broad sense.

Targets: Additions, divisions, combinations, and retired terms are listed in alphabetical order.

- Added the target, *anger management.*

Rationale: Reflects needs in practice settings.

- Added the target, *community outreach worker services.*

Rationale: Reflects adoption in expanded settings and makes term more parallel to other targets.

- Added the target, *continuity of care.*

Rationale: Reflects practitioners' increased responsibilities.

- Added the target, *dietary management,* after combining and retiring two targets, *food* and *nutrition.*

Rationale: Because original targets were too similar, users were confused and resulted in decreased interrater reliability. New target includes foods and fluids.

- Added the target, *end-of-life care.*

Rationale: Reflects practitioners' increased responsibilities.

- Added the target, *genetics.*

Rationale: Reflects new and diverse services providers are offering.

- Added the target, *homemaking/housekeeping,* after retiring the target, *homemaking.*

Rationale: Reflects expanded use in diverse settings.

- Added the target, *infection precautions.*

Rationale: Reflects increase in emerging infectious agents and practitioners' expanded responsibilities.

- Added the target, *interpreter/translator services.*

Rationale: Reflects adoption in expanded settings and makes term more parallel to other targets.

- Added the target, *medication coordination/ordering.*

Rationale: Reflects diverse practitioners' increased responsibilities and needed communication with pharmacists and others who distribute medications.

- Added the target, *medication prescription.*

Rationale: Reflects the increased number and type of providers who have licensed/approved prescriptive authority for certain medications.

- Added the target, *nursing care.*

Rationale: Provides option parallel to *medical/dental care* and *social work/counseling.*

- Added the target, *occupational therapy care.*

Rationale: Provides option parallel to *medical/dental care* and *social work/counseling;* retired the target, *rehabilitation.*

- Added the target, *paraprofessional/aide care* and retired the target, *nursing care, supplementary.*

Rationale: Reflects adoption in expanded settings and makes term more parallel to other targets.

- Added the target, *physical therapy care.*

Rationale: Provides option parallel to *medical/dental care* and *social work/counseling;* retired the target, *rehabilitation.*

- Added the target, *recreational therapy care.*

Rationale: Provides option parallel to *medical/dental care* and *social work/counseling.*

- Added the target, *respiratory care,* after retiring the target, *bronchial hygiene.*

Rationale: Reflects expansion and simplifies term.

- Added the target, *respiratory therapy care.*

Rationale: Provides option parallel to *medical/dental care* and *social work/counseling.*

- Added the target, *speech and language pathology care.*

Rationale: Provides option parallel to *medical/dental care* and *social work/counseling.*

- Added the target, *substance use cessation,* after retiring the target, *substance use.*

Rationale: Reflects expansion and simplifies term.

GUIDELINES FOR USE

Learning to use the Omaha System can be a very challenging yet rewarding experience for both teachers and learners. Most often groups consist of individuals who are at different phases of the novice-to-expert continuum and have different learning styles. Teachers need to be creative and to emphasize and repeat information many times. They can select suggestions from those described throughout this book to develop reasonable planning, orientation, implementation, and maintenance steps and schedules to match the situation. Then user organizations should adopt an ongoing quality improvement approach to evaluate progress and revise the steps and schedules.

Remember that the Omaha System was designed to enhance practice, documentation, and information management. Consider that a client record is a professional and legal communication trail that reflects the information practitioners *and* others need to know about clients and practice. It presents a summary of the pertinent words and ideas that a videotape would capture during a client encounter. Quality documentation is comprehensive, brief, precise, timely, and essential, but it is secondary to service, practitioners' first priority.

While the Omaha System is an organizational framework or tool for sorting and organizing client data, it is only a tool. Users need practical experience and the ability to prioritize information regardless of the type of clients, setting, electronic health records, technology, or manual forms. Practitioners have unique personalities and thought patterns, and sometimes select different Omaha System terms when describing similar situations. The goal of using the Omaha System is not to develop "cookie-cutter practitioners" or "cookie-cutter clients," but to encourage practitioners to respond to and record client data accurately and consistently. Usually there are not "right" and "wrong" choices, but some terms are a better match for the presenting data. Some practitioners tend to be "lumpers" (combining data into a small number of large subdivisions) while others are "splitters" (dividing data into a large number of small subdivisions). A balance is essential; extremes of both approaches lead to low rates of accuracy and interrater reliability. Teachers need to allow learners to be flexible and to encourage creative, critical thinking, especially with new learners. Simultaneously, because other goals of the Omaha System are to encourage standardized, high quality documentation and interrater reliability so that aggregate data are accurate and consistent, teachers must provide positive reinforcement for better answers and help colleagues reinforce each other.

Discussing guidelines and rules is an effective teaching strategy. Guidelines were established during early Omaha System development to facilitate accuracy and consistency; many were published in the 1992 books. User experiences in practice, education, and research settings have helped to refine, elaborate, and add details. Although it is important to introduce novices to the guidelines and rules during orientation, they need to practice using the Omaha System and to develop skills before that information becomes meaningful. Consider scheduling a review and discussion period later, and ask learners to recall examples based on their experiences. Incorporate a guideline and rule discussion into a record audit or other quality improvement activity at periodic intervals. Encourage practitioners to understand the guidelines.

General Use Guidelines

- Recognize that the Omaha System is a series of feedback loops. It can effectively link client problems, professional interventions, and client outcomes, the foundation of evidence-based practice.
- Acknowledge that critical thinking will always be important. The Omaha System gives a context to coding; *it supports, but does not prescribe, practice.*

- Remember the forest and trees introduced in the Preface of this book.Learn to use the details (trees) of the Omaha System well, but do not forget about the bigger picture (forest), the purpose for using the System.
- Use the Omaha System to focus and direct your professional energy.
- Make certain that your practice reflects your belief that you and your clients are partners.
- Recognize that it takes time, commitment, and flexibility to learn correct application. Perfection and 100% interrater reliability or agreement are not reasonable goals; it should be reasonable for the group to achieve at least 80% agreement.
- Note the pattern of capital letters and italics used throughout the book to identify Omaha System terms (i.e., *Income, low/no income, Treatments and Procedures, Status*).
- Note that slashes represent and/or ideas.
- Review the Omaha System terms, definitions, and guidelines regularly. Discuss application with others. Everyone benefits from occasional review that reinforces good habits and reduces bad habits. Often, review and discussion among a diverse group of users decreases the urge to suggest that additions to the Omaha System are needed, because it provides reminders about the entire Omaha System and some lesser-used terms.
- Refine your skills, differentiating between data that are pertinent and those that are not, and document using four words rather than fourteen if those words are adequate. Documentation should be brief and concise.
- Use the structure, terms, and guidelines consistently and accurately. Otherwise, data cannot be compared between providers, disciplines, or clients within a setting or between settings.
- Consider practice and documentation as dynamic, integrated processes. Both should reflect reality. Evaluate problems, care plans, interventions, and ratings at intervals and revise care accordingly. Identify new problems and resolve others when appropriate. NOTE: Practitioners and managers should establish agency or organizational guidelines for the rating intervals based on their clients, staff, and programs.
- Use the term "other" infrequently. When the Omaha System does not seem to accommodate terms or ideas, practitioners should seek assistance from their colleagues and managers who may suggest an alternative. When no standardized terms fit, specify the words (short explanation) for "other."
- Expect to continue using other methods and classifications to document and communicate practice-related data. The Omaha System will not replace all others such as time and mileage documentation, immunization history, Current Procedural Terminology (CPT) codes, or the International Classification of Diseases.
- Accept that the Omaha System is evolving and will not match every client situation perfectly.
- Celebrate successes and laugh regularly.

Problem Classification Scheme Guidelines

- Replace the term "client problem" mentally and in your vocabulary with client need, focus, concern, issue, consideration, care component, interest area, or another synonym if you prefer. If you are part of a group, agency, or organization, select one synonym and use it consistently. However, recognize that the term "problem" appears throughout this book, and continue to use the definition of that term consistently.
- Use the Scheme as the framework or foundation for a holistic, comprehensive assessment. However, consider referral data, client requests, assessment tools, practice

wisdom, and other factors to substantiate your conclusions and predict high-priority problems. When interacting with clients, use your senses of sight, hearing, touch, and smell to further refine your priorities.

- Synthesize related data before reaching a conclusion and documenting that conclusion. For instance, *missing/broken/malformed teeth* is a sign/symptom for the *Actual* problem *Oral health.* Since a client with missing teeth may not need a practitioner to provide interventions, the presence of a single sign/symptom may or may not be sufficient cause for documentation on a problem list. However, such data should be noted in the assessment section of the client record.
- Remember that problems modified by *Health Promotion, Potential*, or *Actual* may be high-priority problems that require interventions *or* may be low-priority problems that do not require interventions. Thus some *Health* or *Potential Promotion* problems may be considered high priority while some *Actual* problems may be considered low priority. For example, *Income* is an *Actual* and low-priority problem when all available resources have been identified. In contrast, *Medication regimen* is a *Potential* and high-priority problem right after hospital discharge when the nurse helps a client and family members understand critical information about new medications and organize a reminder system.
- Choose salient problems for documentation. Select one problem rather than two to reflect client data, distinguish between high- and low-priority problems, refrain from documenting a large number of high-priority problems, and document less about low-priority problems. Neither practitioners nor clients can work on unlimited problems. Remember that problem selection is a dynamic process throughout the duration of client care.
- Document free text (practitioner-generated words or phrases) to provide essential details about client concerns, needs, strengths, risk factors, signs, and symptoms. This text should be pertinent, brief, and focused. Regardless of how many problems or comorbidities exist, free text *should not* be documented for all 42 problems. Free text *should* be documented on occasion even if a *Health Promotion*, *Potential*, or *Actual* problem is not identified. For example, use free text to document strengths.
- Recognize that problems are stated from the client's perspective and are "owned" by the client.
- Consider the reason for referral or start of service as you complete the assessment. Usually those data will be reflected in the identification of one or more problems.
- Note that problem names are intended to be neutral. Exceptions are *Grief*, *Neglect*, *Abuse*, and *Pain.* Regardless if problems are neutral or negative, use the same guidelines for modifiers, signs/symptoms, the Intervention Scheme, and the Problem Rating Scale for Outcomes.
- Differentiate between client problems and medical diagnoses. Medical diagnoses are an essential part of many client records. Because of professional practice acts, many providers do not treat medical diagnoses such as diabetes mellitus, although clinicians including nurse practitioners, nurse midwives, physicians' assistants, and physicians do.
- Remember that a problem statement consists of three parts: a problem name or label and two modifiers (e.g., *Circulation: Actual, Individual*).
- Refer to the User's Guide examples when deciding if the correct modifier is *Health Promotion*, *Potential*, or *Actual.* These examples are based on actual practice and were developed by practitioners to serve as a guide for decision making. NOTE: Since only one example is given for each modifier, the examples may or may not match your clients' data. Practitioners must develop their own examples to serve as a bridge between the examples in the book and their own clients.

- Document signs/symptoms for *Actual* problems only. One or several signs/symptoms will be appropriate to identify an *Actual* problem.
- Note that this book includes clusters of signs/symptoms for *Actual* problems but not equivalent clusters for *Health Promotion* and *Potential* problems. The diversity and number of *Health Promotion* and *Potential* are too great to organize formally and would produce duplicated lists.
- Differentiate signs/symptoms and problems from interventions. For example, inserting a Foley catheter is an intervention designed to address the *Actual* problem *Urinary function.*
- Differentiate the cause or etiology of a problem from the problem itself. Frequently, the etiology involves a medical diagnosis or lack of knowledge. For example, a stroke is the etiology of the *Actual* problem *Neuro-musculo-skeletal function* and the sign/symptom, *gait/ambulation disturbance.* A practitioner may document that a 15-year-old mother or father has an *Actual Caretaking/parenting* problem because he or she does not hold and stimulate the newborn appropriately. The etiology may include lack of experience, knowledge, and positive role models.
- Differentiate risk factors from signs/symptoms. For example, "first experience with parenting" is usually a risk factor (use the modifier, *Potential*) and not a sign/symptom of *Caretaking/parenting.*

Intervention Scheme Guidelines

- Use the Scheme in two ways: to develop a care plan defined as a set of anticipated interventions, and to document health-related actions that were provided. While documentation must be concise, client records are legal documents, and interventions that are not recorded are not considered to have been provided.
- Recognize that although the Scheme is designed for multidisciplinary use, practitioners should provide and document interventions based on their standards of practice and their level of expertise. No practitioner is competent to provide all intervention combinations for all problems.
- Recognize that the time frame for the care plan can vary with the client, the practitioner, and the agency or organization.
- Document care plans and interventions with three parts: a category, target(s), and client-specific information. For example, for the problem *Caretaking/parenting*, a nurse developed a care plan that included the category *Teaching, Guidance, and Counseling*, the target *safety*, and the client-specific information *use the Smith County Poison Control Guide for Mrs. Blue's 2- and 4-year-olds.* For the problem *Neuro-musculo-skeletal function*, a physical therapist documented the category *Treatments and Procedures*, the target *exercises*, and the client-specific information *resistive range of motion to the left shoulder: lateral raises with a 3-pound weight.*
- Refer to the examples in the User's Guide (Section II) when documenting care plans or completed interventions. Because these examples are based on actual practice and represent practitioners' frequently selected options, all targets are not listed in the examples. NOTE: The examples may *or* may not match your documentation needs; you may need to develop your own example or use a target that is not listed.
- Differentiate objective and subjective data from interventions. For example, if the client is an individual who took her/his blood pressure, the numeric reading should be documented with objective/assessment information. If the practitioner takes the blood pressure, the reading should be documented with the category *Surveillance.* If the practitioner calls the nurse practitioner or physician's office and reports significant findings or

changes with blood pressure readings, that action should be documented with the category *Case Management.*

- Discuss categories and targets that are used frequently in your organization. For example, how do your practice patterns compare to your colleagues'?
- Develop pathways (standardized protocols or care planning guides) for high frequency or intensity problems, groups of clients, intervention categories, medical diagnoses, or other parameters. Test and revise as needed. Refer to suggestions about how to use and not use these pathways and practice standards in Chapter 3 so that evidence-based practice becomes a reality.

Problem Rating Scale for Outcomes Guidelines

- Use the Scale to consider goals for client care, intervention alternatives, and measurable changes in client care.
- Select one numeric rating for *Knowledge*, one for *Behavior*, and one for *Status* for high-priority problems to reflect the client's data that are evident before interventions are provided. This approach establishes an admission baseline to compare with ratings at later time intervals and dismissal. Avoid rating low-priority problems.
- Establish a guideline indicating when practitioners are expected to document the next *Knowledge, Behavior,* and *Status* ratings (see Chapters 3 and 4). For example, some educators require their students to use the Scale during each client encounter. Some agencies and organizations select one interval (e.g., weekly, monthly, or every 2 months) for one program and other intervals for other programs.
- Choose the three ratings in isolation and in the order you prefer. For example, determine the *Knowledge* rating; put it aside mentally. Determine the *Behavior* rating; put it aside mentally. Then, determine the *Status* rating. The numeric rating for one concept may or may not be the same numeric rating for either of the other two concepts.
- Rate *Knowledge, Behavior,* and *Status* for all situations. For example, when the client is an infant, child, or dependent adult and the problem is *Neglect*, rate the *Knowledge* of the primary caregiver and document who was being rated. When documenting in computerized or manual records, practitioners should note if the rating is for someone other than the client who "owns" the problem. Follow the rating with a *slash* and a *C* (/C) for caregiver, and then use free text to indicate who the *C* represents.
- Base ratings on existing client *Knowledge*, *Behavior*, and *Status* data that you can explain to others. For example, incorporate the results of the Denver II, PDQ II, Mini-Mental State Examination, or Braden Scale into your conclusions about *Status*. Ratings may improve or deteriorate over time; try to identify why and document appropriately.
- Select a "1-5" rating for the client's *Knowledge* and *Behavior* based on existing data. Do not use all five options for *Status*. When the modifier is *Health Promotion* or *Potential*, the *Status* rating should be a "5" to indicate that no signs or symptoms exist. When the modifier is *Actual*, select "1-4" for the *Status* rating to *indicate that signs or symptoms do exist.*
- Document anticipated ratings (those that are most likely to occur at a later date or discharge) if your agency's or organization's policies require you to do so. The terms "anticipated or expected ratings" are preferable to the term "goal," because most practitioners assume the latter to be a "5" even if that is not realistic or achievable for a given individual, family, or community. Clearly differentiate anticipated ratings from your other ratings.
- Discuss the advantages and disadvantages of using the Scale with a onetime visit or encounter. Proceed cautiously depending on the type of program and desired outcomes.

For example, it may be appropriate to document an increase in *Knowledge* when the purpose of the visit or encounter is to provide the category *Teaching, Guidance, and Counseling* and the client offers evidence that learning occurred. However, it may be more difficult or impossible to identify a change in *Behavior* or *Status*.

- Document a whole number; a range or a fraction of a number such as "2.5" is not acceptable. If you cannot honestly decide between a "2" and a "3," select the lower number. It is better to underestimate the rating and err by selecting the lower rating. In addition, the lower rating results in more room for improvement.
- Select ratings thoughtfully, and consider the universe of clients who have a specific problem. That universe includes diverse clients as well as relatives, friends, and neighborhoods. Recall previous experiences, even remembering names. Try to remember vivid details about clients who were a "1," "2," "3," "4," and "5" for *Knowledge, Behavior*, and *Status* for a particular problem, especially those you use often. These clients will serve as your anchors, improve your consistency, and increase your inter-rater reliability.
- Refer to the examples or patterns in the User's Guide when selecting ratings. These examples are based on actual practice, and were developed by practitioners to serve as a guide for decision making. NOTE: Because only one example (i.e., a continuum of 1 through 5) is included for each problem-specific *Knowledge, Behavior*, and *Status* rating, the examples may or may not match your clients' data. Practitioners must develop their own examples to serve as a bridge between the examples in the book and their own clients.

FREQUENTLY ASKED QUESTIONS

The following are examples of general questions frequently asked by Omaha System users.*

Do I need to buy the Omaha System in order to use it?

No. The structure, terms, definitions, and codes of the Omaha System (Appendixes A and E) are not copyrighted so that they are equally accessible to all potential users. Definitions are also organized by topic in the Glossary. Saunders, an affiliate of Elsevier, is the publisher of the book and holds copyright for the book with the exception of Appendixes A and E. Boxes 2-1 and Figures 2-3 through 2-5 are held under copyright but can be copied without permission for clinical and educational use. Thus, according to copyright law, you must follow the usual steps to obtain permission from Saunders to include text, examples, figures, tables, or boxes from this book in journals, books, conference proceedings, online features, or software. If you purchase software based on the Omaha System, the companies must also follow copyright laws. Vendors charge for software development, maintenance, and related business expenses; they do not charge for the Omaha System per se.

How can I, my agency or organization, my educator colleagues, or my students learn to use the Omaha System successfully?

Learning to use the Omaha System is like learning a new language and should be approached as such. Establish a systematic, incremental, flexible orientation plan that

*Some questions have been adapted from those found on the Omaha System Web site: www.omahasystem.org.

includes clear expectations for learners. Design the introduction to help learners recognize that the Omaha System is intended to describe most client situations, practitioner interventions, and client outcomes. An easy way to convince learners of the power of the Omaha System is to have them summarize a recent client encounter, then ask them to open the User's Guide and search for the words that describe that client and encounter.

Suggest reading assignments such as this book, other Omaha System references listed in this book, and the Omaha System Web site (www.omahasystem.org), so that learners become familiar with general information including the purpose, organization, benefits, and rules. Consider teaching and learning ideas and materials described in Chapters 3 and 4. Then introduce practice-specific client applications. Refer to the 33 diverse case studies in Appendix B and the User's Guide in Section 2 to practice, become familiar with terms and definitions, develop ever increasing skills, and eventually internalize the Omaha System. Although case studies are included in Appendix B and other publications, you and your colleagues can also develop examples involving your clients and your practice, a strategy that will help practitioners develop a sense of "ownership." Case studies help learners understand the "spirit" of the Omaha System and prepare for new application complexities, similar to the experiences in the mastering of a new language. As with learning a new language, "practice makes perfect"; stated another way, it is important to practice, practice, practice. Most learners say the language of the Omaha System is intuitive and easy once they "get the hang of it." According to Henry and LeClair (1987, p. 21):

> Orientation programs and internships are mechanisms for secondary socialization. Through these mechanisms, new information is internalized through new language; we learn a second language by building on our "mother tongue." Exposed for the first time to unfamiliar language, we consciously translate and integrate new words into our existing vocabulary to give the unaccustomed words meaning. As socialization proceeds, we increasingly forego translation and think in our newly acquired language.

Why does it matter if I use the Omaha System or my organization's record in the same way my colleagues use it?

Read this entire chapter, since it attempts to answer that question in multiple ways, some of which will be more important and appealing to you and some to others.

- If you document pertinent, focused, brief, yet comprehensive data consistently, you are more likely to record facts (a data trail) that reflect what actually occurred and that you can use to identify evidence-based practice patterns for yourself and with your colleagues (Young, 2003). Establish personal documentation goals such as making certain your entries reflect your clients' uniqueness, giving yourself credit for your professional accomplishments and using a minimal amount of your time.
- In many or most cases, you are not the only practitioner who provides care to a specific client. Standardized documentation enhances communication between practitioners and increases the probability that clients will receive efficient, effective, and safe care.
- Computers and novels are not a good combination. Standardization is necessary to maximize the benefits of automated clinical information systems.
- Most managers and administrations need data for multiple purposes about clients' needs, practitioners' interventions, and clients' outcomes of care. The ability to maintain staff positions in your organization's budget is one of them.

- Use of the Omaha System or automated or manual records will not be identical in all organizations. Each site must establish guidelines that address its specific practice, documentation, and information management needs.
- Reviewers, accreditors, and third party payers increasingly expect that documentation be accurate, consistent, and easy to read. Reimbursement may be linked to their conclusions.
- It is of little value to analyze aggregate data if your organization's practitioners do not document accurate and consistent client data.

What are the most important predictors of Omaha System success?

Each agency, institution, university program, clinic, and other user has a unique set of circumstances with numerous driving and restraining forces. However, teamwork and the presence of a champion are two of the most important predictors.

> It is a fact that in the right formation, the lifting power of many wings can achieve twice the distance of any bird flying alone.

Without a collective vision and collaboration during the planning, orientation, implementation, and maintenance phases of the entire Omaha System process, difficulties will occur continuously. The steps needed to establish the team, develop action plans and expectations, and implement technology are described in this book and other publications (Larrabee, 1999; *On-line Journal of Nursing Informatics*, 1999; Monsen & Martin, 2002a and 2002b; Barton et al., 2003; Handly et al., 2003; Elfrink & Davis, 2004; Nelson, 2004; Rosebaugh, 2004).

Strong leaders contribute to success. In addition, it is advantageous when at least one person becomes a "superstar" and is designated as a champion or cheerleader. That person must be passionate about the Omaha System and understand the practice, documentation, and information management vision or context. Responsibilities should include reading extra materials and attending educational sessions, encouraging others, conducting orientation and pilot testing, developing guidelines for users, and participating in quality improvement and data analysis activities.

Are there forms, models, graphics, or "cheat sheets" that will help me?

Refer to the Omaha System model (see Figure 1-2) and the associated definitions as a refresher about clients, steps, and the practitioner-client relationship. Personalize the concepts to your memorable clients and events.

The Overview of the Omaha System (Box 2-1) is an abbreviated version of the basic terms. You may print and even reduce and laminate these terms to use as a "cheat sheet" at your desk or beside your computer, or to carry with you.

Understanding the Omaha System (Figure 2-3) and Using the Omaha System (Figure 2-4) are illustrations. They and Figure 1-2 may be helpful because they visually depict the relationships among the Problem Classification Scheme, Intervention Scheme, and Problem Rating Scale for Outcomes; they also emphasize that the Omaha System model is circular and dynamic rather than linear, an approach that is similar to mind-mapping, a recent concept described in the literature. Be creative and develop additional Omaha System graphic illustrations that are meaningful to you and your colleagues and help you remember the terms and relationships.

BOX 2-1 Overview of the Omaha System

PROBLEM CLASSIFICATION SCHEME

Environmental Domain
Income
Sanitation
Residence
Neighborhood/workplace safety

Psychosocial Domain
Communication with community resources
Social contact
Role change
Interpersonal relationship
Spirituality
Grief
Mental health
Sexuality
Caretaking/parenting
Neglect
Abuse
Growth and development

Physiological Domain
Hearing
Vision
Speech and language
Oral health

Physiological Domain (cont'd)
Cognition
Pain
Consciousness
Skin
Neuro-musculo-skeletal function
Respiration
Circulation
Digestion-hydration
Bowel function
Urinary function
Reproductive function
Pregnancy
Postpartum
Communicable/infectious condition

Health-related Behaviors Domain
Nutrition
Sleep and rest patterns
Physical activity
Personal care
Substance use
Family planning
Health care supervision
Medication regimen

PROBLEM RATING SCALE FOR OUTCOMES

Rating	Knowledge	Behavior	Status
1	No knowledge	Not appropriate behavior	Extreme signs/symptoms
2	Minimal knowledge	Rarely appropriate behavior	Severe signs/symptoms
3	Basic knowledge	Inconsistently appropriate behavior	Moderate signs/symptoms
4	Adequate knowledge	Usually appropriate behavior	Minimal signs/symptoms
5	Superior knowledge	Consistently appropriate behavior	No signs/symptoms

Continued

BOX 2-1 Overview of the Omaha System—cont'd

INTERVENTION SCHEME

Categories

Teaching, Guidance, and Counseling
Treatments and Procedures
Case Management
Surveillance

Targets

anatomy/physiology
anger management
behavior modification
bladder care
bonding/attachment
bowel care
cardiac care
caretaking/parenting skills
cast care
communication
community outreach worker services
continuity of care
coping skills
day care/respite
dietary management
discipline
dressing change/wound care
durable medical equipment
education
employment
end-of-life care
environment
exercises
family planning care
feeding procedures
finances
gait training
genetics
growth/development care
home
homemaking/housekeeping
infection precautions
interaction
interpreter/translator services

Targets—cont'd

laboratory findings
legal system
medical/dental care
medication action/side effects
medication administration
medication coordination/ordering
medication prescription
medication set-up
mobility/transfers
nursing care
nutritionist care
occupational therapy care
ostomy care
other community resources
paraprofessional/aide care
personal hygiene
physical therapy care
positioning
recreational therapy care
relaxation/breathing techniques
respiratory care
respiratory therapy care
rest/sleep
safety
screening procedures
sickness/injury care
signs/symptoms-mental/emotional
signs/symptoms-physical
skin care
social work/counseling care
specimen collection
speech and language pathology care
spiritual care
stimulation/nurturance
stress management
substance use cessation
supplies
support group
support system
transportation
wellness
other

The Omaha System Worksheet (Figure 2-5) is a simple, effective form to use with initial case studies and practice sessions. Often learners are less overwhelmed and distracted if they are introduced to the Omaha System terms and definitions with a neutral, paper worksheet than with software screens, copies of software screens, or new manual forms. Some organizations planning to purchase software in 6 to 12 months have transformed this worksheet into a record audit form. Their project implementation teams use it to practice and maintain their skills, and they discuss the audits at monthly meetings or during conference calls. Some use it as printed in this chapter, and others have modified it by adding columns for dates and details.

How long does it take to learn to use the Omaha System?

There are as many answers to that question as there are learners. Some practitioners, educators, and students apply the Omaha System *accurately* and *consistently* within 6 months and others need longer. Each and every learner must become an active participant in the process and invest time, commitment, repetition, and work. There is no magic wand to bypass the basic steps or to have someone else be responsible for the learner's thinking or learning. If learners feel a sense of ownership, their learning curve will become faster and easier.

> Tell me, and I'll forget; show me, and I'll remember; involve me, and I'll understand.
>
> Lao-Tse in 565 BC

> An average listener forgets 40% of information after one-half hour, 60% at the end of the day, and 90% by the end of the week.
>
> Hermann Ebbinghaus, 1885 (German psychologist)

It is essential to schedule frequent, positive practice opportunities to increase objective and decrease subjective use. Practice must be planned, proceed from simple to complex, be relevant to the daily experiences of the learners, and be fun. Learners are grounded and reinforced when a variety of case studies are presented that encourage them to recall memories of previous clients and experiences. They need to discuss ways of describing their work using the Omaha System with their colleagues, to apply the same critical thinking skills that they do when providing care. Continue practice sessions when Omaha System implementation officially begins. The discussion that experienced users have about a case study is more sophisticated and very different than the type of discussion they had when they were novices. Research findings regularly describe data drift and the need for repetition and reinforcement to maintain interrater reliability.

Other important variables for learners include their previous education, experience, and exposure to the Omaha System; knowledge about the concepts and benefits of standardized terminologies in general; use of literature and audiovisual resources; computer skills when documentation is automated; mentoring and feedback; support systems; attitudes; and motivation. Because adult learning styles are so varied, it is important to present information in many ways and at different times, rather than assuming that all learners will understand and retain equally (Carty, 2000; Englebardt & Nelson, 2002; Nightingale Tracker Clinical Field Test Nurse Team, 2000; Monsen & Martin, 2002a; Barton et al., 2003; Oermann & Heinrich, 2003; Leonardo et al., 2004; Monsen & Kerr, 2004). Practitioners' documentation experiences with their current and former employers are another critical variable. For practitioners or agencies whose records are accurately described as "novels," the change to a structured, more streamlined documentation system that includes guidelines and expectations is a major transition. These practitioners or agencies may

Understanding the Omaha System

Problem Classification Scheme

Level 1
Domains (4)
- Environmental (includes Income)

Level 2
Problems (42)
- Income

Level 3
Modifiers (2 sets)
- [Individual (who owns the problem) / Family / Community]
- [Health Promotion (most+) / Potential / Actual]

Level 4
Signs/symptoms
(low/no income)
(uninsured)
⋮
(each problem has a cluster of s/s that are unique to that problem and 1 "other")

- Sanitation
- Residence
⋮
- Psychosocial (includes Spirituality)
- Physiological (includes Circulation)
- Health-related Behaviors (includes Substance use)

Intervention Scheme

Level 1
Categories (4)
- Teaching, Guidance, and Counseling (i.e., range)

Level 2
Targets (75 actions and 1 "other")
- Anatomy/physiology
- Anger management
- Behavior modification
- Bladder care
⋮

Level 3
Client-specific information
(not included in the Scheme itself)

- Treatments and Procedures (i.e., direct care, technical)
- Case Management (i.e., referral, coordination)
- Surveillance (i.e., monitor care over time, compare change)

Problem Rating Scale for Outcomes

When
- Admission
- Interim
- Discharge

What

	low				high	
• Knowledge	1	2	3	4	5	(what the client knows)
• Behavior	1	2	3	4	5	(what the client does)
• Status	1	2	3	4	5	(how the client is)

Figure 2-3 Understanding the Omaha System. May be reproduced for instructional and clinical use. From Martin K.S.: *The Omaha System* (Reprinted 2nd ed.). Adapted from work of Chia-Yi Chen, RN, MA, MS, Doctoral Student, University of California-Los Angeles.

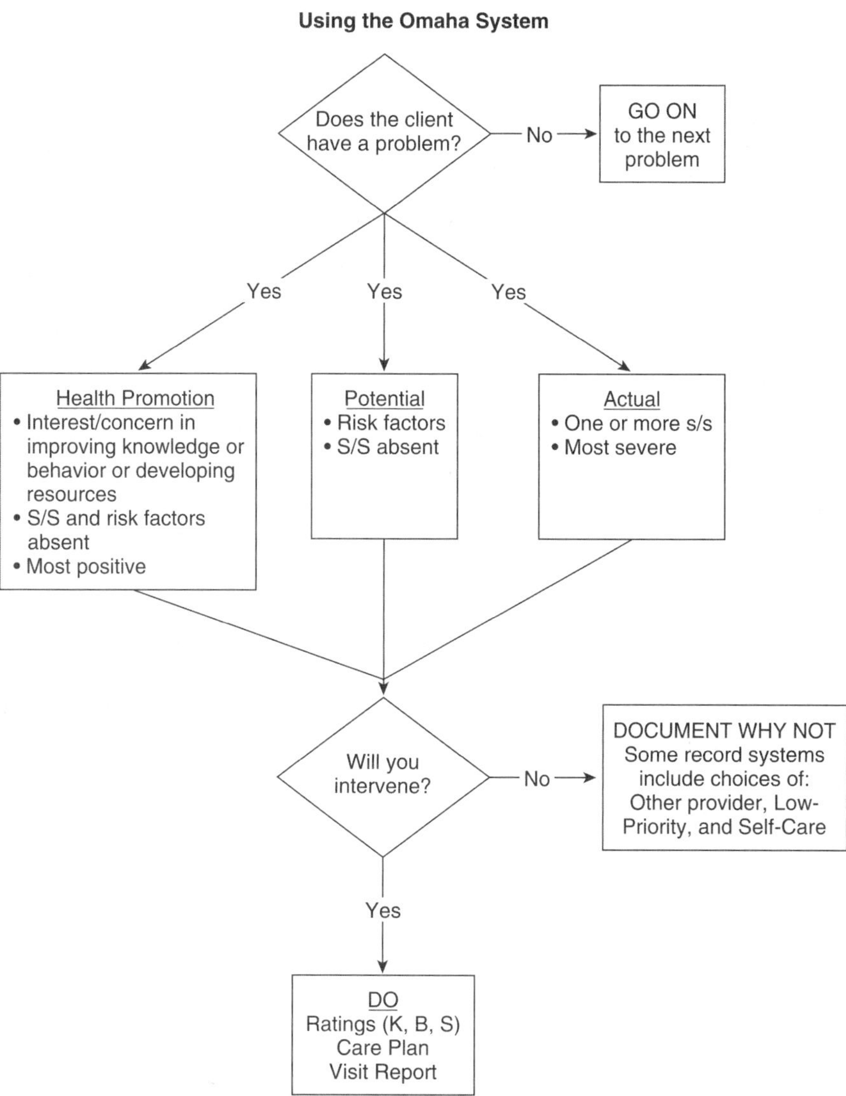

Figure 2-4 Using the Omaha System. May be reproduced for instructional and clinical use. From Martin, K. S.: *The Omaha System* (Reprinted 2nd ed.).

Omaha System Worksheet

1. Problem	2. Modifier (I, F, or C)	3. Modifier (A, P, or H)	4. S/S (only A)	5. Intervention		6. Admission Rating		
				Category	Target	K	B	S

1. Problem Classification Scheme: Problem
2. Problem Classification Scheme: I = Individual, F = Family, C = Community modifier
3. Problem Classification Scheme: A = Actual, P = Potential, or H = Health Promotion modifier
4. Problem Classification Scheme: Sign/symptom
5. Intervention Scheme: Category and target
6. Problem Rating Scale for Outcomes: Admission rating for Knowledge, Behavior, and Status

Figure 2-5 Omaha System Worksheet. Developed by Karen S. Martin. May be reproduced for instructional and clinical use. For all other uses, contact Karen S. Martin for permission.

have more difficulty letting go of old habits and adjusting to a system based on "more is not necessarily better."

What are the benefits of using the Omaha System?

The answers depend on your perspective and responsibilities. Users need to anticipate and experience personal benefits if they are going to be motivated. As a general summary, the System helps practitioners and students improve their practice skills and make documentation easier and faster. Managers expect the Omaha System to improve communication, make documentation more legible, and increase productivity. When surveyors, accreditors, third party payers, and attorneys review client records, managers want them to be considered acceptable. The Omaha System is designed to help administrators, educators, and researchers obtain accurate and consistent clinical data that can be evaluated, aggregated, presented, and published; they want statistics that demonstrate the impact of services. Many health care providers are incorporating benchmarking and report cards into their quality improvement programs. They compare their practitioners' client statistics across time and their information with other providers (Braveman & Wright, 2003; Whitman, 2003; Wilson & Nathan, 2003). Computer vendors want to offer features in electronic health records and information systems that groups, agencies, and organizations will purchase.

All groups want a relatively simple, easy to use, practice-oriented method to recognize data patterns, quantify client data, and identify best practices, as well as transform data into information, knowledge, and wisdom. Chapters 1 through 6 describe numerous Omaha System benefits in detail; Chapters 3 through 6 focus on specialized applications, settings, clients, and health care personnel.

Can clients be involved with the Omaha System?

Practitioners must develop partnerships with clients and document pertinent details in the record. Practitioners begin the process when they ask clients about their expectations and preferences regarding services, are clear about the aims of service, inform clients about the care they should expect to receive, provide mutually acceptable interventions, and evaluate and discuss the client's and practitioner's satisfaction. For example, Michael, his mother, and the school nurse discussed the Omaha System terms and ratings in the case study entitled, Michael O.: A Teen Who Had Diabetes (Appendix B). Several years ago, home care practitioners at the St. Joseph's Area Health Services Home Care and Hospice, in Park Rapids, Minnesota, began to discuss the Problem Rating Scale for Outcomes with selected clients. Although they discussed it in a different way than they did with their colleagues, they talked to clients about their *Knowledge*, *Behavior,* and *Status* ratings. The purpose was to help clients understand their current ratings, evaluate their interest and willingness to improve the ratings, and track changes over time. Some practitioners, agencies, and organizations share portions of records with their clients. While this can be a valuable strategy, it is important to first consider the client, the actual portion of the record, the policies of the setting, and potential ramifications.

Where can the Omaha System be used?

The Omaha System can be used in a variety of settings and with diverse client groups. Since the early 1970s, the goal of those developing and testing the Omaha System was that the structure, terms, and definitions would be valuable to interested practitioners when they provided care to clients who represent the entire health-illness continuum, regardless of their ages, medical diagnoses, cultures, ethnicities, races, spiritual beliefs, and economic strata. Simultaneously, the assumption was that these practitioners would provide care in the community rather than acute or long-term settings. Over time, the location and type of users has expanded dramatically (see Chapter 1) so that users now represent all types of settings.

What will happen when the revised Omaha System is released?

This new edition has been widely publicized to encourage users to update their documentation and information management systems to reflect twenty-first century practice. Users need to adopt the terms and definitions as they are listed in Appendix A. Individuals or groups who have manual forms are urged to revise those forms. Most vendors that incorporate the Omaha System in their electronic health records and information systems are planning to make the necessary programming changes and release revised software soon after this book is published. When any data system is updated, two sets or vintages of data result. Users need to be cautious when comparing or analyzing client data that is in both systems, whether comparison is internal (within their group, agency, or organization) or external (with other manual or automated systems).

How are the Omaha System and quality improvement related?

Quality improvement is a systematic evaluation process to measure how well health care and social services meet specific expectations and standards, and to identify ways in which care can be improved through evidence-based practice. Practice sites should evaluate their needs at least annually and tailor their comprehensive and multifaceted quality improvement program to meet those needs.

The Omaha System serves as one important component of a quality improvement program. As a strategy to develop practice and documentation standards, the public health nurses at Saint Paul-Ramsey County Department of Public Health, in St. Paul, Minnesota, selected several of their clients' highest frequency problems, discussed the rating examples in the pocket guide (Martin & Scheet, 1992b), and developed more detailed examples that reflected their clients' *Knowledge*, *Behavior*, and *Status*. They shared their work with the nurses at a neighbor agency, Washington County Department of Public Health and Environment, in Stillwater, Minnesota, whose staff completed more examples (E. Hodkinson, B. Lescenski, A. Lytton, & J. Timm; Personal communication, October 29, 2003).

Another strategy involves periodically evaluating documentation of each practitioner, and comparing it to verbal reports from that practitioner, supervisory or observational visits, client satisfaction surveys, productivity and time reports, and other sources of data. Consider conducting record audits so that documentation from groups of practitioners is compared and contrasted. If data are analyzed, the most frequently occurring client problems, practitioner interventions, and client outcomes will be identified. Such data becomes the basis for evidence-based practice, development of guidelines for high frequency areas of practice, and continuing education for practitioners. Aggregate data about agency or institutional trends can be compared to similar and different provider organizations if all are using the Omaha System consistently as it is presented in this book.

How can I contact others about the Omaha System?

Chapter authors for this book have provided contact information. Additional links and information are available on the Omaha System Web site (www.omahasystem.org) and listserv. Karen Martin (martinks@tconl.com) facilitates networking among those interested in the Omaha System, and offers consultation services to prospective, new, and experienced users. Biennial conferences provide an excellent opportunity for networking, as does the Minnesota User Group mentioned in Chapter 1.

Are there other ways I can participate? If you and your practice, educational, or research setting have not completed an Omaha System survey, please do so. The survey is in Appendix F and on the Omaha System Web site. Information from recent surveys is an essential source of data about users and is summarized in Chapter 1. You may complete the survey as a way to share your experiences and suggest revisions, or you may contact Advisory Board members.

There are limitless opportunities to participate in Omaha System activities. For example, you may help develop and implement best practice and quality improvement programs at your agency or organization. Also consider conference presentations or panels, poster sessions, research, publications, and the listserv. You do not have to wait until you have been using the Omaha System for years and consider yourself an expert. It is very important for novices and advanced beginners to ask questions and share their experiences as a way to encourage others, expand the base of knowledge, and develop personal and professional skills.

SUMMARY

This chapter serves as a bridge to help learners and teachers focus on pertinent information. All practitioners need to understand the fundamental concepts, basic guidelines, and new terms in order to implement the Omaha System structure, terms, and definitions accurately and consistently. It is not sufficient to use the terms without understanding the "what, why, how, and when" or the context of the terminology. Although teaching and learning styles, sequences, and priorities vary dramatically among practice, education, and research settings, those who emphasize a team approach and have strong leaders are likely to be more successful.

REFERENCES

Barton, A.J., Gilbert, L., Erickson, V., Baramee, J., Sowers, D., & Robertson, K.J. (2003, May/June). A guide to assist nurse practitioners with standardized nursing language. *CIN: Computers, Informatics, Nursing, 21*(3):128-133.

Benner, P.A. (1984). *From Novice to Expert: Excellence and Power in Clinical Nursing Practice.* Menlo Park, California, Addison-Wesley.

Benner, P., Tanner, C.A., & Chesla, C.A. (Eds.). (1996). *Expertise in Nursing Practice: Caring, Clinical Judgment, and Ethics.* New York, Springer.

Braveman, C. & Wright, K. (2003, June). Total turnaround: How to use national benchmarks, an operational review, and focus change strategies to totally turn an agency around, *Caring, XXII*(6):12-16.

Carty, B. (Ed.). (2000). *Nursing Informatics Education for Practice.* New York, Springer.

Donabedian, A. (1966, July). Evaluating the quality of medical care.*Milbank Memorial Fund Quarterly, 44*(2): 166-206.

Dreyfus, H.L. (1979). *What Computers Can't Do: The Limits of Artificial Intelligence.* New York, Harper & Row.

Elfrink, V.L. & Davis, L.S. (2004, April). Using Omaha System data to improve the clinical education experiences of nursing students: The University of Cincinnati Project. *Home Health Management and Practice, 16*(3):185-191.

Englebardt, S.P. & Nelson, R. (Eds.). (2002). *Health Care Informatics: An Interdisciplinary Approach.* St. Louis, Mosby.

Handly, M.J., Grubb, S.K., Keefe, N.A., & Martin, K.S. (2003, January). Essential activities for implementing a clinical information system in public health nursing. *Journal of Nursing Administration, 33*(1):14-16.

Henry, B. & LeClair, H. (1987, January). Language, leadership, and power. *Journal of Nursing Administration, 17*(1):19-25.

Keller, L.O., Strohschein, S., Lia-Hoagberg, B., & Schaffer, M. (1998, June). Population-based public health nursing interventions: A model from practice. *Public Health Nursing, 15*(3):207-215.

Keller, L.O., Strohschein, S., Lia-Hoagberg, B., & Schaffer, M. (in press). Population-based public health interventions: Practice-based and evidence-supported (Part I). *Public Health Nursing.*

Keller, L.O., Strohschein, S., Schaffer, M., & Lia-Hoagberg, B. (in press). Population-based public health interventions: Innovations in practice, teaching, and management (Part II). *Public Health Nursing.*

Larrabee, S.B. (1999, August). Benner's Novice to Expert Nursing Theory applied to the implementation of laptops in the home care setting. *Home Health Care Management and Practice, 11*(4):41-47.

Leonardo, M.E., Resick, L.K., Bingman, C.A., & Strotmeyer, S. (2004, April). The alternatives for wellness centers: Drown in data or develop a reasonable electronic documentation system. *Home Health Care Management and Practice, 16*(3):177-184.

Martin, K.S. & Scheet, N.J. (1992a). *The Omaha System: Application for Community Health Nursing.* Philadelphia, Saunders.

Martin, K.S. & Scheet, N.J. (1992b). *The Omaha System: A Pocket Guide for Community Health Nursing.* Philadelphia, Saunders.

Martin, K.S., Norris, J., & Leak, G.K. (1999, January/March). Psychometric analysis of the Problem Rating Scale for Outcomes. *Outcomes Management for Nursing Practice, 3*(1):20-25.

Monsen, K.A. & Kerr, M.J. (2004, April). Mining quality documentation data for golden outcomes. *Home Health Management and Practice, 16*(3):192-199.

Monsen, K.A. & Martin, K.S. (2002a, April/June). Developing an outcomes management program in a public health department. *Outcomes Management, 6*(2):62-66.

Monsen, K.A. & Martin, K.S. (2002b, July/September). Using an outcomes management program in a public health department. *Outcomes Management, 6*(3):120-124.

Nelson, R.M. (2004, April). Measuring outcomes in home health care: Beyond the OASIS data set. *Home Health Care Management and Practice, 16*(3):200-205.

Nightingale Tracker Clinical Field Test Nurse Team. (2000, May/June). A comparison of teaching strategies for integrating information technology into clinical nursing education. *Nurse Educator, 25*(3):136-144.

Oermann, M.H. (1998, November/December). How to assess critical thinking in clinical practice. *Dimensions of Critical Care Nursing, 17*(6):322-327.

Oermann, M.H. & Heinrich, K.T. (2003). *Annual Review of Nursing Education*, New York, Springer.

On-line Journal of Nursing Informatics, *3*(1). (1999, Winter). 5 Omaha System articles. Retrieved March 8, 2004 from the Internet: http://www.eaa-knowledge.com/ojni/ni/dm/ojni/html.

Rosebaugh, D.L. (2004, April). Getting ready for the software in your future. *Home Health Care Management and Practice, 16*(3):228-234.

Whitman, G.R. (2003, January/March). Making the grade. *Outcomes Management, I7*(1):4-7.

Wilson, A. & Nathan, L. (2003, February). Understanding benchmarks. *Home Healthcare Nurse, 21*(2):102-107.

Young, K.M. (October, 2003). Where's the evidence? *American Journal of Nursing, 103*(10):11.

CHAPTER 3

3

USE OF THE OMAHA SYSTEM IN PRACTICE

Karen A. Monsen

The Omaha System appeals to a wide variety of provider organizations and multidisciplinary practitioners (Martin & Scheet, 1992; Shuttleworth-Diaz, 1995; Wills & Sloan, 1996; Jacobson & Eckstrom, 1997; Bednarz, 1998; Slack & McEwen, 1999; Westra & Solomon, 1999; Plowfield & Raymond, 2001; Monsen & Martin, 2002b; Martin, Baisch, & Bell-Calvin, 2003). Early users were community health practice organizations located in the United States. Adoption in practice, education, and research settings has expanded nationally and internationally (Jonkergouw, 1991; Huang, 1994; Martin & Scheet, 1997; Martin, Bessho, & Saito, 1999; Park, Kim, & Cho, 2000; Clark et al., 2001; Wilson, 2002).

Examples of organizations now using the Omaha System include public health departments, home care agencies, school health services, community-oriented clinics, hospital-based and managed care case management programs, long-term care facilities, and parish nursing programs. Many have purchased clinical information software based on the Omaha System. The Omaha System has been used in rehabilitation facilities, and research was conducted successfully in acute care settings, although it is not known if any of these organizations have computerized records (Shuttleworth-Diaz, 1995; Doran et al., 1997; Sampson & Doran, 1998; Bowles, 1999; Bowles, 2000). A large long-term care center–chronic illness hospital is in the process of implementing an automated clinical information system based on the Omaha System.

Among those who use the Omaha System are social workers, home care nurses, hospice nurses, public health nurses, parish nurses, paraprofessionals, case managers, nutritionists and registered dieticians, occupational therapists, physical therapists, speech and language pathologists, probation officers, physicians, police officers, and consultants. Although nurses were the primary users initially and continue to predominate, the diversity of practitioners is expanding as organizations employ more multidisciplinary staff members. The hospice program in Crookston, Minnesota, exemplifies a team approach to practice, documentation, and information management, as presented in Omaha System Box 3-1.

Motivation for using the Omaha System varies. Reasons that appear to be universal include the need to improve practice, standardize documentation, convert to an automated clinical information system, link clinical data to other information, and track the quality of health care. Internationally, the primary reasons are to measure outcomes of care and prove the effectiveness of provider services. In the United States, sites need to increase fiscal efficiency and produce meaningful reports for board members, community

OMAHA SYSTEM BOX 3-1

Omaha System Experiences in Practice: Applying the Omaha System in a Hospice Program

Danielle M. Conrad, MSW
Social Worker and Family Service Coordinator
Riverview Homecare and Hospice Agency
Crookston, Minnesota

When I was employed by the hospice team of our Medicare-certified home care agency, I learned to use the computerized method of Omaha System documentation fairly quickly, in part because I was familiar with computers. Our terminally ill clients range from infants to elders and are often on our caseload for more than a month. We maintain contact with families for 13 more months after the client's death. I, as the hospice coordinator, and my nurse colleagues use the Omaha System to plan, document, and evaluate care. Physicians, clergy, and volunteers are also team members; when they want to document care, I complete their entries. We meet on a regular basis to discuss our clients and review documentation. Often the client's condition changes rapidly, so we must document soon after we complete visits or phone calls, limit the quantity of recording, have access to user-friendly records, and maintain phone contact. I have started to type brief notes to show my rationale for my rating choices. Often the nurses' ratings are accompanied by objective data that readily supports their decisions.

As a social worker, I focus on problems such as *Grief*, *Spirituality*, *Mental health*, *Interpersonal relationship*, and *Social contact*. In order of frequency, my interventions are *Teaching, Guidance,* and *Counseling; Surveillance*; *Case Management*; and *Treatments and Procedures*. Often clients do not begin hospice services until late in the disease process, when they have progressed through early stages of grief. Therefore I do not observe frequent or dramatic rating changes. The nurses focus on physiological problems and are more likely to provide *Case Management* and *Treatments and Procedures*. The ratings they document also fluctuate more. When clients achieve pain control, ratings related to *Pain* improve. Ratings often decrease for problems such as *Respiration* or *Skin* that reflect the causes and effects of terminal illness.

The ability to streamline and increase the precision of documentation and improve communication are definite benefits of using the Omaha System and automation in our hospice program.

residents, third party payers, auditors, and accreditation personnel (Weidmann & North, 1987; Martin & Scheet, 1988; Jorgensen & Young, 1989; Clark & Lang, 1992; Martin & Norris, 1996; Martin & Gorski, 1998; Walker, 1998; Mallard, 2000; Martin, Baisch, & Bell-Calvin, 2003). Public health departments have implemented the Omaha System to describe populations at risk, health disparities, and client outcomes. Home care agencies need to determine the appropriate level of client care, assure that practitioners perform standard interventions, and demonstrate outcomes of care. School health nurses use the Omaha System to monitor the health of students in a standardized way and communicate with other providers as needed. Parish nurses use the Omaha System to collect basic information about the interrelated health care and spiritual needs of parish members. Community clinics track outpatient client progress over time and gather statistics about the most common health problems addressed with clients; these are described in detail in Chapter 4.

THE OMAHA SYSTEM AND OTHER MODELS

Practice settings use and comply with various data sets, classification schemes, and models. The Omaha System helps organizations articulate their compliance, demonstrate practice outcomes, and develop linkages (Westra, 1996; Marek & Rantz, 2000; Madigan, 2002). While other models are described in Chapters 1 and 5, the Outcome and Assessment Information Set (OASIS), *Healthy People 2010*, and the Core Functions of Public Health are delineated below.

Outcome and Assessment Information Set (OASIS)

Documentation is an essential responsibility of Medicare-certified home care practitioners in the United States (Croke, 2003; Duckett, 2003). The Outcome and Assessment Information Set (OASIS) is a standardized data set that these practitioners must complete at designated intervals for reimbursement and for outcomes measurement purposes. The Problem Classification Scheme offers a comprehensive standardized assessment designed to address the spectrum of health needs and problems for all clients. Home care practitioners use the Omaha System to organize and document a holistic client assessment, and the OASIS data set for reporting as described by the Kenosha, Wisconsin, VNA in Omaha System Box 3-2, in Chapter 5, and elsewhere (Martin, Scheet, & Stegman, 1993; Scoates, Fishman, & McAdam, 1996; Westra & Solomon, 1999, McGourthy, 1999; Martin, 2000; Gaskell & McGourthy, 2002; Madigan, 2002; Zuber, 2002; Nelson, 2004).

Healthy People 2010

Healthy People 2010 is a set of health objectives from the U.S. Department of Health and Human Services that is designed to help states, communities, and professional organizations develop health improvement programs. The Problem Classification Scheme is a structure of discrete terms that complement the Healthy People 2010 objectives. Public health departments can collect, aggregate, and analyze Omaha System data about their populations, and convert those data to information in relation to selected objectives. Table 3-1 compares examples of selected categories of the *Healthy People 2010* objectives and Omaha System problems (Healthy People 2010, 2000).

Core Functions of Public Health

Three core public health functions—assessment, policy development, and assurance—were established by the U.S. Department of Health and Human Services and several partner organizations (Public Health Functions Steering Committee, 1994). Local, county, and state public health departments carry out these core functions by providing ten essential services. The Omaha System can be used to describe these core functions and services. It serves as an assessment model to collect information about specific populations, providing valuable population-based assessment data that are easily understood by administrators and policy makers. Using these data for decision making facilitates the policy development process. The Omaha System also provides the terms to document practitioner services and measure client outcomes. Doing so yields data to demonstrate that services provided were appropriate for the population and client needs (Table 3-2). Several public health nursing organizations are developing competencies for public health nurses that are compatible with the Omaha System, the core functions, and the essential services.

OMAHA SYSTEM BOX 3-2
Omaha System Experiences in Practice: Integrating the Omaha System and OASIS

Rochelle M. Nelson, RN, MS, CNS
Former Clinical Education Coordinator
Kenosha Visiting Nurse Association
Kenosha, Wisconsin
Rosemary T. Trotta, RN-C, MSN
Former Director of Home Care Services
Kenosha Visiting Nurse Association
Kenosha, Wisconsin

The Omaha System and the Outcome and Assessment Information Set (OASIS) generate quantifiable client outcome data. Our home care nurses collect both types of data at similar times during the course of care: start of care, resumption of care, recertification, significant change in client condition, and discharge. Nurses use an automated documentation system that includes the Omaha System and OASIS in an effort to decrease their documentation burden.

As part of a comprehensive intake assessment, our nurses consider and use a list that consists of 20 Omaha System problems frequently encountered in home care. Concurrently, nurses answer the OASIS questions and select responses as they document the corresponding problem's signs and symptoms. The exception involves functional status dimension elements, which are competed separately.

The nature of OASIS creates a number of challenges. Our nurses try to answer OASIS questions accurately and consistently, but the available multiple-choice answers sometimes do not match clients' needs and situations and the care provided. The quality of our data needs to be excellent because the clinical, functional, and service utilization dimensions of OASIS determine our clients' home care resource group, which in turn determines our agency's level of reimbursement for the episode of care. In addition, we are required to submit OASIS data as a quality of care measure. We do not receive outcomes reports from our fiscal intermediary for 4 to 6 months, so results are not available to nurses when they plan or evaluate care.

In comparison, our nurses find that their Omaha System documentation results in an accurate data trail about their clients' needs and care. They use it to create individualized care plans and monitor client progress, and can actually track improvement over time through their documentation. Our future plans are to evaluate the interrater reliability of our Omaha System documentation so we can use our outcomes data more effectively.

PLANNING

The majority of organizations that implement the Omaha System develop an immediate or short-range automation plan. Many find that the benefits of improved communication and automated data collection dramatically exceed the effort required for orientation and conversion as well as the financial investment in hardware and software. All practice settings should develop a plan for retrieving data and information, whether the plan is based on automation or data entry from a manual record system into a database.

In an ideal world, organizations would have the time and resources to thoughtfully select the Omaha System for their documentation model, educate practitioners to use it, and then select and implement software. Separating learning about the Omaha System from learning about the software decreases confusion that is inherent when a learner is introduced to two new systems at the same time. However, there are many organizations in which the Omaha

Table 3-1 Comparison of Selected *Healthy People 2010* Objectives and the Problem Classification Scheme

Healthy People 2010 Objective	Omaha System Problem
1. Access to Quality Health Services	Health care supervision
9. Family Planning	Family planning
12. Heart Disease and Stroke	Circulation
18. Mental Health and Mental Disorders	Mental health
19. Nutrition and Overweight	Nutrition
26. Substance Abuse	Substance use

Based on data from *Healthy People 2010* (2000, January). *Table of Contents.* Retrieved March 16, 2004, from the Internet: http://www.healthypeople.gov/Document/tableofcontents.htm#parta.

System and a software system have been successfully implemented together. Implementation timelines vary by organization and depend on the software system selected, the hardware and orientation needs, resource availability, and the number of practitioners.

Personnel

Regardless of the size or type of the organization, administrators and managers set the tone. Positive, committed, and informed leadership is fundamental to the success of implementing a new practice, documentation, and information management system. Practitioners, managers, and administrators must share the vision that changing to standardized documentation is necessary.

Most organizations establish an Omaha System automation project committee during this stage of the process. Typical committees consist of managers, multidisciplinary practitioners, information technology staff, and support staff. As described in Chapters 2 and 4 and other publications, practitioners need to participate in the planning process from the beginning to develop a sense of ownership (Martin & Scheet, 1992; Monsen & Martin, 2002a). They are the originators and most frequent users of the client record. Committee responsibilities often include recommending a software product or manual record forms; developing a budget, orientation plan, and timeline for implementation; and ensuring buy-in by the entire staff. Usual activities include meeting with software vendors, discussing data needs and technological capabilities, planning a strategy for empowering practitioners to change systems, and identifying unique practical considerations that could influence implementation.

Personnel at all organizational levels face challenges during the transition to Omaha System documentation. Practitioners' primary challenge is learning to correctly use a new language to document salient facts about client characteristics, their services, and client outcomes. Managers must understand the Omaha System in depth, helping practitioners discern how to standardize, collect, and interpret practice data. Reluctant practitioners and frustrated managers challenge administrators when the learning curve is steep, but success will result if leaders hold to the original vision and do not waiver from it.

Technical support offered by software vendors will not meet all the needs of system implementation and ongoing maintenance. Information technology staff members or

Table 3-2 Describing the Ten Essential Services of Public Health Using Omaha System Data

Ten Essential Services of Public Health	Omaha System
1. Monitor health status to identify community health problems	Identify and analyze problem frequency, including those with community modifiers
2. Diagnose and investigate health problems and health hazards in the community	Identify problems in the *Environmental Domain* and investigate health hazards in the community
3. Inform, educate, and empower people about health issues	Analyze *Teaching, Guidance*, and *Counseling* interventions and related targets to demonstrate diverse educational efforts of public health personnel
4. Mobilize community partnerships to identify and solve health problems	Aggregate data to inform community partners about population problems
5. Develop policies and plans that support individual and community health efforts	Aggregate data and use for outcomes-based decision making
6. Enforce laws and regulations that protect health and ensure safety	(Not applicable)
7. Link people to needed personal health services and ensure the provision of health care when otherwise unavailable	Summarize *Case Management* interventions to demonstrate links to resources
8. Assure a competent public health and personal health care workforce	Provide infrastructure for quality improvement program within public health department
9. Evaluate effectiveness, accessibility, and quality of personal and population-based health services	See Number 8
10. Research new insights and innovative solutions to health problems	Use Problem Rating Scale for Outcomes to measure effectiveness of new programs

Based on data from Public Health Functions Steering Committee (1994, Fall). *Essential Public Health Services.* Retrieved March 16, 2004, from the Internet: http://www.health.gov/phfunctions/public.htm.

contract personnel must be included in the organization's project committee. These technology personnel must understand the responsibilities of practitioners; approve specifications for servers, networks, and workstations or laptop computers that will be required for the software; and determine that the software can coexist with or be integrated into existing networks. They work collaboratively with managers and practitioners to ensure that equipment and software function well. Ongoing technology support is needed throughout the life of the software. Technology personnel should address problems promptly so that practice continues without interruption.

Automation

Because of the costs involved with automated information systems, funds must be budgeted in advance, sometimes over a period of several years. Administrators, managers, and project committee members must consider costs for software, computers, servers, licenses, orientation, books, and maintenance fees. Manual documentation based on the Omaha System appears to cost less, but data retrieval from a manual system is labor intensive, time consuming, and a barrier to data analysis. Agencies should anticipate that practitioners will need time to learn to use the new software. Expect and plan for short-term decreased productivity to allow for the long-term gain of accessible documentation data.

Clinical software that collects private data about clients is by nature highly complex, and few organizations have the capacity to develop a viable product on their own. The advent of the Health Insurance Portability and Accountability Act of 1996 (HIPAA) has increased the pressure on health care providers in the United States to adopt automated records and carefully control access to those records (Centers for Medicare and Medicaid Services, 2003). Commercial software that is based on the Omaha System is increasingly popular, and has helped promote Omaha System dissemination. Keys to a successful automation search include comparing several products and involving information technology personnel in the process (Westra & Raup, 1995; Bowles, 1997; Geraci, 1997; Androwich et al., 2003; Handly et al., 2003; Rosebaugh, 2004).

Software based on the Omaha System must:

- Protect private data.
- Fully incorporate the Omaha System's Problem Classification Scheme, Intervention Scheme, and Problem Rating Scale for Outcomes.
- Enable the three components of the Omaha System to interact.
- Produce a working care plan based on assessments and planned interventions.
- Extract and aggregate data.
- Generate a variety of outcomes reports by dates, demographics, or other variables.
- Have reasonable hardware requirements.
- Integrate with existing systems.
- Make documentation simple for users.

Ideally, the Omaha System will be intact within the software. Altered or "customized" versions of the Omaha System will not generate reliable data or information. The three components should interact to make care planning and outcomes measurement simple for the user. Outcomes and productivity reports should be easily accessible according to date, client, program, or practitioner. No software works well when hardware is inadequate; computers must be powerful enough to handle large software applications. It is unrealistic to expect that one software program will meet all of the organization's documentation, billing, and productivity needs, but it is important to investigate potential compatibility with other essential programs before choosing a product.

Pilot Testing

While all practitioners can implement the Omaha System at the same time in smaller organizations, larger organizations will increase their success by starting with a pilot test phase. Groups of eight to twelve practitioners can easily attend orientation, work together, and communicate well while learning to use the Omaha System and then the software. When they are successfully using their new system, they will become excellent teachers and mentors for new groups of practitioners. An important responsibility of pilot test groups is to draft procedures for the use of software, as well as Omaha System practice and documentation standards. Some project committee members should be part of the initial pilot test group to increase continuity and share the long-range vision.

IMPLEMENTATION

A period of at least 3 and no more than 6 months usually works well to complete the transition to an automated or manual version of the Omaha System. It is important to allow adequate time for change, but it is equally important to establish an end date for orientation and to avoid prolonging the process unnecessarily. Managers must decide the extent to which old records have to be converted to the new system, and they must give support staff time to enter existing client data or find a way to convert existing electronic data that can be "dumped into" the new system. It is important to allow adequate time for learning to navigate the new system. It is helpful to prioritize practitioners' work time so that they are able to comply with implementation time lines. Finally, be sure to acknowledge progress and completion of goals.

Orientation

Orienting practitioners to the Omaha System involves four steps that are also described in Chapters 2 and 4 (see Table 4-1) (Martin & Scheet, 1992; Omaha System Web site, 2004). First, practitioners must recognize that they will benefit from this potentially challenging change to Omaha System documentation. They need to develop an appreciation for using the Omaha System to capture their practice expertise and translate it into data for the benefit of clients and their organization. Second, practitioners deserve adequate education about the Omaha System, including materials and methods designed to meet the needs of diverse learning styles. Retention increases when information is introduced incrementally and is repeated in a variety of ways. Third, practitioners need ample opportunities to practice using the Omaha System. This book includes examples of using videotaped role plays and written case studies for practice and discussion. The public health nursing program in the state of Maine used this strategy successfully, as is detailed in Omaha System Box 3-3. Fourth, practitioners benefit from frequent interaction while building and maintaining documentation skills, and from discussing the appropriate use of the Omaha System in their particular settings. To foster improvement in documentation, practitioners need time for problem solving, question-and-answer sessions, and consensus building (Monsen & Martin, 2002a). Organizations that restrict the orientation process are likely to have frustrated practitioners and difficulties with data.

Practitioners' attitudes and skills are predictors of the successes or difficulties that occur during implementation. Like the Marion County (Indiana) Health Department (Handly et al, 2003) (Omaha System Box 3-4), practitioners in many organizations find the process of implementing a new automated or manual documentation system frustrating regardless of whether it includes the Omaha System (Stricklin et al., 2000; Hockenjos & Wharton, 2001; Larrabee et al., 2001; Souther, 2001; Tressa & Barber, 2001). When the need for change is presented positively, practitioners appreciate the potential benefits that result. Several strategies can decrease any resistance that remains, for example allowing opportunities for "buddies" to help others practice and learn, and scheduling group documentation sessions. It is important to recognize individual improvement and achievements at all levels, such as learning to turn on a computer for the first time, or successfully entering existing client demographics into the new system. Committed leaders, realistic expectations, support, and encouragement help even reluctant practitioners achieve the desired results.

EVALUATION AND MAINTENANCE

A successful transition to a new Omaha System record is reinforced by incorporating the Omaha System into the organization's structure. Typically, the project committee and

CHAPTER 3

OMAHA SYSTEM BOX 3-3

Omaha System Experiences in Practice: Using Videotapes of Role-plays for Public Health Nurse Orientation

Beth B. Patterson, RN, MN
Director of Public Health Nursing Program
State of Maine
Augusta, Maine

Maine is a rural state with long winters that make travel challenging. Sixty-one public health nurses who provide maternal-child health and communicable disease services and their supervisors are located in 18 offices throughout the state. We identified the need for a documentation system based on the nursing process and decided to implement an automated system despite major budget constraints. We selected the Omaha System because it is amenable to community nursing practice, describes client needs, and generates nurse-sensitive client outcomes.

A core group of public health staff nurses, supervisors, and consultants began using a manual version of the Omaha System about 18 months before converting to an automated system. The group provided ongoing orientation for colleagues in their offices, using case discussion as a teaching and learning tool. We developed and videotaped role-play scenarios of familiar client situations to help nurses become more proficient using the Omaha System. Nurses wrote, acted, and taped five role-play situations, each about 15 minutes in length: a mother who was at high risk for parenting problems and her baby, a pregnant woman, a normal newborn, a refugee with active tuberculosis, and a woman with latent tuberculosis. The group members decided what the most appropriate Omaha System answers were for each situation. We then showed the videotapes to their nurse colleagues who independently completed answer sheets (worksheets) based on the Omaha System. The discussion time that followed was designed to establish group consensus and increase learners' ability to generalize their decision making skills to additional client situations. This standardized approach ensured that all nurses received the same information, yet did not have to travel long distances to meet. As our budgetary situation deteriorated, we used videoconferencing equipment to show the tapes to several offices simultaneously, view and discuss the videotape together, and eliminate expensive travel. This allowed practitioners and managers to learn from each other in a nonthreatening environment and to improve their Omaha System documentation, accuracy, and consistency.

managers are responsible for monitoring the quality of documentation to determine if it is accurate and consistent, revising practice and documentation guidelines, providing ongoing education and encouragement for practitioners, and proceeding with plans to use aggregate data. If organizations expect to have accurate and consistent reports, these activities must continue on an ongoing basis.

Quality Improvement

A standardized classification such as the Omaha System provides organizations with an inherent quality improvement infrastructure (Martin & Scheet, 1992; Westra, Martin, & Swan, 1996; Martin & Gorski, 1998; Ingersoll, 2000; Institute of Medicine, 2000; Institute of Medicine, 2001; Institute of Medicine, 2004). Practitioners must understand and agree upon definitions of terms for assessments, interventions, and outcomes. Practice and documentation guidelines based on Omaha System terms help organizations create

OMAHA SYSTEM BOX 3-4

Omaha System Experiences in Practice: Implementing a Clinical Information System in a Large County Health Department

Nancy A. Keefe, RN, BSN
Administrator, Community-Based Care
Health and Hospital Corporation
Marion County Health Department
Indianapolis, Indiana

In 1998 our nursing administrator and managers developed an action plan to implement an Omaha System-based point-of-care clinical information system. During the next 4 years, nurses at all levels participated in planning and implementation activities, many of which are described here and in a journal article. Although we expected progress to be slow as a result of our nurses' limited computer skills and our division's large size and complexity, several unexpected technical and scheduling challenges caused extended delays. Nurses became frustrated and reluctant to continue with the action plan.

Early in 2002 the nursing managers and administrator evaluated options. Returning to a manual record was not possible, given the increasing need for accessible clinical data and quantitative outcomes. Instead, division leaders encouraged a core team of 14 staff nurses and managers to renew efforts for implementation. During initial meetings the core team reviewed barriers and accomplishments to date, and developed an action plan with three primary components:

1. *Attitude.* Members of the core team established a collective "can do" attitude. They developed a sense of ownership for the clinical information system instead of viewing it as an adversary.
2. *Tutorial.* The core team created a customized tutorial based on the software company's manual that was compatible with their responsibilities and expectations. They used this tutorial as they began to teach other colleagues.
3. *Mentoring.* Nurses worked together as they practiced using the Omaha System and software. When they were comfortable with one type of client record, they proceeded to a new one. In time, members of the core team used the buddy approach with their colleagues who were new to the process.

Core team members have been rewarded for their successful efforts in various ways. Four members described their experiences in presentations at the Indiana State Public Health meeting and at the 2002 American Public Health Association meeting.

standards of care and reporting. When client records have a standardized structure and decreased narrative, the problem solving process depicted in Figure 1-1 is more visible and record audits are completed more effectively. In addition, organizations may decide to require standardized assessments for specific client populations: for example, assess all pregnant clients for signs and symptoms of a minimum of five problems (e.g., *Pregnancy*, *Income*, *Substance use*, *Abuse*, and *Family planning*), or assess all clients with chronic obstructive pulmonary disease for signs and symptoms of a minimum of three problems (e.g., *Respiration*, *Circulation*, and *Medication regimen*). Likewise, organizations may establish standard ways to document common activities for specific problems. For example, when practitioners are expected to complete a home safety checklist after admitting a family to service, they identify the problem, *Residence*; then the intervention category, target, and client-specific information may be listed as follows: *Surveillance: safety-presence of hazards/home safety checklist.*

There are several approaches for ensuring that practitioners meet practice and documentation quality standards:

- Provide frequent opportunities for practitioners to discuss documentation terms, definitions, and procedures. Informal question-and-answer sessions help practitioners understand the organization's data needs and the necessary procedure modifications.
- Set a regular schedule for record audits. Have one person volunteer to provide copies of a short, recently completed client record. Ask practitioners to review the record together, taking turns identifying areas that were documented well and questions they have about documentation that could be done differently.
- Establish interrater agreement among practitioners and with the Omaha System as described by Washington County, Minnesota, public health nurses (Omaha System Box 3-5) and others (Monsen & Martin, 2002a and 2002b; Monsen and Kerr, 2004).
- Give practitioners feedback about services and client outcomes as described by their documentation.

Standardized Care Plans and Pathways

The three components of the Omaha System complement each other elegantly and provide an integrated approach for developing customized care plans and pathways. When used appropriately, care plans and pathways are valuable resources. They are excellent orientation tools, can be used as client assessment templates, save time by eliminating cumbersome repetition, and document required data consistently for all clients. Section II of this book is a User's Guide that provides suggested care planning and intervention guides for clients in general. Organizations can use those guides as a basis for developing standardized care plans for specific client groups.

Many organizations use pathways, a more structured type of care plan for specific types of clients. Pathways articulate best practices for client assessment and care planning in Omaha System terms. Practitioners who follow these pathways consistently and effectively complete required assessments and data fields, and begin the process of developing a best practices approach. The three steps to create a new pathway are:

1. Identify the client population for which the pathway will be used.
2. Choose only the most salient and common problems experienced by that population for required assessment.
3. Add typical interventions related to those problems.

Practitioners assess all problems included in a pathway to determine if the problem should be addressed with that client and, if so, which modifiers should be selected. The practitioner's decision to address the problems is based on the presence of client interest *(Health Promotion),* risk factors *(Potential),* or signs and symptoms *(Actual)* as defined by the Omaha System for each of the problems. In addition to considering the problems listed in a pathway, practitioners use their assessment skills and identify additional pertinent problems when they exist. Practitioners add interventions to pathways to meet client needs. If pathways are customized appropriately, they are unique to each client while facilitating evidence-based practice and documentation.

Although pathways often make documentation faster and more consistent, they also have several potential pitfalls. If practitioners rely completely on pathways, they may have more difficulty learning to use the Omaha System and accurately describing unique client situations and services provided. Client care plans will not be individualized, and data

OMAHA SYSTEM BOX 3-5

Omaha System Experiences in Practice: Establishing and Maintaining Interrater Reliability

Ellie K. Hodkinson, RN, MPH
Public Health Nurse II
Washington Country Department of Public Health and Environment
Stillwater, Minnesota
Jill Timm, RN, JD
Public Health Nurse II
Washington County Department of Public Health and Environment
Stillwater, Minnesota

Washington County public health nurses provide home visiting services to clients who are pregnant, new parents, or those who have difficulties with parenting. In response to increasing demands for data that demonstrates the effectiveness of nursing services, the department has implemented automated documentation that includes the Omaha System.

To ensure consistency with the new documentation system, the public health nurses and manager created two valuable tools: a policy manual that guides nurses as they document client assessment with the Omaha System, and a user's manual to assist staff in agency-specific implementation of the software.

Two of the team's eight public health nurses agreed to serve as Omaha System and software "experts." To establish expert status, the public health nurses studied articles about the Omaha System, reviewed and discussed each others' records, and met with an Omaha System consultant 3 times over a 7-month period. During the consultations, specific questions about the Omaha System were discussed. The two nurses watched and independently documented a simulated visit scenario. The nurses' and consultant's answers were compared to establish interrater reliability. Since that time, the public health nurses have verified interrater agreement with the consultant annually.

The two public health nurse experts established a peer mentoring system with their team members. Mentoring activities included monthly team discussions about specific Omaha System topics and documentation situations. Quarterly reviews of a sample record allowed all team members to participate in critiquing documentation practice. The team members helped each other with documentation questions as they arose. Using the Omaha System experts to mentor team members has provided a method to ensure that data are accurate and reliable, a prerequisite for sharing reports with board members and the public. Through this process, the entire team developed a sense of personal ownership and pride in demonstrating the effectiveness of the department's public health nursing services.

integrity will be sacrificed. Organizations should exercise caution in the use of pathways developed by others because they may not reflect agency practice or the particular needs of local clientele. Organizations that maximize the potential of pathways use a few core pathways to standardize assessments for all clients and then use additional problem-specific pathways for special circumstances. Core pathways should reflect the most common problems identified in the population served, and the additional pathways should reflect typical interventions for specific problems that are identified regularly but less frequently and have a common intervention response.

Care plans and pathways must be reevaluated regularly to ensure that they meet client, practitioner, and data collection needs. When practitioners become experienced using Omaha System documentation, they will further develop their skills in collecting assessment data, developing care plans and pathways, choosing interventions, and evaluating clients' outcomes. Their insight will guide pathway revisions and ensure that they reflect current best practices and agency standards (Humphrey, 2002a and 2002b).

Figures 3-1 and 3-2 are examples of pathways that demonstrate the versatility of the Omaha System for diverse populations. Figure 3-1 is a pathway used during the admission assessment of all adult family health clients at Washington County Public Health and Environment, in Stillwater, Minnesota. Figure 3-2 is a pathway used during the admission assessment of home care clients who have congestive heart failure at Fairview Lakes HomeCaring and Hospice, in Chisago City, Minnesota.

Personnel

Managers should expect a temporary decrease in practitioner productivity while implementing a new documentation system. Before and after changing to automated systems, organizations have compared productivity and documentation time and report little difference. However, managers save time when they retrieve information from an automated system, monitor practitioner activity, and aggregate, analyze, and report data.

When turnover occurs, organizations face the challenge of helping newly employed practitioners gain competence and experience a seamless transition to their responsibilities with the Omaha System record. Establishing a solid infrastructure for this process is essential. Clear, step-by-step procedures, practice and documentation guidelines, and agency-specific pathways provide excellent orientation tools. Experienced practitioners and managers serve as coaches for new employees. Frequent review of the new employees' records prevents them from forming misguided documentation habits. Using these strategies ensures new and existing employee satisfaction and promotes data integrity. As noted in Omaha System Box 3-1, orientation is easier for some employees than others and may relate to a variety of factors, including computer science experience, practice experience, attitude, and insight into potential benefits of change.

Experienced Omaha System users benefit from opportunities to learn more about the Omaha System, to interact with other practitioners who use it, and to share their expertise with other potential users. They can develop educational materials for team meetings and lead team discussions. Attending conferences and multi-agency users' sessions offers exposure to new information about Omaha System applications with different programs and populations.

The ongoing role of the information technology staff is to ensure that network systems and hardware continue to have the capability to support the software. In some organizations, these staff members provide direct individual support to practitioners and managers. In others, support staff members fulfill that role. Most software companies offer continuing technical support to their customers. Designating one information technology or support staff person to communicate with the software company and to serve as the primary contact for practitioners and managers is helpful in preventing duplication of effort and increasing the organization's internal capacity to resolve issues.

Software Vendors

Practitioners become frustrated if software does not function properly. It is important to maintain close communication with software vendors and closely monitor software performance issues. Vendors may offer services to their customers including workshops, newsletters, news releases, and upgrades. Initial and ongoing software orientation may or may not be included in the purchase price of the software (Rosebaugh, 2004).

Admission Assessment Pathway With Standard Interventions for Adult Family Health		
Clients		
Income		
TGC	Finances	Use of community resources
TGC	Finances	Long-range planning/decision making
TGC	Finances	Income versus expenses
CM	Finances	Facilitate use of community support services
Residence		
TGC	Safety	Home safety checklist
TGC	Home	Use of community resources
CM	Home	Facilitate use of community support services
S	Safety	Presence of hazards
Abuse		
TGC	Support system	How to access
CM	Social work/ counseling care	Facilitate use of community support services
S	S/Sx-emotional	Assess signs/symptoms of emotional abuse
S	S/Sx-physical	Assess signs/symptoms of physical abuse
Substance Use		
TGC	Substance use cessation	Effects of use on others
TGC	Substance use cessation	Effects of use on self
TGC	Behavior modification	Decrease/discontinue substance use
CM	Other community resource	Facilitate use of community support services
S	Substance use cessation	Monitor change in substance use
Family Planning		
TGC	Family planning care	Methods
TGC	Anatomy/physiology	Reproductive system
CM	Family planning care	Sources of care
S	Family planning care	Compliance with method

Figure 3-1 Example of a family health pathway.

(Courtesy Washington County Department of Public Health and Environment, Stillwater, Minnesota.)

Admission Assessment Pathway With Standard Interventions for Clients Who Have Congestive Heart Failure		
Respiration		
S	S/Sx-physical	Respiratory status: Lung sounds, cough, shortness of breath with exertion
Circulation		
TGC	Cardiac care	Prescribed diet: 2-3 gram sodium diet, foods to avoid, fluid restriction, daily weights
TGC	Cardiac care	Self assessment, precipitating behaviors, preventive measures, symptoms of exacerbation
TGC	Anatomy/physiology	Circulatory system: All aspects of disease process, energy conservation, and exercise guidelines
S	Cardiac care	Vital signs, weight, jugular-venous distention, abdominal girth, edema, adherence to care plan
S	Cardiac care	Activity tolerance, need for other providers (therapies, paraprofessional, social worker, spiritual)
S	Dietary management	Appetite, fluid intake and bowel/bladder function, adherence to diet
Medication Regimen		
TGC	Medication action/ side effects	Medication regimen, actions, side effects, precautions, interactions
S	Medication administration	Adherence to prescribed medications

Figure 3-2 Example of a congestive heart failure pathway.
(Courtesy Fairview Lakes HomeCaring and Hospice, Chisago City, Minnesota.)

Software upgrades are required to accommodate new regulations, technology, and improvements. Each software update creates added expenses for the organization and a new learning curve for practitioners. Managers need to provide a supportive environment by making time available to adapt to program changes and adjust procedures.

DATA ANALYSIS AND MANAGEMENT

For too long, clinical data from client record systems have been relegated to data cemeteries. Although practitioners collect and document information, no useful reports are produced. Data are essentially "buried." The advent of automated records provides practice settings with the ability to aggregate, analyze, and apply their clinical data routinely

(Martin & Monsen, 2002; Monsen, 2002; Monsen & Martin, 2002a and 2002b). In order to use Omaha System clinical data, organizations need to have the capacity to use simple databases and statistical software tools (*Home Health Care Management and Practice,* 2004). Usually, practice settings assign the primary data management responsibilities to a data analyst (manager, practitioner, planner, or statistician). Some organizations are fortunate and employ one person who has the needed skills. In many organizations, consultants are needed to work with an agency employee. All data analysts need a working knowledge of the Omaha System so that they understand the implications of the analysis and use appropriate statistical tests. Responsible data analysts monitor the data sets closely and remove test cases and other inaccurate information, an editing process sometimes referred to as "cleaning the data." It is essential that data analysts verify interpretations with practitioners on a regular basis. Practitioners' insight into the meaning of data they generate can prevent data analysts from making mistakes when they interpret it (Westra, Martin, & Swan, 1996; Martin, Norris, & Leak, 1999; Martin & Monsen, 2002; Monsen, 2002; Monsen & Martin, 2002a and 2002b; Monsen & Kerr, 2004).

Practitioners skilled in documentation generate meaningful and integrated assessment, intervention, and outcomes data when they use the Omaha System. This chapter describes how those data can be converted into information and reports. For more details about collecting and analyzing data in research settings, see Chapter 5. An essential prerequisite before sharing reports based on Omaha System information is to confirm that data are reliable and valid. Interrater reliability is addressed in Omaha System Box 3-6 and elsewhere (Martin & Scheet, 1992; Martin, Norris, & Leak, 1999; Monsen & Martin, 2002a and 2002b; Monsen & Kerr, 2004).

Omaha System data generated by practitioners can be converted to information and provide answers to organizations' questions about clients and services such as:

1. What are the primary needs of the client populations we serve?
2. Are the needs of group A different from the needs of group B or group C?
3. How can we describe our service populations' needs to the public?
4. What interventions did we use to address these problems?
5. Which interventions were used most frequently when successful outcomes were described within this population?
6. How can we describe our program's services to the public?
7. Did clients' *Knowledge, Behavior*, and/or *Status* improve following intervention?
8. With which groups are our services most successful?
9. Which of our services were most cost effective?
10. What is the value and impact of providing prevention services?
11. What is the optimal length of time to serve a particular client group?
12. How can we describe the impact of our program to the public?

Each organization should consider its unique information needs when beginning to analyze demographic characteristics, problems, modifiers, signs and symptoms, interventions, and rating scale data.

Describing Client Populations with the Problem Classification Scheme

The Problem Classification Scheme provides information about client needs. Problem data gathered as an unduplicated list of problem numbers addressed with clients answer questions 1-3.

1. What are the primary needs of the client population(s) we serve?

A frequency test applied to problem data reveals which problems are most commonly addressed by practitioners. Splitting data between groups based on a particular client characteristic, such as age, race or ethnicity, address, or diagnosis yields information about the most commonly addressed problems with each group.

2. Are the needs of group A different from the needs of group B or group C?
A test of differences between problems by client groups yields information about whether the needs of groups differ. For example, differences in needs are expected between clients served in family health care or home care, and between those who live in high income or low income neighborhoods.

3. How can we describe our service populations' needs to the public?
A simple list of the most commonly addressed Omaha System problems describes a service population's needs effectively and succinctly. Translating the list into a bar graph provides a convincing illustration of those needs. As presented in Omaha System Box 3-6 and Figure 3-3, practitioners from the Eau Claire City-County (Wisconsin) Health Department used this strategy when they converted their data to information and presented it to county administrators.

Describing Service Delivery with the Intervention Scheme

The Intervention Scheme provides information about program services. Intervention data are gathered as lists of problem-specific categories and targets, and answer questions 4 to 6.

OMAHA SYSTEM BOX 3-6

Omaha System Experiences in Practice: Describing Client Needs to Decision Makers

Kathleen M. Rahl, RN, MS
Director of Nursing
Eau Claire City-County Health Department
Eau Claire, Wisconsin

Our public health nursing records have been based on the Omaha System for many years. When we developed a new grant-funded program to promote healthy living for families who were at risk for child abuse and neglect, we used the Omaha System in our program evaluation plan. The plan was designed to measure the specific client needs our program addressed and to determine if our public health nursing efforts made a difference.

The fact that we have a manual documentation system was not a deterrent to collecting the data. Nurses designed a record audit tool to retrieve problem-specific outcomes data simply and quickly. An audit of 16 family records showed that a total of 48 problems had been opened for intervention. The most commonly addressed problems in order of frequency were *Caretaking/parenting, Growth and development, Health care supervision, Income, Nutrition, Residence, Sleep and rest patterns, Antepartum/postpartum* (now divided into two problems–*Pregnancy* and *Postpartum*), *Sanitation, Interpersonal relationship, Mental health, and Communication with community resources.* Figure 3-3 depicts these problems and frequencies in a graph so that they can be easily understood by department staff, administrators, and the public.

OMAHA SYSTEM BOX 3-6

Omaha System Experiences in Practice: Describing Client Needs to Decision Makers—cont'd

Additional analysis was conducted on 41 problems documented in family records that had been open to service for at least 2 months. Families' *Knowledge* improved on 10 problems, *Behavior* improved on 11 problems, and *Status* improved on 13 problems. A range of 22 to 27 problems showed unchanged ratings for *Knowledge*, *Behavior,* or *Status*, a positive finding in a program addressing needs of moderate risk to high risk families. Only two to three problems showed ratings reflecting regressed *Status* while the families received program services.

Omaha System data effectively described the needs of the families we served and the impact that public health nursing intervention had on them. These results were convincing when presented to the Human Services Board Long-term Support Committee. From these and other data reported about the program, the Committee concluded that the program had resulted in positive outcomes for high risk families and should be continued.

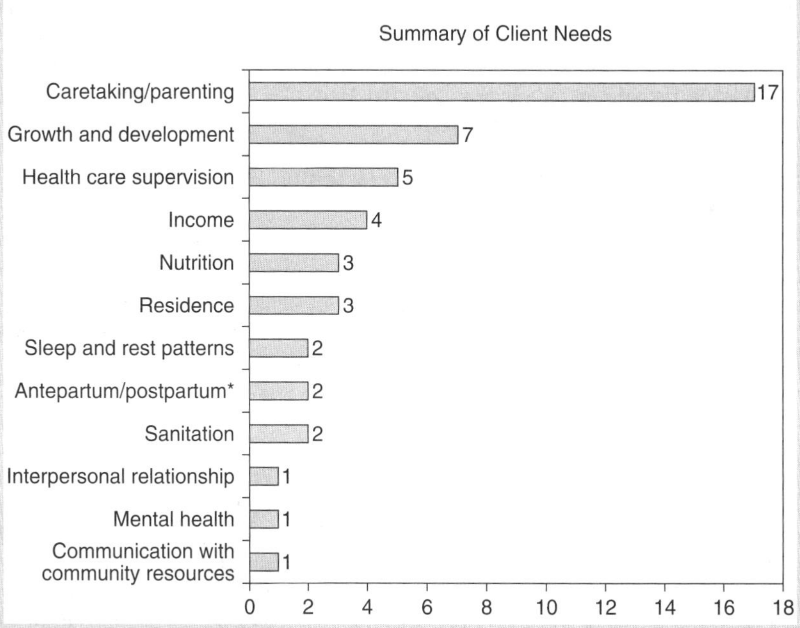

Figure 3-3 Graph depicting the most common Omaha System problems addressed with high-risk parents at Eau Claire (Wisconsin) City-County Health Department (n=16 families). *Divided into two problems: Pregnancy and Postpartum.

(Courtesy Eau Claire City-County Health Department, Eau Claire, Wisconsin.)

4. What interventions did we use to address these problems?

A frequency test of intervention categories describes the most common types of interventions performed by practitioners. Home care agencies would expect interventions such as *Treatments and Procedures* to be very common, while public health agencies would expect more *Teaching, Guidance, and Counseling* and *Surveillance*. Splitting the data file by problem, category, and target and applying a frequency test yields information about which specific interventions addressed particular problems.

5. Which interventions were used most frequently when successful outcomes were described within this population?

Answering this question requires splitting the intervention data according to an outcomes indicator, such as a particular final *Status* rating, weeks of gestation at delivery, or fewer hospitalizations. Risk factors of each group must also be considered as a part of the analysis and discussion. While a causal relationship between interventions and outcomes cannot be shown definitively by these data, they provide an opportunity to explore services provided in light of problems addressed, client risk factors, and client outcomes.

6. How can we describe our program's services to the public?

A basic summary of practitioner services can be provided in written or graphic form. If reports contain Omaha System terms for interventions, it is helpful to include definitions for readers' reference. It may be necessary to simplify some of the Omaha System language, depending on the audience for the report. The Dakota County (Minnesota) Public Health Nursing Department graphically depicted *Medication regimen* interventions in its final grant report (Omaha System Box 3-7).

Describing Client Outcomes with the Problem Rating Scale for Outcomes

The Problem Rating Scale for Outcomes provides information about client *Knowledge, Behavior*, and *Status* at particular points in time. Rating scale data gathered as lists of initial, interim, and final *Knowledge*, *Behavior*, and *Status* ratings answer questions 7-12.

When initiating this analysis, the organization must define desirable outcomes for client groups served. For example, for hospice clients who have the problem *Pain,* an improvement in the status rating from a "2" (severe signs/symptoms) to a "3" (moderate signs/symptoms) might be commendable and demonstrate successful interventions. Complete relief of signs and symptoms ("5") may be the goal, but may not be possible. For chronically ill clients, it may be appropriate to select a 6-month interval for comparing the initial and interim *Knowledge*, *Behavior*, and *Status* ratings for problems such as *Personal care* and *Circulation*. Success for chronically ill clients may mean maintaining ratings at the initial assessment level. For high-risk family health clients, desirable outcomes would be improvement from initial to final *Knowledge*, *Behavior,* and *Status* ratings. For clients at risk who receive prevention services, *Status* ratings should remain unchanged at "5" (no signs/symptoms) for initial and final ratings.

7. Did clients' *Knowledge, Behavior,* and/or *Status* improve following intervention?

To answer this question, it is necessary to aggregate *Knowledge, Behavior,* and *Status* ratings for two points in time. Data from each of the three rating scales for *Knowledge, Behavior*, and *Status* should be analyzed separately. Split the information by problem before analysis to show problem-specific outcomes. Split the information by client, compute average *Knowledge*, *Behavior*, and *Status* ratings for each client's problems, and then analyze to show client-specific overall outcomes for the client population.

Applying a statistical test to compare means (for example, pair initial and final mean *Knowledge* ratings) yields information about the significance of changes.

8. With which client groups are our services most successful?

Splitting files by client groups and comparing *Knowledge, Behavior,* and *Status* outcomes ratings yields information for discussion about this question.

9. Which of our services were most cost effective?

Combining number of visits and case management time to compute the cost of services provided with outcomes information yields information about cost-effectiveness of services.

OMAHA SYSTEM BOX 3-7

Omaha System Experiences in Practice: Using Data to Link Interventions and Outcomes

Carol A. Fish, RN, MSN
Public Health Supervisor
Dakota County Public Health Department
West St. Paul, Minnesota

When our home care team initially analyzed Omaha System data abstracted from client records, we noted that the most frequently occurring problem was *Medication regimen.* This finding validated our perception that successful medication management was a key to helping senior citizens live independently in their homes.

We wanted to know the underlying causes of senior citizens' difficulties with medication management and to identify which interventions were most effective. Based on Omaha System data, we successfully obtained a grant to investigate these questions. Grant funds were used to complete three primary objectives: (1) provide interrater reliability orientation and consultation to ensure the quality of public health nurses' Omaha System documentation, (2) provide software enhancements to abstract and aggregate client signs and symptoms from the existing documentation, and (3) develop educational materials about medication management for client and family education.

Nurses provided 2296 interventions to 44 clients over a period of 4 years. Analysis of Omaha System documentation data allowed us to describe the client problems, nursing services, and client outcomes. The majority of clients (79%) deviated from prescribed dosage/schedule. Nearly half of the clients (46%) had an inadequate system for taking medications and failed to obtain refills appropriately (44%). Intervention categories and targets documented for medication problems were *Treatments and Procedures* to set up and administer client medications, *Teaching, Guidance, and Counseling* to teach and reinforce medication management, *Case Management* to order and reorder medications, and *Surveillance* to monitor medication compliance and side effects. Figure 3-4 depicts targeted interventions by category.

Continued

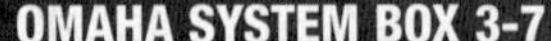

CHAPTER 3

OMAHA SYSTEM BOX 3-7

Omaha System Experiences in Practice: Using Data to Link Interventions and Outcomes—cont'd

Clients' *Knowledge* and *Status* for the *Medication regimen* problem improved significantly with interventions, but *Behavior* did not. We concluded that the nursing interventions successfully addressed the underlying causes of the problem, even though client behavior did not change. Data indicated that a high percentage of clients had other identified problems, including *Cognition*, which probably limited clients' ability to change *Behavior* related to *Medication regimen*.

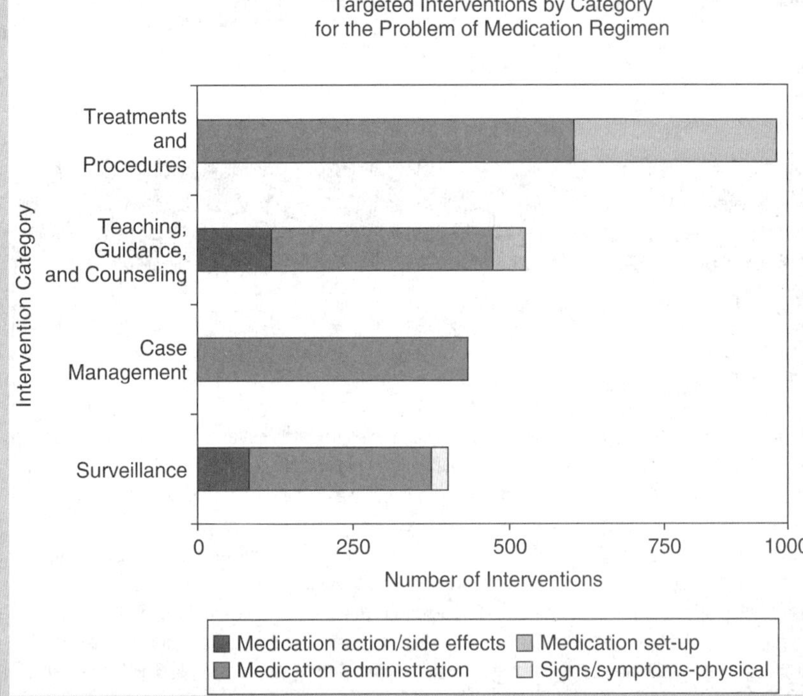

Figure 3-4 Graph depicting the types of interventions used by public health nurses addressing the *Medication regimen* problem at Dakota County (Minnesota) Public Health Department (n = 2296 interventions).

(Courtesy Dakota County Public Health Department, West St. Paul, Minnesota.)

10. What is the value and impact of providing prevention services?

Separating data by *Actual* problems (initial status ≤ "4") and *Potential* or *Health Promotion* problems (initial status = "5") provides a mechanism for examining prevention activities and their outcomes.

11. What is the optimal length of time to serve a particular client group?

Comparing outcomes for clients served according to length of time served may reveal an optimal duration of service for achieving a particular outcome.

12. How can we describe the impact of our program to the public?

Simply stating that clients' *Knowledge*, *Behavior*, and/or *Status* improved significantly during the specified service interval powerfully describes the impact of services. Limitations of the data include not having a control or comparison group, and not knowing whether circumstances besides service interventions also contributed to the outcome.

Line and bar graphs comparing initial and subsequent *Knowledge*, *Behavior*, and *Status* ratings depict client change and are easily understood and appreciated by practitioners, managers, administrators, and the public. The Sure Start Program in Wales provides an example of such an approach and includes details about their history, present, analysis, and future plans (Omaha System Box 3-8) (Clark et al., 2001; Christensen, 2003).

OMAHA SYSTEM BOX 3-8

Omaha System Experiences in Practice: Documenting Sure Start Services in Wales

Jean R. Christensen, RN, RHV, BSc (Hons)
Project Manager
Welsh Assembly Government
Cardiff, Wales, United Kingdom

Chris E. Koukos, RN, BSc (Hons), RM, RHV
Sure Start Manager
Swansea National Health Service Trust
Swansea, Wales, United Kingdom

Dame June Clark, RN, PhD, RHV, FRCN
Professor of Community Nursing
University of Wales, Swansea
Swansea, Wales, United Kingdom

Sure Start is a government-initiated United Kingdom-wide health visiting service designed to break the cycle of disadvantage experienced by young children. Health visitors are public health nurses who provide generalized services to families in their communities, with a special focus on children under the age of 5 years. In targeted Sure Start geographic areas, public health nurses visit families at home and in other community settings to promote children's physical, intellectual, and social development.

To obtain continued funding, Sure Start managers must submit annual reports to the government and provide evidence that the program is effective. It has been difficult to document this effectiveness and to measure the outcomes of health visitors' services. Because the Omaha System had been successfully pilot tested, a Sure Start manager in the Swansea National Health Service Trust decided to initiate its use in 2000. When Omaha System data were analyzed, problem frequencies demonstrated that the home visiting service was accurately targeting its objectives, and paired *t* tests on *Knowledge, Behaviour,* and *Status* ratings demonstrated highly significant results for those problems that matched the government targets. Figure 3-5 depicts the significant change in client *Knowledge, Behaviour,* and *Status* related to the problem, *Nutrition*.

Continued

CHAPTER 3

OMAHA SYSTEM BOX 3-8

Omaha System Experiences in Practice: Documenting Sure Start Services in Wales—cont'd

During two previous pilot tests, health visitors had requested modifications to the Omaha System terms because they wanted to make it more comprehensive for their health visiting practice. Following each pilot, many of the amended terms were changed back to original Omaha System terms. The health visitors learned that for the most part, the original Omaha System terms and definitions met their needs. It remained necessary to expand two problems, *Neglect* and *Abuse,* to correlate with the four categories of the United Kingdom's Child Protection Register.

Use of the Omaha System produced clear evidence of the efficacy of Sure Start, and helped to secure continued funding for its future development. Health visitors reported that an unexpected advantage of using the Omaha System was that visits became more focused on the problems that needed to be addressed.

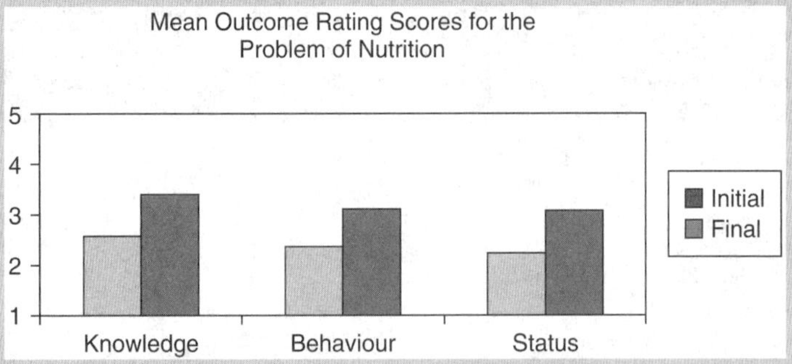

Figure 3-5 Graph depicting change in *Knowledge, Behaviour,* and *Status* ratings from the Problem Rating Scale for Outcomes for clients who had the *Nutrition* problem (n = 61 clients, $p<0.001$ for all) in the Sure Start Program, Swansea, Wales, United Kingdom.
Knowledge ratings: 1, no knowledge; 2, minimal knowledge; 3, basic knowledge; 4, adequate knowledge; 5, superior knowledge. *Behaviour* ratings: 1, not appropriate behaviour; 2, rarely appropriate behaviour; 3, inconsistently appropriate behaviour; 4, usually appropriate behaviour; 5, consistently appropriate behaviour. *Status* ratings: 1, extreme signs/symptoms; 2, severe signs/symptoms; 3, moderate signs/symptoms; 4, minimal signs/symptoms; 5, no signs/symptoms.
(Courtesy Sure Start Program, Swansea, Wales, United Kingdom.)

SUMMARY

Implementing the three components of the Omaha System in health care and social service organizations has far-reaching implications. While changing to Omaha System documentation presents financial barriers and a formidable learning curve, the benefits far outweigh the challenges. Use of the Omaha System promotes evidence-based practice and documentation, generates data, and creates information management opportunities.

When Omaha System data are analyzed, practitioners, managers, and administrators can describe their clients, service delivery, and related client outcomes.

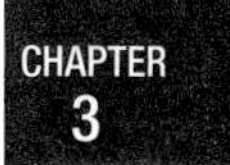

REFERENCES

Androwich, I.M., Bickford, C.J., Button, P.S., Hunter, K.M, Murphy, J., & Sensmeier, J. (2003). *Clinical Information Systems: A Framework for Reaching the Vision.* Washington, DC, ANA Publishing.

Bednarz, P.K. (1998, August). The Omaha System: A model for describing school nurse case management. *Journal of School Nursing, 14*(3):24-30.

Bowles, K.H. (1997, July/August). The barriers and benefits of nursing information systems. *Computers in Nursing, 15*(4):191-196.

Bowles, K.H. (1999, Winter). The Omaha System: Bridging hospital and home care. *On-Line Journal of Nursing Informatics, 3*(1):7-11. Retrieved March 8, 2004 from the Internet: http://www.eaa-knowledge.com/ojni/ni/dm/ojni.html.

Bowles, K.H. (2000, April). Patient problems and nurse interventions during acute care and discharge planning. *Journal of Cardiovascular Nursing, 14*(3): 29-41.

Centers for Medicare and Medicaid Services. (2003). *Conditions of Participation: Home health agencies.* Retrieved September 1, 2003 from the Internet: http://www.cms.hhs.gov/.

Christensen, J. (2003). A language for health visiting. In Clark, J. (Ed.), *Naming Nursing: Proceedings of the First ACENDIO Ireland/UK Conference* (pp. 241-248). Bern, Switzerland, Hans Huber.

Clark, J. & Lang, N.M. (1992, July/August). Nursing's next advance: An international classification for nursing practice. *International Nursing Review, 39*(4):109-111, 128.

Clark, J., Christensen, J., Mooney, G., Davies, P., Edwards, J., Fitchett, L., Spowart, B., & Thomas, P. (2001, March). New methods of documenting health visiting practice. *Community Practitioner, 74*(3):108-112.

Croke, E.M. (2003, September). Nurses, negligence, and malpractice. *American Journal of Nursing, 103*(9): 54-64.

Doran, K., Sampson, B., Staus, R., Ahern, C., & Schiro, D. (1997, January). Clinical pathway across tertiary and community care after an interventional cardiology procedure. *Journal of Cardiovascular Nursing, 11*(2):1-14.

Duckett, K.K. (2003, May). 10 Ways to lose your Medicare certification. *Home Healthcare Nurse, 21*(5):318-324.

Gaskell, S.M. & McGourthy, R. (2002, May/June) Is OASIS a mirage? *The Remington Report, 10*(3):16-18.

Geraci, E.P. (1997, July/August). Computers in home care: Application of change theory. *Computers in Nursing, 15*(4):199-203.

Handly, M.J., Grubb, S.K., Keefe, N.A., & Martin, K.S. (2003, January). Essential activities for implementing a clinical information system in public health nursing. *Journal of Nursing Administration, 33*(1):14-16.

Healthy People 2010 (2000, January). *Table of Contents.* Retrieved September 1, 2003 from the Internet: http://www.healthypeople.gov/Document/tableofcontents.htm#parta.

Hockenjos, G.J. & Wharton, A. (2001, December). Point-of-care training: Strategies for success. *Home Healthcare Nurse, 19*(12):766-773.

Home Health Care Management and Practice, 16(3). (2004, April). Entire issue.

Huang, L.H. (1994, September). The Omaha System application in home health nursing. *Journal of Nursing of the Republic of China, 41*(3):14-17.

Humphrey, C.J. (2002a, October). The current status of home care nursing practice, Part 1. *Home Healthcare Nurse, 20*(10):677-684.

Humphrey, C.J. (2002b, November). The current status of home care nursing practice, Part 2. *Home Healthcare Nurse, 20*(11):741-747.

Ingersoll, G. (2000, July/August). Evidence-based nursing: What it is and what it isn't. *Nursing Outlook, 48*(4):151-152.

Institute of Medicine. (2000). *To Err is Human: Building a Safer Health Care System.* Kohn, L.T., Corrigan, J.M., & Donaldson, M.S. (Eds.). Washington, DC, National Academies Press.

Institute of Medicine. (2001). *Crossing the Quality Chasm.* Committee on Quality of Health Care in America. (Ed.). Washington, DC, National Academies Press.

Institute of Medicine. (2004). *Keeping Patients Safe: Transforming the Work Environment of Nurses.* Page, A. (Ed.). Washington, DC, National Academies Press.

Jacobson, J.M. & Eckstrom, D.L. (1997, February). Assessing homeless veterans using the Omaha System assessment tool in a nontraditional home care setting. *Home Care Provider, 2*(1):22-29.

Jonkergouw, P.H. (1991). Computerisation of the nursing process. In Hovenga, E.J.S., Hannah, K.J., McCormick, K.A., & Ronald, J.S. (Eds.), *Nursing Informatics '91: Proceedings of the Fourth International Conference* (pp. 457-463). New York, Springer.

Jorgensen, C.K. & Young, B.A. (1989, May/June). The supervisory shared home visit tool. *Home Healthcare Nurse, 7*(3):33-36.

Larrabee, J.H., Boldreghini, S., Elder-Sorrells, K., Turner, Z.M., Wender, R.G., Hart, J.M., & Lenzi, P.S. (2001, March/April). Evaluation of documentation before and after implementation of a nursing information system in an acute care hospital. *Computers in Nursing, 19*(2):56-68.

Madigan, E.A. (2002, September). The scientific dimensions of OASIS for home care outcome measurement. *Home Healthcare Nurse, 20*(9):579-583.

Mallard, C.O. (2000). Nursing informatics in the home health care environment. In Carty, B. (Ed.), *Nursing Informatics: Education for Practice* (pp. 252-270). New York, Springer.

Marek, K.D. (1996, June). Nursing diagnoses and home care nursing utilization. *Public Health Nursing, 13*(3): 195-200.

Marek, K.D. & Rantz, M.J. (2000, Spring). Aging in place: A new model for long-term care. *Nursing Administration Quarterly, 24*(3):1-11.

Martin, K.S. (2000, January/February). Home health care, outcomes management, and the Land of Oz. *Outcomes Management for Nursing Practice, 4*(1):7-12.

Martin, K.S., Baisch, M.J., & Bell-Calvin, J. (2003, January). Data mining produces gold. *Nursing Matters, 14*(1): 6-7.

Martin, K.S., Bessho, Y., & Saito, Y. (1999, April). The introduction to the Omaha System. *The Japanese Journal of Total Care, 9*(4):64-72.

Martin, K.S. & Gorski, L.A. (1998, Fall). Managed care: Effects on home health providers and stroke survivors. *Topics in Stroke Rehabilitation, 5*(3):11-24.

Martin, K.S. & Monsen, K.A. (2002, November). Communicating public health nursing outcomes to the public. 130th Annual Meeting of the American Public Health Association. Philadelphia.

Martin, K.S. & Norris, J. (1996, October). The Omaha System: A model for describing practice. *Holistic Nursing Practice, 11*(1):75-83.

Martin, K.S., Norris, J., & Leak, G.K. (1999, January/March). Psychometric analysis of the Problem Rating Scale for Outcomes. *Outcomes Management for Nursing Practice, 3*(1):20-25.

Martin, K.S. & Scheet, N.J. (1988, May-June). The Omaha System: Providing a framework for assuring quality of home care. *Home Healthcare Nurse, 6*(3):24-28.

Martin, K.S. & Scheet, N.J. (1992). *The Omaha System: Applications for Community Health Nursing.* Philadelphia, Saunders.

Martin, K.S. & Scheet, N.J. (1997). *The Omaha System: A Pocket Guide for Community Health Nursing.* Tokyo, Ishiyaku. (Reprinted.)

Martin, K.S., Scheet, N.J., & Stegman, M.R. (1993, December). Home health clients: Characteristics, outcomes of care, and nursing interventions. *American Journal of Public Health, 83*(12):1730-1734.

McGourthy, R.J. (1999, February). Omaha and OASIS: A comparative study of outcomes in patients with chronic obstructive pulmonary disease. *Home Care Provider, 4*(1):21-25.

Monsen, K.A. (2002). Using the Omaha System to describe outcomes of clients receiving public health nurse home visiting services. (Unpublished master's thesis, University of Minnesota, Minneapolis, Minnesota.)

Monsen, K.A. & Kerr, M.J. (2004, April). Mining quality documentation for golden outcomes. *Home Health Care Management and Practice, 16*(3):192-199.

Monsen, K.A. & Martin, K.S. (2002a, April/June). Developing an outcomes management program in a public health department. *Outcomes Management, 6*(2):61-66.

Monsen, K.A. & Martin, K.S. (2002b, July/September). Using an outcomes management program in a public health department. *Outcomes Management, 6*(3):120-124.

Nelson, R.M. (2004, April). Measuring outcomes in home health care: Beyond the OASIS data set. *Home Health Care Management and Practice, 16*(3):200-205.

Omaha System Web site (2004). Retrieved March 8, 2003 from the Internet: http://www.omahasystem.org.

Nursing Outlook, 52(1). (2004, January/February). Entire issue.

Park, H.A., Kim, J.E., & Cho, I. (2000). *Nursing Diagnoses, Interventions, and Outcomes Classification.* Seoul, Korea: Seoul National University.

Plowfield, L.A. & Raymond, J.E. (2001, July 30). Capturing nursing interventions and patient outcomes. *Greater Philadelphia Advance for Nurses, 3*(15):21-22, 34.

Public Health Functions Steering Committee (1994, Fall). *Essential Public Health Services.* Retrieved March 8, 2004 from the Internet: http://www.health.gov/phfunctions/public.htm.

Rosebaugh, D.L. (2004, April 1). Getting ready for the software in your future. *Home Health Care Management and Practice, 16*(3):228-234.

Sampson, B.K. & Doran, K.A. (1998, May/June). Health needs of coronary artery bypass graph surgery patients at discharge. *Dimensions of Critical Care Nursing, 17*(3):158-164.

Scoates, G.H., Fishman, M., & McAdam, B. (1996, August). Health care focus documentation: More efficient charting. *Nursing Management, 27*(8):30-32.

Shaughnessy, P.W. & Richard, A.A. (2002, November). Performance benchmarking. *Caring, XXI*(11):12-18.

Shuttleworth-Diaz, R. (1995, September). The use of the Omaha Information System in a multidisciplinary outpatient rehabilitation program for frail older persons. *Topics in Geriatric Rehabilitation, 11*(1):67-74.

Slack, M.K. & McEwen, M.M. (1999, October). The impact of interdisciplinary case management on client outcomes. *Family and Community Health, 22*(3):30-48.

Souther, E. (2001, March/April). Implementation of the electronic medical record: The team approach. *Computers in Nursing, 19*(2): 47-55.

Stricklin, M.L.V., Niles, S.A., Struk, C., & Jones, S. (2000, September). What nurses and managers expect from point of care technology. *Home Healthcare Nurse, 18*(8):514-523.

Tressa, S.S. & Barber, D.A. (2001, September). Home care automation: An agency looks back. *Caring, XX*(9): 36-38.

Walker, P.H. (1998, January/March). Costs of interdisciplinary practice in a school-based health center. *Outcomes Management for Nursing Practice, 2*(1):37-44.

Weidmann, J. & North, H. (1987, December). Implementing the Omaha Classification System in a public health agency. *Nursing Clinics of North America, 22*(4):971-979.

Westra, B. (1996, November/December). Making the right choice: Computerizing clinical information. *The Remington Report, 4*(6):32-35.

Westra, B.L. & Raup, G. (1995, August). Computerized charting: An essential tool for survival. *Caring, XIV* (8):57-61.

Westra, B.L., Martin, K.S., & Swan, A.R. (1996, August). Recognizing the need for standardized documentation and classifying patient needs. *Home Health Care Management and Practice, 8*(5):24-31.

Westra, B. & Solomon, D. (1999, Winter). The Omaha System: Bridging home care and technology. *On-line Journal of Nursing Informatics, 3*(1):12-14. Retrieved March 8, 2004 from the Internet: http://www.eaa-knowledge.com/ojni/ni/dm/ojni/html.

Wills, E.M. & Sloan, H.L. (1996, September). Assessing peripheral arterial disorders in the home: A multidisciplinary clinical guide. *Home Healthcare Nurse, 14*(9):669-682.

Wilson, S. (2002). Development of a personal digital assistant (PDA) as point-of-care technology in nursing education. *Journal of Mobile Informatics.* Retrieved October 20, 2003 from the Internet: http://www.pdacortex.com/pda_nursing_education.htm.

Zuber, R.F. (2002, November). OASIS data quality needs attention. *Home Healthcare Nurse, 20*(11): 756.

4

CHAPTER 4

USE OF THE OMAHA SYSTEM IN EDUCATION

Victoria L. Elfrink

Changes in today's health care system influence the way that practitioners need to be educated. Educators must prepare graduates to function effectively in diverse and rapidly changing settings, apply new methods to record and manage clinical data, and understand the potential value of clinical data (Elfrink & Martin, 1996; Carty, 2000; Elfrink & Martin, 2000; Hamner & Wilder, 2001; Moritz & Barton, 2001; Barton et al., 2003; Institute of Medicine, 2003; Elfrink & Davis, 2004). Designing a curriculum to meet the needs of the present and the future is daunting.

If health care educators are to prepare students for the future, they must be innovative and move beyond reacting to change to anticipating future practice requirements. In other words, they need to critically assess the emerging needs of practice. When addressing nursing education, Tanner (1995) described the urgency of developing a responsive nursing curriculum and suggested that educators are obligated to continuously and critically reevaluate their programs in light of health care trends. Educators who accomplish this task provide students with the skills they need to practice successfully; of equal importance, they send graduates into service settings who are prepared to diffuse their knowledge and make positive changes in the delivery of care.

Converging trends, such as the expanded nursing shortage, increased need for timely data, growth of community care, and intensified interest in faculty practice, are prompting the use of innovative documentation solutions including standardized terminologies and automated information systems (Hanson, 1996; National Advisory Council, 1997; Tagliareni & Marckx, 1997; Travis & Brennan, 1998; American Association of Colleges of Nursing, 1999; Marek & Rantz, 2000; Buerhaus & Norman, 2001; Elfrink et al., 2001; Clemen-Stone, McGuire, & Eigsti, 2002; Ervin, 2002; Turley, 2002; Androwich et al., 2003; Martin, Baisch, & Bell-Calvin, 2003; Oermann & Heinrich, 2003; *Healthcare Informatics,* 2004; Marek et al., 2004; *Nursing Outlook,* 2004). The Institute of Medicine published a report specific to the education of health care professionals (2003). The report identified five critical core competencies: provide client-centered care, participate as members of a multidisciplinary team, use evidence-based practice, apply quality improvement approaches, and utilize informatics. In regard to informatics, the report stated that graduates should use informatics technology to communicate, manage knowledge, mitigate error, and support decision making.

Preparing students to develop sound decision making skills, document care, and manage information using standardized terminologies has become an increasingly significant strategy in education. Because the Omaha System encourages communication and documentation of care that is clear, evidence-based, and capable of being compared and used for research, educators, especially nursing educators, are introducing it into their curricula. Thus the Omaha System creates a unity between education, practice, and research that is responsive and meaningful.

ADOPTION IN CURRICULA

Students began using the Omaha System in the mid-1970s (Tully & Bennett, 1992; Martin & Scheet, 1992a). Since then the student population has grown to include many nursing programs in the United States and some schools internationally. Students and educators from diploma, associate degree, baccalaureate, masters, and doctoral programs use the Omaha System. As mentioned in this and other chapters, selected nurse educators have introduced their colleagues from other disciplines to the Omaha System. Multidisciplinary student use is increasing, although slowly.

The first essential step for all educators and students is learning about the structure, terms, and definitions of the Omaha System. However, that learning is very different from the second step, learning how to use it, or the third step, learning how to use it accurately and consistently. Although these progressive steps were described in the previous chapters, they present unique challenges in regard to educators and students. For some educators the appropriate goal is basic knowledge, so they can introduce the Omaha System to students in a single course that focuses on the problem solving process, information systems, or standardized terminologies. Although students will likely graduate from these programs with a limited knowledge of the Omaha System, they should develop a respect for the value of clinical data and information technology. For other educators the goal is intermediate knowledge, so they can teach students to apply the Omaha System reliably as they complete manual or automated records in clinical settings. For yet another group of educators the goal is proficient knowledge, because they provide direct client care in community-oriented clinics and nurse-managed centers, case management programs, or other clinical sites. As indicated in Chapter 5, these educators serve as role models for students and may be conducting research based on their data. A number of schools have established ongoing programs of Omaha System research.

INSTRUCTIONAL RESOURCES AND STRATEGIES

Many educators have not used the Omaha System previously in practice settings. Their particular challenge is to function as educators and learners simultaneously, and to acknowledge that some students may have more Omaha System skills than they have. As cognitive learning theory indicates, gaining knowledge that moves beyond "knowing about" to "knowing how" requires Omaha System users to develop new skills and behaviors to provide care (Reilly & Oermann, 1985). Learning different ways to organize and think about clinical documentation is a multitasked process, involving the organization and filtering of new information, and the generation and testing of hypotheses (Gagne & Briggs, 1979; Turley, 2002). The diverse resources and strategies described in this section address understanding clinical phenomena in new ways and structuring data entry.

General guidelines for successful Omaha System use were described in Chapter 2, and include simplicity, repetition, triangulation, and positive reinforcement. However, novice Omaha System educators and students need a special combination of resources and strategies to progress along Benner's novice-to-expert continuum (Benner, 1984; Benner,

Tanner, & Chesla, 1996). One strategy, often overlooked but essential to success, is to *have a positive attitude*. Educators who introduce the Omaha System to their colleagues or students need an affirmative approach that includes the expectation that learners will be successful and develop a commitment to their learning. Another useful strategy is to *use a consistent teach/reteach approach*. For example, if the Omaha System is introduced in a junior level theory course, the educator who teaches a senior level community assessment course should not assume that students retained basic details about terms, structure, definitions, or rationale. Yet another strategy is to *attend Omaha System workshops*. Educators or students who plan to become proficient Omaha System users should attend a basic workshop, followed by adoption of other resources and strategies. Once Omaha System basics have been mastered, discussion with others and practice using case studies help to take the learner to a higher level of proficiency (Elfrink & Martin, 2000; Elfrink & Davis, 2004).

Publications

Publications are essential Omaha System instructional resources. Fortunately, the number and diversity of books, journals, and Web sites continues to increase, including those designed for diverse students and educators. Some have a general education and national focus (Martin & Bowles, 2002; Lowry & Martin, 2004; Martin, in press) while others have an international focus (Huang, 1994; Murashima et al., 1997; Chen, 1998; Martin, Bessho, & Saito, 1999; Park, Kim, & Cho, 2000; Wilson, 2002). Some national and international publications address specific areas such as research (see Chapter 5), case management (Slack & McEwen, 1999; Mahn & Zazworsky, 2000), curriculum restructuring (Merrill, et al., 1998), or the use of technology (Elfrink & Martin, 1996; Elfrink, Martin, & Davis, 1997; Connolly, Huynh, & Gorney-Moreno, 1999; Elfrink, 1999; Nightingale Tracker Field Test Nurse Team, 1999; Carty, 2000; Connolly & Novak, 2000; Elfrink & Martin, 2000; Nightingale Tracker Clinical Field Test Nurse Team, 2000; Thomas, Coppola, & Feldman, 2001; Connolly & Elfrink, 2002; Englebardt & Nelson, 2002; Wilson, 2002; Sloan & Delahoussaye, 2003). A number of publications describe the Omaha System, faculty practice, and community-oriented clinics or nurse-managed centers (Mundt, 1988; Reilly, Grier, & Blomquist, 1992; Lundeen, 1993; Coenen, Marek, & Lundeen, 1996; Frenn et al., 1996; Jacobson & Eckstrom, 1997; Lundeen, 1997; Zachariah & Lundeen, 1997; Anderko, Uscian & Robertson, 1999; Glick, Thompson, & Ridge, 1999; Resick, 1999; Anderko & Kinion, 2001; Moritz & Barton, 2001; Schoneman, 2002a and 2002b; Barton et al., 2003a and 2003b; Neff et al., 2003; Barton, Clark, & Baramee, 2004; Leonardo et al., 2004; Marek et al., 2004).

This book is designed as a basic reference for educators and students. It replaces the previous comprehensive book designed for instructors in all settings and the pocket guide designed for users in all settings (Martin & Scheet, 1992a; Martin & Scheet, 1992b). How to answer the question "Do students need to purchase copies of this book?" depends on the extent that the Omaha System is included in the curriculum. For those programs that include the Omaha System in various classes or for documentation in clinical settings, the answer is yes. Educators can select from the numerous references and assign those that match their students' needs. For example, some references describe educational strategies and "user champions" (Martin & Scheet, 1992a; Elfrink, Martin & Davis, 1997; Elfrink, 1999; Connolly, Huynh, & Gorney-Moreno, 1999; Nightingale Tracker Field Test Nurse Team, 1999; Pearce, Castleman & Elfrink, 1999; Martin & Bowles, 2002, Sloan & Delahoussaye, 2003; Elfrink & Davis, 2004; Lowry & Martin, 2004; Martin, in press).

Videotapes

FITNE Inc. (FITNE Inc. Web site, 2004) developed orientation videotapes for academic and service settings. The videotapes, *The Omaha System: Basics for Community-Focused Practice* (tape 1) and *The Omaha System: Applications for Community-Focused Documentation* (tape 2) (1996), offer new users the opportunity to learn more about the Omaha System from authoritative experts. In tape 1, DeLanne Simmons, former CEO of the Visiting Nurse Association of Omaha, and Karen Martin and Nancy Scheet, the principal investigators of the Omaha System research, discuss the history and foundation of the Omaha System. Tape 2 contains two community-focused health care video scenarios, with Martin and Scheet offering suggestions about the correct use of the Omaha System for each scenario. These videos and others that are planned facilitate a valid and consistent approach for use with educators and students.

Omaha System Web Site

The Omaha System Web site (http://www.omahasystem.org) is a recently developed instructional resource on the Internet. Representatives from practice, education, and research settings and software vendors provided suggestions to make the site a trustworthy source for essential Omaha System information. The site includes:

- An overview, including the components of the Omaha System
- Case studies
- Comprehensive reference list
- Links to related Web sites
- Conference and newsworthy items
- Survey for users to complete
- Frequently asked questions
- Link to the Omaha System listserv

The Omaha System listserv can be a valuable instructional resource for educators and students. Operated by an educator at the University of Florida, the listserv is a convenient way for novices and experienced users to meet electronically and share relevant information. New users can join the list to learn more tips for educating others about the Omaha System, strategies for increasing the reliability, validity, and usability of data, recent publications or presentations, and opportunities for future publications or abstract submission.

Case Studies

Case studies offer an ideal venue for educators and students to practice and master the Omaha System. Case studies that model relevant clinical situations are effective and efficient strategies to facilitate the development of higher order problem solving skills (Elfrink & Martin, 2000). When conducted in group settings by leaders who are flexible and have a positive attitude and a good sense of humor, practice encourages learners to accurately and consistently make the most reasonable decisions about clinical data, apply the Omaha System rules, and accept feedback from colleagues. Educators can use case studies to promote discussion about holistic practice; practitioners' and clients' expectations and responsibilities; ethical issues; similarities and differences between the Omaha System and other standardized terminologies; and generating data to enhance practice, documentation, and information management. Specifically, when learners are repeatedly immersed in case studies that replicate actual experiences, they will develop useful skills that they can apply in practice settings. In contrast, if educators cannot tolerate ambiguity and have limited experience in practice settings, case studies will not be an effective strategy. Benner (1994) noted that this form of learning is most efficiently mastered when clinical exemplars are provided to help learners distinguish the attributes of the problem, generate scenarios where there are multiple possibilities for classifying the phenomena, and evaluate or validate clinical hunches with others.

Case studies can be obtained or developed from multiple sources. The FITNE videotapes were described previously. The 18 case studies in this book are based on the revised Omaha System terms. The case studies should be useful for educators and students because they offer differing complexities, diverse settings, and a wide range of clients, including individuals, families, and communities. As indicated in the Appendix B guidelines, it is important to select the most appropriate case study (entire or portion) to meet the learners' needs. Case studies were also included in textbook chapters written for students (Martin & Bowles, 2002; Lowry & Martin, 2004; Martin, in press) and in the previous Omaha System book (Martin & Scheet, 1992a). The Omaha System Web site includes four case studies. The first part of each case study is a story that includes a referral profile, client data obtained by students or practitioners during the visit, and clues about interventions provided by students or practitioners. The second part of each case study is designed to help the reader apply the Omaha System to document the findings and care provided. This section includes the "best answers" or terms from the Problem Classification Scheme (domains, problems, modifiers, and signs/symptoms), Intervention Scheme (categories, targets, and client-specific information/details), and Problem Rating Scale for Outcomes (*Knowledge, Behavior*, and *Status* ratings).

Students are also an excellent source of their own case studies, and they develop a sense of ownership in the process. They can select a real client situation and modify it for confidentiality purposes or create a client situation that is a composite of others. Depending on their skills, they may need guidance to focus the content and identify the most appropriate Omaha System choices for their answer list. They can present their case studies as a handout, with overhead projection or PowerPoint equipment, a role play, or a videotape. Often, role plays are the easiest, least expensive, and the most fun strategy. After presenting the case study, the student group and the educator should spend about an hour discussing Omaha System choices. More details are included in Chapter 2.

The Nightingale Tracker

Information technology is permeating academia. Increasingly educators recognize that students need diverse hands-on experiences in learning laboratories and clinical sites. The automated information systems available at clinical sites may not match the students' knowledge and skill levels. In addition, clinical sites may not permit students and educators to enter client data because of cost, time, access, and security issues. Therefore, educators are considering many alternatives for students that are described in this chapter and Chapter 6. Although the Nightingale Tracker® was the first Omaha System–based point-of-care technology developed explicitly for student use, others are in progress, including the electronic versions described in Omaha System Boxes 4-9 and 6-5.

Findings from a 1997 national clinical field test of the Nightingale Tracker described the effectiveness of instructional resources and strategies when using automated client records (Nightingale Tracker Clinical Field Test Team, 2000; Elfrink & Davis, 2004). The findings and suggestions are also pertinent when students use manual records or other terminologies. The field test was conducted in five schools of nursing. Included was an attitudinal survey questionnaire designed to measure students' acceptance of the Tracker at the beginning and the end of the trial. When scores were compared, students demonstrated similar levels of acceptance at the beginning of the field test, but varied significantly at the end of their experience. Factors such as gender, age, education level, type of program, and computer experience did not account for the variance. The only variable that was significant was "program identity." Two schools of nursing scored significantly higher in acceptance as compared to the remaining three. Although the two highest scoring schools differed on all other variables, they were similar in their teaching approaches for preparing students to use the automated version of the Omaha System. Specifically, educators at these two schools:

1. Presented the Omaha System as a framework for documentation before introducing the technical features of the Tracker.
2. Practiced documenting videotape case studies using manual forms.
3. Used these same manual forms to document care with clients during actual visits.
4. Integrated the automated version of the Omaha System with the Tracker's associated screens and menu options as the final step in learning how to use the technology.

Evidence indicated that the students from the two schools who followed instructional sequencing gained a greater degree of expertise using the Omaha System terms and taxonomic rules before being introduced to the complexities of the information technology system (Table 4-1). Students followed a pattern of mastering skills as these progressed from simpler to more complex. They developed basic Omaha System proficiency as a prerequisite to the more complex task of either manual or automated documentation competency. As a result of these findings, instructional best practices for teaching were developed. The schedule was designed for use during two class days, preferably within a week's time.

OMAHA SYSTEM EXPERIENCES IN EDUCATION

Many more educators and students are using the Omaha System nationally and globally. Nine examples have been selected for inclusion in this chapter. While the educators and students in these examples share a common goal of embracing the Omaha System within their curricula, each experience is unique and represents a specific level and type of inclusion.

Rogers's Diffusion of Innovation model (1995; Hilz, 2000) addresses the unique qualities of user experiences and can be applied to integrating the Omaha System into the learning experiences of students. An innovation can be an idea, a product, or a process that is perceived as new to the social system. Applying this definition to the Omaha System, the set of standardized terms, structure, and rules represents a documentation innovation that is unique to each educational setting. Rogers's theory indicates that the adoption of an innovation occurs in stages and the outcome or diffusion occurs during an extended period of time, usually many years. Adoption of the innovation is hastened when it includes a relative advantage, is compatible with the current environment, can be used in trials, and is observable. Adoption is slowed when the innovation is complex. These characteristics reflect the Omaha System and the educational settings described in this chapter. In time, the Omaha System will be integrated extensively throughout the curricula in some schools. In others, its use will be more focused and limited. There will continue to be some educator skeptics who question the value of standardized terminology and even question if computers are a passing fad (Carty, 2000; Pesut, 2002).

The experiences of the nine programs illustrate the diversity of locations, the continuum of focused to expansive use, and the range of ways that nursing and other educators introduce the Omaha System to their diverse undergraduate and graduate students. In addition, the descriptions demonstrate the impact of practice, education, and research trends on health care education, and the potential for conducting practice-based research

CHAPTER 4

Table 4-1 Summary of Omaha System Teaching Methods, Rationale, and Time Frames

Teaching Methods	Rationale	Time Frames
I. Present structure, terms, definitions, and rules with discussion and videotape.	Introduce in a simple and consistent manner.	45 minutes
II. Present text-based case study.	Introduce an inconsistent narrative, similar to many novice practitioners' documentation.	10 minutes
A. Select problems, interventions, and outcome ratings independently.	Identify extent of learners' skills.	30 minutes
B. Discuss case study, answers, and rationale for answers.	Use group validation to encourage concrete thinking.	60 minutes
C. Gain consensus for priority problems and rationale.	Discuss concepts, rules, and the complex process of distinguishing the priority of data.	40 minutes
D. Identify problems to be placed on a "to be considered later" list.	Apply newly learned rules by making decisions with higher-ordered rules and problem solving to help the group arrive at consensus about the priorities for future service.	45 minutes
E. Discuss rationale for teaching methods.	Synthesize learning goals, process, and rationale.	20 minutes
III. Present a videotaped case study and repeat the previous steps, II A-D, but use actual form(s) from an agency's automated or manual record.	Repeat II A-D; use of forms adds complexity to the problem solving process.	Time frame varies, but decision making and consensus occur more rapidly than previously.
IV. Use the same videotaped case study and apply the same Omaha System rules, but use a computerized version of the Omaha System.		
A. Move through screens and menus while explaining the rationale behind user screens.	Use clinical data, defined concepts, rules, and higher-ordered rules to indicate how data are entered and represented.	90 minutes
	Use clinical data and problem solving to practice data management procedures.	90 minutes
B. Demonstrate screen-by-screen data management procedures (reports, data repository, email) while users have a hands-on experience.		

Adapted from Elfrink, V.L. (1998). Nightingale Tracker® Orientation Materials. FITNE, Inc. Athens, Ohio.

(Hamner & Wilder, 2001; Turley, 2002; Androwich et al., 2003; Martin, Baisch, & Bell-Calvin, 2003). Although not depicted as an example, it is typical for the Omaha System to be introduced into a curriculum as an innovation in an even simpler way. One educator makes the decision to assign one or several Omaha System references to students in one class. In time, this educator's effort leads to more extensive use. Regardless of the approach educators select, students gain skills applying the problem solving process and a standardized clinical terminology that is robust and has nonambiguous rules. These skills are valued by service administrators because they help new practitioners organize their assessments, plan care, document interventions, and measure outcomes and use terms that are reliable, valid, and capable of being compared across settings.

Dr. Sally Lundeen had extensive experience as a practitioner and manager in a primary care center when she and her University of Wisconsin-Milwaukee colleagues established the Silver Spring Community Nursing Center in 1986. Although their primary goal was to provide high quality services that matched the needs of their target population who live in the Silver Springs neighborhood, their secondary goals included establishing a repository that faculty and students could use to integrate clinical, financial, and statistical data. The faculty had formidable goals for the repository. They needed to generate diverse statistics and reports that would satisfy current and potential sources of funding, stimulate educator and student research, and allow the Silver Springs Community Nursing Center to be financially viable. Many nurse-managed centers and multidisciplinary primary care clinics have been established since 1986 and have closed. The University of Wisconsin-Milwaukee efforts continue to thrive and expand (Lundeen, 1993; Coenen, Marek, & Lundeen, 1996; Frenn et al., 1996; Lundeen, 1997; Zachariah & Lundeen, 1997; Anderko & Kinion, 2001; Schoneman, 2002a and 2002b; Hildebrandt et al., 2003; University of Wisconsin-Milwaukee IUHP, 2004). Details about their instructional resources and their strategies involving the Omaha System, their records, and the data analysis procedures they developed are described in Omaha System Box 4-1.

The University of Wisconsin-Oshkosh and the Virginia Appalachian Tricollege Nursing Program used the Omaha System with specific programs and targeted populations (Omaha System Boxes 4-2 and 4-3). Both schools wanted to introduce students to innovative practice patterns (Tagliareni & Marckx, 1997; Turley, 2002; Androwich et al., 2003; Oermann & Heinrich, 2003). The University of Wisconsin-Oshkosh is a baccalaureate program located in an urban area. Students applied the Omaha System in a manual documentation format, although the school has plans for automated use, too. Virginia Appalachian Tricollege is an associate degree program in a rural area. Students used technology to document the Omaha System in that setting.

The University of Louisiana-Lafayette, San Jose State University, and the University of Oklahoma Omaha System Boxes illustrate an expanded use of the Omaha System across a continuum of students and extensive educator dedication (Omaha System Boxes 4-4 to 4-6). Nursing students at the University of Louisiana-Lafayette visit a wide range of clients with diverse needs. Details of their clinical experiences have been published (Sloan, 2000; Sloan & Delahoussaye, 2003). San Jose State University nursing and speech pathology students have the opportunity to collaboratively develop practice, documentation, and information management skills. Data from the project have been analyzed and published (Connolly & Novak, 2000; Connolly & Elfrink, 2002), as well as results of related research and projects (Kataoka-Yahiro et al., 1998; Connolly, Huynh, & Gorney-Moreno, 1999; Cohen et al., 2000; Barrera et al., 2003). The San Jose effort to link clinical data, quality improvement, technology, and research represents a definite trend in academic settings (Marek & Rantz, 2000; Institute of Medicine, 2001; Moritz & Barton, 2001; Barton et al.,

OMAHA SYSTEM BOX 4-1

Omaha System Experiences in Education: Developing Consistent Learning Resources and Strategies

Bev Zabler, RN-C, FNP, CMT, PhDc
Clinical Assistant Professor
School of Nursing
University of Wisconsin, Milwaukee
Milwaukee, Wisconsin

The Omaha System has provided the structure for documentation at the Silver Spring Community Nursing Center since it was established by the university's College of Nursing. Use of the System has expanded to three other nursing center sites, the practitioners who provide service in the four centers, nursing students who are introduced to the Omaha System early in their baccalaureate education, first-through fourth-year medical students, and graduate social work students.

Initially orientation to the Omaha System varied from a basic introduction to a more intense orientation designed to help nursing center practitioners develop skills needed for their practice. Historically, the practitioners who possessed the most knowledge and experience conducted the orientation sessions, approaching the content with little uniformity and using varied instructional methods.

To correct this situation, we developed an orientation plan to meet the diverse orientation needs and increase the probability of interrater reliability. Presenting uniform information in a simple and standardized format was viewed as one way to achieve both goals. We developed a versatile approach, designed to cover basic information as well as the steps for using the manual nursing center forms to document and code accurately and consistently. Teaching methods included integrated approaches such as interactive practice exercises, incorporating self-learning, group activities, and a self-paced PowerPoint slide presentation. After developing and testing our PowerPoint slides, we referred to the slide presentation as "The Omaha System—The Basics."

The standardized approach to orientation produced numerous benefits. Practitioners who are responsible for orientation and have a range of Omaha System experience reported greater comfort when they used the standardized instructional materials. They indicated that the materials helped clarify their understanding of the Omaha System and enhanced their own skills. We used the PowerPoint presentation successfully with students who have various needs. It provides introductory information for novice baccalaureate and graduate students and in-depth information for senior baccalaureate students who go on to document client services during their 16-week semester clinical experience. The senior students need to develop user skills near or beyond the intermediate level. In addition, students who use the materials independently have demonstrated verbal understanding and a readiness for further documentation orientation.

If students or practitioners need details or practice other than that offered by the standardized materials, we have books, articles, videos, and case studies with more information about Omaha System history, research, theoretical framework, and applications in various settings. Based on student and practitioner responses, we will revise our standardized instructional materials to become even more effective and efficient while maintaining simplicity.

OMAHA SYSTEM BOX 4-2

Omaha System Experiences in Education: Providing Community-level Services

Vicki A. Moss, RN, DNSc
Associate Professor
College of Nursing
University of Wisconsin-Oshkosh
Oshkosh, Wisconsin

A major assignment for our senior nursing students enrolled in a five-credit clinical course, Family and Community Nursing, was to use the Omaha System for planning and implementing a project at the aggregate or community level that emphasized primary and secondary prevention. After students met with the personnel from two county health departments and reviewed recent community assessment documents and the Omaha System, they decided to focus on the smoking behaviors of middle and high school students at two schools. Their goals were to investigate these smoking behaviors and develop interventions to inform the youths about the dangers of smoking and ways to stop.

The nursing students planned and conducted a health fair at two high schools. They used the Omaha System as their assessment and documentation guide, and identified the problem, *Substance use.* At School 1, the modifier was *Potential.* Although nursing students assumed some students were smoking, they needed to collect data about the extent and so focused on the intervention, *Surveillance.* At School 2, they already had access to data about smoking patterns and decided to emphasize the intervention, *Teaching, Guidance, and Counseling.* Thus, they selected different interventions to obtain appropriate outcomes for the same problem at each school.

By incorporating the Omaha System in this field project, nursing students were encouraged to develop and apply critical thinking skills as they identified an aggregate or community health problem, and assessed and planned interventions appropriate for their specific aggregate group. Although the Omaha System is a classification that has specific rules for use, it was easy for students to understand and apply. Their enthusiasm was evident as they presented their projects to their peers and educators. As one of the students said, "For once, care planning was fun!"

2003a and 2003b; Institute of Medicine, 2003; Elfrink & Davis, 2004; Leonardo et al., 2004; Marek et al., 2004). Numerous examples are included in Chapter 5. The University of Oklahoma is the first school to integrate the Omaha System in theory and clinical courses throughout their undergraduate curriculum. Note that they continue to introduce other standardized terminologies, recognizing that their graduates need to be multilingual (Merrill et al., 1998).

The innovation strategies used by educators at the University of Rochester and Bethel College involve extensive community collaboration, an important educational trend (Omaha System Boxes 4-7 and 4-8) (Tagliareni & Marckx, 1997; Moritz & Barton, 2001). The Rochester experience is unique. It is based on a corporate wellness model and represents close integration of education and service. It is designed to be an income-generating program or revenue stream for the school, an approach that other schools may use in the near future. Educators traditionally collaborate with local service providers so that students observe and participate in direct care provided by experienced practitioners.

CHAPTER 4

OMAHA SYSTEM BOX 4-3

Omaha System Experiences in Education: Introducing Practice in Rural Communities

Kathy J. Mitchell, MSN, RN
Professor of Nursing
Virginia Appalachian Tricollege Nursing Program at Southwest Virginia Community College
Richlands, Virginia

To adequately prepare the associate degree nursing students from our three campuses for their changing practice roles, we initiated a series of increasingly complex clinical experiences in local, rural communities. The Nightingale Tracker®, with its automated version of the Omaha System, was an essential part of our plan. The area served by our campuses is about 1,800 square miles and has a population of only 118,000. Students were introduced to the Tracker and the Omaha System during the last semester of their program, and they used both to communicate about client care from distant sites.

Working as partners with the senior citizen associations in three local communities, students provided home visits to many economically disadvantaged seniors. During these visits, the students used the Omaha System to complete thorough assessments of individual clients, their families, and their environments. Based on these assessments, the students provided teaching related to health care, evaluated the need for referral to available community resources, and facilitated those referrals.

When clinical experiences were completed, students sent completed visit documentation reports to us, their clinical instructors, and to the senior citizens' organizations. Case managers, even those who were not nurses, could easily understand the Omaha System-based documentation. It was evident that students provided services that many seniors had not previously been able to obtain.

Introducing nursing students to the Omaha System and using the Nightingale Tracker provided an opportunity to establish meaningful clinical experiences in an extensive geographic area. Benefits extended beyond an understanding of diverse clients' diagnoses and treatment plans. Students had a new level of responsibility for planning care and evaluating the results of that care. They gained experience with the referral process and community dynamics. Because students witnessed the influence of family support and the home environment on prognoses, they developed a new appreciation of a holistic approach to care, even when it is delivered in acute or long-term care settings. By using the Omaha System, students actually applied the nursing process.

The Bethel experience is also unique and represents a first for the Omaha System. During their clinical experience at a home care agency, Bethel students used a computer and Omaha System software while practitioners used a different type of computer and different Omaha System software. Despite the differences in the computer systems, the experience was very beneficial for students, and the agency used the students' documentation for their records.

Information technology is causing dramatic changes for health care students, educators, and educational institutions (Katz, 1999; Englebardt & Nelson, 2002). Usually, these changes are complex, difficult, and expensive. UNITEC Polytechnic Institute of New Zealand progressed from introducing the Omaha System to students for limited use, to expanding use and then initiating a large-scale information technology development effort (Omaha System Box 4-9). Nursing educators formed partnerships with others who had informatics expertise to develop new technology and test the Omaha System in combina-

Text continued on p. 100

OMAHA SYSTEM BOX 4-4

Omaha System Experiences in Education: Learning to Provide Evidence-based Practice

Helen L. Sloan, RN, CS, DNS
Assistant Professor, Hamilton Endowed Professor
Gerontological Nurse Practitioner
College of Nursing and Allied Health Professions
University of Louisiana-Lafayette
Lafayette, Louisiana

As part of our Comprehensive Nursing course, 60 baccalaureate-nursing students visit older adult clients in their homes. Since many clients have chronic illnesses, students provide interventions designed to promote self-care management. We selected the Omaha System to organize documentation because it is community-oriented and encourages students to promote health and to focus on self-care management interventions. When students were initially introduced to the Omaha System, they used a manual client record. Beginning in 1999, students used the Nightingale Tracker®, a personal digital assistant device that includes an electronic version of the Omaha System. This combination helps students effectively apply the nursing process and address the issues and problems of the target population.

We have identified numerous benefits. When students view the Problem Classification Scheme screens during client assessment, the screens often provide a trigger, reminding them to collect and record complete data. The same triggers occur with the Intervention Scheme and Problem Rating Scale for Outcomes. As students use the Rating Scale, they critically evaluate their clients' problem-specific *Knowledge, Behavior*, and *Status*, a process that emphasizes clients' needs and progress over time.

Client reports generated from the Nightingale Tracker showed a dramatic improvement compared to previous documentation. Students now receive legible records from the previous students who were assigned to their clients, and can track the progression of identified problems. By consistently using Omaha System terms, students and educators communicate efficiently with less text. The standard reports make it easier for me, the only supervising educator, to read and critique documentation during the semester; an important consideration, since each of the 60 students submits six home visit reports.

Students reacted favorably to the Omaha System, and often refer to its clarity. Educators indicated that it is easy to teach the Omaha System. The automated version of the Omaha System helps us accomplish two valued objectives: using point-of-care technology and documenting client care with a research-based terminology.

OMAHA SYSTEM BOX 4-5

Omaha System Experiences in Education: Promoting Collaboration Among Multidisciplinary Students

Phyllis M. Connolly, APRN, BC, CS, PhD
Professor
School of Nursing
San Jose State University
San Jose, California

Baccalaureate nursing and graduate speech pathology students provided care to clients who had mental illness and resided in the community. We initiated this collaborative program to provide holistic services to underserved clients. Research indicates that people who have serious mental illness may have limited access to necessary health care services, suffer from chronic physical problems, neglect their physiological and self-care needs, and refuse to seek treatment for their physical disorders.

The experience involved a partnership between students not only to provide client care, but also to use the Omaha System to document that care. For example, the problem, *Speech and language*, with the modifier, *Actual*, was identified for a client. The Omaha System provided a method for the nursing and speech pathology student partners to assess and describe the client's signs and symptoms, coordinate their respective therapeutic interventions, and document their care. The specific outcomes included an increase in social interactions, adjustments in the rate and volume of speech, and an increase in self-expression and self-esteem. The Problem Rating Scale for Outcomes was used when the client was admitted to service. Ratings were *Knowledge* = 2, *Behavior* = 2, and *Status* = 2. The ratings at the end of the school term increased to *Knowledge* = 4, *Behavior* = 4, and *Status* = 4.

Data analysis revealed that 34 of the 40 Omaha System problems were identified at least once and that outcome ratings for the physical problems improved by the end of 1 or more semesters. Note that the extent of positive change described in the previous example did not occur for all problems and all clients.

During the collaborative program, use of the Omaha System improved problem identification, team communication, and coordination of multidisciplinary health care for clients who had chronic mental illness. Because subsequent students have access to the client records of both the nursing and the speech pathology teams, they can enhance the continuity of care.

OMAHA SYSTEM BOX 4-6

Omaha System Experiences in Education: Focusing on the Community in Baccalaureate Nursing Courses

Ann S. Merrill, RN, MA, MS
Assistant Professor
College of Nursing
University of Oklahoma
Oklahoma City, Oklahoma

We decided to revise our curriculum because we recognized that community clinical experiences had to be increased and integrated throughout the program, rather than concentrated in one semester. After comparing four terminologies recognized by the American Nurses Association, we selected the practice-based Omaha System to guide course content reorganization. The Omaha System is consistent with our university mission, our college philosophy, and current health care trends.

When we began to integrate the Problem Classification Scheme, Intervention Scheme, and Problem Rating Scale for Outcomes in our biopsychosocial theory and clinical courses, we were able to complete the process quite easily. Educators who taught theory courses discovered that the Problem Classification Scheme identified content gaps and redundancies both within a course and across semesters. The Scheme became the basis for course assignments, such as case study papers and presentations. In clinical courses, the Omaha System is the foundation of the client assessment form that students complete in the acute care setting. The Intervention Scheme and Problem Rating Scale for Outcomes are used only in clinical courses. The Intervention Scheme is the basis for the skills that students learn in the professional practice laboratory. We developed an additional use for the Problem Rating Scales for Outcomes. After revising the Scale to address cognitive, affective, and psychomotor performance under each of the curriculum's specified abilities (critical thinking, caring, communication, and citizenship), we began using it as our clinical evaluation tool. We expanded the ratings to a 0-10 scale to more clearly discriminate performance level.

Our experience has included challenges and benefits. Challenges include the inability to find adequate textbooks that organize content based on the Omaha System and to apply the System to some specific course content. We resolved application of the Omaha System in the acute care setting by using "other" for targets in the Intervention Scheme. Using the Omaha System has produced definite benefits. It links our nursing program's needs to emerging health care trends and demonstrates that this practice-based classification is an effective teaching tool in an academic setting.

CHAPTER 4

OMAHA SYSTEM BOX 4-7

Omaha System Experiences in Education: Helping Consumers Manage their Care

Patricia A. Chiverton, RN, EdD, FNAP
Dean and Professor
School of Nursing
University of Rochester
Vice President, Strong Health
Rochester, New York

Kathryn M. Votava, PhD, RN
Director of Research, Community Nursing Center
School of Nursing
University of Rochester
Rochester, New York

Donna M. Tortoretti, RNC, BSN, BA, CMAC
Chief Operating Officer, Community Nursing Center
School of Nursing
University of Rochester
Rochester, New York

We incorporated the Omaha System into our program called Health Checkpoint™. The program is unique because it offers consumers access to quality health promotion and anticipatory guidance interventions through the integrated use of nursing care, standardized documentation, and information technology.

The consumers served during the beta test were recruited through diverse community organizations. At the time of enrollment, they met with a nurse and completed a health risk appraisal to identify their health-promoting goals. The nurse then provided consumers with the technology to facilitate wireless remote monitoring of human vital signs including basic temperature, pulse, respiration, oxygen saturation, blood pressure, and weight. These data were transmitted via wireless technology to the central monitoring station to be trended and reviewed by the nurse. The consumers and nurse maintained communication and focused on achieving their individualized health-promoting goals.

During the beta test, we used the Omaha System to describe problems, interventions, and outcome ratings and as one of the structures for comparing data and analyzing findings. We selected the Omaha System because we had previously used it in a case management program and knew nurses could understand it and produce data that could be aggregated and analyzed. As a result of findings from beta site testing, Health Checkpoint is now being developed for implementation on a national level. We believe that integrating cutting edge information technology tools with the Omaha System offers the potential for providing interventions that can decrease health care costs and increase efficiency. Nurses can care for large groups of consumers in multiple locations with a relatively small nursing work force.

OMAHA SYSTEM BOX 4-8

Omaha System Experiences in Education: Advancing Partnerships between Service and Education

Ann Jones, RN, DNSc
Director of Undergraduate Studies
School of Nursing
University of Minnesota
Minneapolis, Minnesota
David Muhovich, RN, MS
Assistant Professor of Nursing
Bethel College
St. Paul, Minnesota
Elizabeth A. Peterson, RN, MA, MS
Director, Preprofessional Nursing Program
Bethel College
St. Paul, Minnesota

Several interrelated factors led to our decision in 1998 to teach the Omaha System to baccalaureate nursing students. First, we wrote and received a grant to purchase Nightingale Tracker®, for use in clinical experiences. Second, we wanted to expose students to multiple terminologies, innovative health care technology, and computerized documentation systems.

We wanted to form a partnership with a clinical agency that used the Omaha System and was willing to provide a unique student clinical experience. Fairview Lakes HomeCaring and Hospice not only welcomed students into their hospital-based, nonprofit home care agency, but used the Omaha System in their automated clinical information system. Educators introduced students to the Omaha System as a part of their orientation to the clinical agency. That information was reinforced as the students made joint visits with the agency nurses and as they used their Trackers. Students learned to complete their assessment, plan of care, and visit summary in an efficient, yet meaningful and complete way.

There were several important benefits to the collaboration for students and educators. Educators saved time reading assignments because they were systematic, organized, and brief. An arrangement between Bethel College and the home care agency allowed students to submit their Tracker summaries as the record of their visits, avoiding the need to complete "duplicate documentation." Students had practical experience working with an automated documentation system. More importantly, they learned to use and value the Omaha System because they saw nurses use it daily. Educators never needed to convince students that the Omaha System was relevant to clinical practice.

OMAHA SYSTEM BOX 4-9

Omaha System Experiences in Education: Developing International Alliances

Shona K. Wilson, RGON, BHSC, MA
Informatics Lecturer and Consultant
School of Health Science
Ngaa Kaawai Oranga Faculty of Health and Environmental Sciences
UNITEC Polytechnic Institute
Auckland, New Zealand

Nursing students in New Zealand rarely or never observe electronic documentation during their clinical experiences, yet need to have attained associated competencies before obtaining their nurse registration. We made a commitment to offer opportunities to our 350 baccalaureate students to achieve these competencies. In 1998, we evaluated existing automated documentation processes and chose the Omaha System as the foundation for a data management system that provides the basis for care planning and automation during community clinical experiences.

An electronic version of the Omaha System, referred to as KIWIN™, is used in conjunction with an automated adaptation of the New Zealand National Health Index, National Minimum Data Set, and National Medical Warning System. This data management system runs on desktop computers and personal digital assistants (point-of-care) that are connected to a clinical data repository located on a server at our school. When students enter the nursing programme, they are introduced to the Omaha System in conjunction with assessment frameworks, specific to the context of their clinical experiences throughout their education. Initially, they use desktop computers and then use point-of-care technology in their final year, demonstrating the progressive steps of our integrated technology approach.

Students use the data management system to plan care, document services, and generate comprehensive electronic reports from their community clinical nursing visits. The reports include details about the client (demographics, generic initial assessment details, and baseline recordings) and details about care planning and delivery (based on the Omaha System). Students can use text to clarify their documentation and can analyze their own records.

As educators, we are conducting evaluation research that focuses on our data management system and plan to apply our findings in exciting ways. We have plans for using the analysis of the aggregate problem, intervention, and problem rating scale data created by the records from a particular student, a student cohort, or students across time in further curriculum development. Analysis of student opinions and use experiences will be used for future revision of the data management system.

tion with other national databases. In addition, UNITEC educators are testing the documentation capabilities of the electronic device with both students and community nurses and are expanding its use to other schools (Wilson, 2002; Wilson & Roy, 2003).

SUMMARY

In the evolving health care delivery system, it is vital that multidisciplinary students and educators be prepared to conceptualize and document clinical data in ways that are compatible with automated information systems. Integrating the Omaha System into the educational experiences of students provides an important foundation on which to build toward this goal. System is a practice-based classification and adheres to nonambiguous rules, it is user-friendly and robust. Today's educators face unprecedented decisions about which learning opportunities to include in their curricula. The use of standardized languages to document and manage information must, however, remain a significant education strategy. The ultimate global benefits—the potential to improve the outcomes of care and use comparable data to drive health care decisions and shape health policy—make these educational investments worthwhile.

REFERENCES

American Association of Colleges of Nursing. (1999, January-February). A vision of baccalaureate and graduate education: The next decade. *Journal of Professional Nursing, 15*(1):59-65.

Anderko, L., & Kinion, E. (2001, November). Speaking with a unified voice: Recommendations for the collection of aggregated outcome data in nurse-managed centers. *Policy, Politics, and Nursing Practice, 2*(4):295-303.

Anderko, L., Uscian, M., & Robertson, J.F. (1999, June). Improving client outcomes through differentiated practice: A rural nursing center model. *Public Health Nursing, 16*(3):168-175.

Androwich, I.M., Bickford, C.J., Button, P.S., Hunter, K.M., Murphy, J., & Sensmeier, J. (2003). *Clinical Information Systems: A Framework for Reaching the Vision.* Washington, DC, ANA Publishing.

Barrera, C., Machanga, M., Connolly, P.M., & Yoder, M. (2003, October/December). Nursing care makes a difference: Application of the Omaha System. *Outcomes Management, 7*(4):181-185.

Barton, A.J., Baramee, J., Sowers, D., & Robertson, K.J. (2003b, December). Articulating the value-added dimension of NP care. *Nurse Practitioner, 28*(12):34-40.

Barton, A.J., Clark, L., & Baramee, J. (2004, April). Tracking outcomes in community-based care. *Home Health Care Management and Practice, 16*(3):171-176.

Barton, A.J., Gilbert, L., Erickson, V., Baramee, J., Sowers, D., & Robertson, K.J. (2003, May/June). A guide to assist nurse practitioners with standardized nursing language. *CIN: Computers, Informatics, Nursing, 21*(3):128-133.

Benner, P.A., Tanner, C.A., & Chesla, C.A. (Eds.), (1996). *Expertise in Nursing Practice: Caring, Clinical Judgment, and Ethics.* New York, Springer.

Benner, P. (1984). *From Novice to Expert: Excellence and Power in Clinical Nursing Practice.* Menlo Park, California, Addison-Wesley.

Buerhaus, P.I., & Norman, L. (2001, March/April). It's time to require theory and methods of quality improvement in basic and graduate nursing education. *Nursing Outlook, 49*(2):67-69.

Carty, B. (Ed.). (2000). *Nursing Informatics: Education for Practice.* New York, Springer.

Chen, C-M. (1998). Nursing diagnosis and the Omaha System. In Chen, C-M. (Ed.), *Community Health Nursing* (pp. 243-279). Taipei, Taiwan, Weyfar.

Clemen-Stone, S., McGuire, S.L., & Eigsti, D.G. (2002). *Comprehensive Community Health Nursing* (6th ed.). St. Louis, Mosby.

Coenen, A. Marek, K.D., & Lundeen, S.P. (1996, October). Using nursing diagnoses to explain utilization in a community nursing center. *Research in Nursing and Health, 19*(5):441-445.

Cohen, J., Saylor, C., Holzemer, W.L., & Gorenberg, B. (2000, October). Linking nursing care interventions with client outcomes: A community-based application of an outcomes model. *Journal of Nursing Care Quality, 15*(1):22-31.

Connolly, P.M., & Elfrink, V. (2002, August). Using information technology in community-based psychiatric nursing education: The SJSU/NT project. *Home Health Care Management and Practice, 14*(5):344-352.

Connolly, P.M., Huynh, M-P.T., & Gorney-Moreno, M.J. (1999, Winter). On the cutting edge or over the edge? Implementing the Nightingale Tracker. *On-line Journal of Nursing Informatics. 3*(1):20-30. Retrieved March 8, 2004 from the Internet: http://www.eaa-knowledge.com/ojni/ni/dm/ojni.html.

Connolly, P.M., & Novak, J.M. (2000, December). Teaching collaboration: A demonstration model. *Journal of American Psychiatric Nurses Association, 6*(6):183-190.

Elfrink, V.L. (1999, Winter) The Omaha System: Bridging nursing education and information technology. *On-line Journal of Nursing Informatics, 3*(1):15-19. Retrieved March 8, 2004 from the Internet: http://www.eaa-knowledge.com/ojni/ni/dm/ojni.html.

CHAPTER 4

Elfrink, V., Bakken, S., Coenen, A., McNeil, B., & Bickford, C. (2001, February). Standardized nursing vocabularies: A foundation of quality care. *Seminars in Oncology Nursing, 17*(1):18-23.

Elfrink, V.L., & Davis, L.S. (2004, April). Using Omaha System data to improve the clinical education experiences of nursing students: The University of Cincinnati Project. *Home Health Care Management and Practice, 16*(3):185-191.

Elfrink, V.L., & Martin, K.S. (1996, Summer). Educating for community nursing practice: Point of care technology. *Healthcare Information Management, 10*(2):81-89.

Elfrink, V.L., & Martin, K.S. (2000). Effective teaching methods for preparing to use standardized vocabularies in automated information management systems. In Saba, V., Carr, R., Sermeus, W., & Rocha, P. (Eds.), *One Step Beyond the Evolution of Technology and Nursing* (pp. 96-101), Auckland, NZ, Adis International.

Elfrink, V.L., Martin, K.S., & Davis, L.S. (1997). The Nightingale Tracker: Information technology for community nursing education. In *Nursing Informatics: The Impact of Nursing Knowledge on Health Care Informatics,* Gerdin, U., Tallberg, M., & Wainwright, P. (Eds.). 46:364-369. Washington, D.C., IOS Press.

Englebardt, S.P., & Nelson, R. (2002). *Health Care Informatics: An Interdisciplinary Approach.* St. Louis, Mosby.

Ervin, N.E. (2002). *Advanced Community Health Nursing Practice.* Upper Saddle River, NJ, Prentice Hall.

FITNE, Inc. Web site. (2004). Retrieved March 18, 2004 from the Internet: http://fitne.net/.

Frenn, M., Lundeen, S.P., Martin, K.S., Reisch, S.K., & Wilson, S.A. (1996, February). Symposium on nursing centers: Past, present, and future. *Journal of Nursing Education, 35*(2): 54-62.

Gagne, R.M., & Briggs, L.J. (1979). *Principles of Instructional Design* (pp. 60-73) 2nd ed. Chicago, Holt Rinehard and Winston.

Glick, D.F., Thompson, K.M., & Ridge, R.A. (1999, January). Population-based research: The foundation for development, management, and evaluation of a community nursing center. *Family and Community Health, 21*(4):41-50.

Hamner, J., & Wilder, B. (2001, May/June). A new curriculum for a new millennium. *Nursing Outlook, 49*(3): 127-131.

Hanson, S.M.H. (1996). *Family Health Care Nursing.* Philadelphia, Davis.

Healthcare Informatics. (2004, February). Retrieved February 28, 2004 from the Internet: http://www.healthcare-informatics.com.issues/2004/02_04/cover.htm.

Hildebrandt, E., Baisch, M.J., Lundeen, S.P., Bell-Calvin, J., & Kelber, S. (2003, September). Eleven years of primary health care delivery in an academic nursing center. *Journal of Professional Nursing, 19*(5):279-288.

Hilz, L.M. (2000, November/December). The informatics nurse specialist as change agent: Application of Innovation-Diffusion Theory. *Computers in Nursing, 18*(6):272-278.

Huang, L.H. (1994, September). The Omaha System application in home health nursing. *Journal of Nursing Research (Republic of China),* 41(3):14-17.

Institute of Medicine. (2001). *Crossing the Quality Chasm.* Committee on Quality of Health Care in America (Ed.). Washington, DC, National Academies Press.

Institute of Medicine. (2003). *Health Professions Education: A Bridge to Quality.* Greiner, A.C. & Knebel, E. (Eds.). Washington, DC, National Academies Press.

Jacobson, J.M. & Eckstrom, D.L. (1997, February). Assessing homeless veterans using the Omaha System assessment tool in a nontraditional home care setting. *Home Care Provider, 2*(1):22-29.

Kataoka-Yahiro, M., Cohen, J., Yoder, M., & Canham, D. (1998, November-December). A learning-service community partnership model for pediatric student experiences. *Nursing and HealthCare Perspectives, 19*(6): 274-277.

Katz, R.N. (1999). *Dancing with the Devil.* San Francisco, Jossey-Bass.

Leonardo, M.E., Resick, L.K., Bingman, C.A., & Strotmeyer, S. (2004, April). The alternatives for wellness centers: Drown in data or develop a reasonable electronic documentation system. *Home Healthcare Management and Practice, 16*(3):177-184.

Lowry, L.W., & Martin, K.S. (2004). Organizing frameworks applied to community-oriented nursing. In Stanhope, M. & Lancaster, J. (Eds.), *Community and Public Health Nursing* (6th ed.). (pp. 194-219). St. Louis, Mosby.

Lundeen, S.P. (1993, July). Comprehensive, collaborative, coordinated, community-based care: A community nursing center model. *Family and Community Health, 16*(2):57-65.

Lundeen, S.P. (1997, March). Community nursing centers: Issues for managed care. *Nursing Management 28*(3):35-37.

Mahn, V.A. & Zazworsky, D. (2000). The advanced practice nurse case manager. In Hamric, A.B., Spross, J.A., & Hanson, C.M. (Eds.), *Advanced Nursing Practice: An Integrated Approach* (2nd ed.) (pp. 549-606). Philadelphia. Saunders.

Marek, K.D., Jenkins, M.L., Stringer, M., Brooten, D., & Alexander, G.L. (2004, April). Classifying perinatal advanced practice data with the Omaha System. *Home Healthcare Management and Practice, 16*(3):214-221.

Marek, K.D., & Rantz, M.J. (2000, Spring). Aging in place: A new model for long-term care. *Nursing Administration Quarterly, 24*(3):1-11.

Martin, K.S. (in press). Home healthcare. In Black, J.M., & Hawks J.H. (Eds.). *Medical-Surgical Nursing: Clinical Management for Positive Outcomes* (7th ed.). Philadelphia, Saunders.

Martin, K.S., Baisch, M.J., & Bell-Calvin, J. (2003, January). Data mining produces gold. *Nursing Matters, 14*(1): 6-7.

Martin, K.S., Bessho, Y., & Saito, Y. (1999, April). The introduction to the Omaha System. *The Japanese Journal of Total Care, 9*(4):64-72.

Martin, K.S., & Bowles, K.H. (2002). Nursing diagnoses, interventions, and outcomes of care: The Omaha System. In Martinson, I.M., Widmer, A.G., & Portillo, C.J. (Eds.), *Home Health Care Nursing* (2nd ed.) (pp. 104-113). Philadelphia, Saunders.

Martin, K.S., & Scheet, N.J. (1992a). *The Omaha System: Applications for Community Health Nursing.* Philadelphia, Saunders.

Martin, K.S., & Scheet, N.J. (1992b). *The Omaha System: A Pocket Guide for Community Health Nursing.* Philadelphia, Saunders.

Merrill, A.S., Hieber, V., Moran, M., & Weatherby, F. (1998, May/June). Curriculum restructuring using the practice-based Omaha System. *Nurse Educator, 23*(3):41-44.

Moritz, P., & Barton, A.J. (2001, July/August). Linking remote practice to research: Technology in action. *Nursing and Health Care Perspectives, 22*(4):189-193.

Mundt, M.H. (1988, Spring). An analysis of nurse recording in family health clinics of a county health department. *Journal of Community Health Nursing, 5*(1):3-10.

Murashima, S., Hukui, S., Kim J-I., & Kanagawa, K. (1997, October). Outcome-oriented home care documentation systems and their comparison. *Japanese Journal of Nursing Research, 30*(5):47-63.

National Advisory Council on Nurse Education and Practice. (1997, December). *A national informatics agenda for nursing education and practice—Report to the Secretary of the Department of Health & Human Services.* U.S. Department of Health and Human Services Health Resources and Services Administration. December 1997: 1-32.

Neff, D.F., Mahama, N., Mohar, D.R.H., & Kinion, E. (2003, April/June). Nursing care delivered at academic community-based nurse-managed center. *Outcomes Management, 7*(2):84-88.

Nightingale Tracker Field Test Nurse Team. (1999, March/April). Designing an information technology application for use in community-focused nursing education. *Computers in Nursing, 17*(2):73-81.

Nightingale Tracker Clinical Field Test Nurse Team. (2000, May/June). A comparison of teaching strategies for integrating information technology into clinical nursing education. *Nurse Educator, 25*(3):136-144.

Nursing Outlook, 52(1). 2004, January/February). Entire issue.

Oermann, M.H., & Heinrich, K.T. (2003). *Annual Review of Nursing Education.* New York, Springer.

Omaha System Web site. Retrieved March 8, 2004 from the Internet: http://www.omahasystem.org.

Park, H.A., Kim, J.E., & Cho, I. (2000). *Nursing Diagnoses, Interventions, and Outcomes Classification.* Seoul, Korea, Seoul National University Press.

Pearce, K., Castleman, J., & Elfrink, V. (1999, June). One nurse's experience with technology. *Home Healthcare Nurse, 17*(6):361-372.

Pesut, D.J. (2002, January-February). Nursing nomenclatures and eye-rolling anxiety control. *Journal of Professional Nursing, 18*(1):3-4.

Reilly, D., & Oermann, M. (1985). *The Clinical Field: Its Use in Nursing Education.* Norwalk, Connecticut, Appleton-Century-Crofts.

Reilly, F.E., Grier, M.R., & Blomquist, K. (1992, Summer). Living arrangements, visit patterns, and health problems in a nurse-managed clinic for the homeless. *Journal of Community Health Nursing, 9*(2):111-121.

Resick, L.K. (1999, August). Challenges in measuring outcomes in two community-based nurse-managed wellness clinics: The development of a chart auditing tool. *Home Health Care Management and Practice, 11*(5):52-59.

Rogers, E.M. (1995). *Diffusion of Innovation* (4th ed.). New York, The Free Press.

Schoneman, D. (2002a, Spring). Surveillance as a nursing intervention: Use in community nursing centers. *Journal of Community Health Nursing, 19*(1):33-47.

Schoneman, D. (2002b, October-December). The intervention of surveillance across classification systems. *International Journal of Nursing Technologies and Classifications*, *13*(4):137-147.

Slack, M.K. & McEwen, M.M. (1999, October). The impact of interdisciplinary case management on client outcomes. *Family and Community Health, 22*(3):30-48.

Sloan, H.L. (2000). Visiting nursing for health promotion within a college of nursing. In Poirrier, G. (Ed.), *Service Learning and Community-based Nursing Education* (pp. 103-110). Boston, Jones & Bartlett.

Sloan, H.L. & Delahoussaye, C.P. (2003, January/February). Clinical application of the Omaha System with the Nightingale Tracker. *Nurse Educator, 28*(1):15-17.

Tagliareni, M.E. & Marckx, B.B. (1997). *Teaching in the Community: Preparing Nurses for the 21st Century.* New York: National League for Nursing.

Tanner, C.A. (1995, September) The times they are a-changing. *Journal of Nursing Education, 34*(6):247.

Thomas, B.A., Coppola, J.F., & Feldman, H. (2001, Spring/Summer). Adopting handheld computers for community-based curriculum: Case study. *Journal of the New York State Nurses Association*, *32*(1):4-6.

Travis, L., & Brennan, P.F. (1998, April). Information science for the future: An innovative nursing informatics curriculum. *Journal of Nursing Education*, *37*(4):162-167.

Turley, J.P. (2002). The future of health care informatics education. In Englebardt, S.P. & Nelson, R. (Ed.), *Health Care Informatics: An Interdisciplinary Approach* (pp. 479-503). St. Louis, Mosby.

Tully, M., & Bennett, K. (1992, March). Extending community health nursing services. *Journal of Nursing Administration*, *22*(3):38-42.

University of Wisconsin-Milwaukee School of Nursing Institute of Urban Health Partnerships (IUHP) Silver Spring Community Nursing Center (SSCNC). (2004). Retrieved March 18, 2004 from the Internet: http://www.cfprod.imt.uwm.edu/nursing/community/urban_health.cfm.

Wilson, S. (2002). Development of a personal digital assistant (PDA) as point-of-care technology in nursing education. *Journal of Mobile Informatics.* Retrieved November 3, 2003, from the internet http://www.pdacortex.com/pda_nursing_education.htm.

Wilson, S.K., & Roy, D. (2003). KIWIN: An automated documentation solution for nursing education. In Marin, H.D.F., Marques, E.P., Hovenga, E., & Goossen, W. (Eds.), *NI 2003: 8th International Conference in Nursing Informatics* (p. 707). Rio de Janeiro, Brazil: E-papers Servicos Editorials Ltd.

Zachariah, R., & Lundeen, S.P. (1997, Third Quarter). Research and practice in an academic community nursing center. *Image: Journal of Nursing Scholarship*, *29*(3):255-259.

5

USE OF THE OMAHA SYSTEM IN RESEARCH

Kathryn H. Bowles

A rich history of Omaha System research has produced a useful body of knowledge that yields many lessons. As described in earlier chapters, an important benefit of terminologies is that they enable the coding and subsequent retrieval of important data about clients, health care services, and the outcomes of care. Many studies demonstrate the value of standardized data that is converted into information and subsequently to knowledge and wisdom that informs and improves care.

RESEARCH HISTORY

The Omaha System had its origins in research and continues to support a rich, diverse research agenda that is growing in sophistication. As described in Chapter 1, the System was defined, developed, validated, and tested through a program of federally-funded research conducted between 1975 and 1993 (Martin & Scheet, 1992; Martin, Scheet, & Stegman, 1993; Martin, Norris, & Leak, 1998).

Many researchers in clinical and academic settings have used the Omaha System to advance the science of practice, especially nursing practice, and generate findings of practical, economic, and professional value. The published Omaha System research includes varying sample sizes and types of clients, study designs and methods, and degrees of scholarly rigor.

This chapter provides a review of studies that incorporated the Omaha System, identifying their design and methodologies, major findings, implications for practice, and areas for future research. Given the years of the studies, the research spans several versions of the Omaha System, although most studies are based on the version published in 1992. The study designs reviewed in this chapter were labeled based on the major types identified by Burns and Grove (2001), including descriptive, correlational, quasi-experimental, experimental, and nontraditional designs. Students, educators, practitioners, and researchers can use the content of this chapter in their literature reviews to determine areas for future research, plan health care services, and encourage others to conduct Omaha System research.

LESSONS LEARNED: CATEGORIES OF RESEARCH

A computerized search of the research literature using CINAHL, MEDLINE, and Dissertation Abstracts databases for the years 1982 to 2003 on the keyword Omaha System, along with hand searches of reference lists and verbal communication with Omaha researchers, found more than 40 unique studies. Nursing studies predominate. The studies do the following: (1) describe client problems; (2) describe clinical practice; (3) describe client outcomes; (4) explain health care resource utilization; (5) advance classification research; (6) involve students; (7) report on the Community Nurse Organization project; and (8) report on unpublished master's and doctoral dissertations. This chapter's text and tables are organized according to these major themes. Studies are summarized and implications for practice and research identified where appropriate.

Studies That Describe Client Problems

In seven studies, practitioners and researchers successfully used the Omaha System to describe the needs of clients (Table 5-1). The Problem Classification Scheme is used to label client problems based on corresponding signs and symptoms. The information generated helps to determine priorities for client teaching, care planning, and future evaluation of progress using the Problem Rating Scale for Outcomes.

Mundt (1988) conducted one of the earliest studies that used a precursor of what are now the Problem Classification and Intervention Schemes. Findings indicated that 40% to 66% of the maternal-child clients were healthy, with no identified problems, and 29% to 36% had problems in the *Physiological Domain*. Health promotion types of interventions predominated. The results helped practitioners identify the health-related concerns of their clients and areas where they needed to focus their expertise.

Reilly, Grier, and Blomquist (1992) tracked Omaha System problems, living arrangements, and visit patterns by age and gender for 18 months at a nurse-managed clinic serving the homeless. Five problems were common across all age and gender groups: *Circulation, Income, Skin, Respiration,* and *Pain. Nutrition* was a primary problem for three of four age and gender groups. Interestingly, *Substance use* was identified as a secondary problem. The authors suggest that clients may not report *Substance use* for a variety of reasons and that nurses must make decisions about how to best assess for and address *Substance use* in the homeless population. While 62% of the problems for older clients were considered chronic, 61% of the visits for younger clients (age <50) were for acute problems such as *Genito-urinary.* Younger men had the largest number of problems judged as extremely severe and overdue, and represented the largest percentage of street dwellers, which had implications for their health and safety. The investigators could have taken this study a step further by testing for significant differences among the age and gender groups for types of problems.

Rose (1993) made a unique contribution to the literature by describing the needs of women with HIV; most prior studies focused on men. The Omaha System worked well as a framework for content analysis of interviews to organize the needs of women into descriptive categories. Study results demonstrated the complex impact of HIV on the lives of women, with many problems described across all four domains. Although it had a small sample size, practitioners may find this study helpful to develop plans of care focused on the most common health-related concerns of HIV-infected women.

A descriptive, correlational study by Hays and Willborn (1996) has several important implications for practice. They studied the differences between clients receiving registered nurse-only care and those receiving nurse and home health aide care. Study findings suggest that the clients most likely to require home health aide services are women who are significantly older, and that they require more hours of registered nurse care and visits than clients with registered nurse care only. They also had longer lengths of stay in home care and greater intensity of care scores. The results indicate the importance of focusing home health aide education on the care of the "old, old." In addition, aides must understand the special needs related to women's health and be skilled in providing assistance with personal hygiene.

Jacobson and Eckstrom (1997) used the Omaha System to document care of a homeless population and highlighted individual health problems. During the study, practitioners and clients established mutually accepted goals followed by multidisciplinary rehabilitation services. They also used the Problem Rating Scale for Outcomes to quantify the benefits of shelter activities and justify federal, state, and private funding.

Kane and Mahoney (1997) used content analysis to describe the most common client problems and their outcomes from the home care records of 145 drug-exposed infants. They reported that *Caretaking/parenting* was the most frequent client problem, but felt the problem label lacked specificity and accuracy for describing the unique needs of drug-exposed infants. The authors discussed several issues raised by the use of standardized language, including how the incomplete or incorrect use of standardized language can lead to misleading or unclear results. The client records were generated from a mixture of different styles of documentation, including minimal use of the Omaha System that required the investigators to code interventions by key words instead of the standard Intervention Scheme labels. The resulting interventions were labeled nutrition, physical assessment, education, growth and development, and assessing parenting skills. It was difficult to link the interventions to the client problems, and the Problem Ratings Scale for Outcomes was not used. The discontinuity between problems, interventions, and outcomes reinforced the need for adequate training and consistent use of standardized languages and the importance of establishing Omaha System documentation before data collection. This study could serve as a model for further research in this important area. An important lesson learned from this study is that to obtain this useful data, the investigators had to complete a lengthy, time-consuming, retrospective content analysis of their medical records. To avoid this it is suggested that agencies establish their clinical documentation with the Omaha System before beginning service delivery so that the clinical information is in a usable format from the start.

Sampson and Doran (1998) described the health concerns of hospitalized patients after coronary artery bypass graft (CABG). Most patients reported problems with *Sleep and rest patterns* while in the hospital. Findings also indicated the need to improve teaching regarding smoking, diet, and pain control. The authors suggested that postoperative anxiety may interfere with knowledge retention, indicating the need to continue the education after the patient is discharged by allowing patients to take educational materials and videos home. This study demonstrated that 74% of the CABG patients should be referred to cardiac rehabilitation to help them progress toward independence and continued healthy lifestyle changes. Most had a need for increases in activity and stamina that would be promoted and monitored by a cardiac rehabilitation program.

This group of seven studies used the Omaha System very effectively to describe the needs of the clients served. However, the samples were adult clients (age 18 and older) in all but one study, the majority had small sample sizes, and there were very limited client types studied. Two of the studies required retrospective content analysis to extract the data that demonstrated the value of establishing Omaha System documentation before data analysis. In future studies, researchers should address the following: increase the diversity of populations so comparisons can be made across studies to look for similarities and differences among groups, use larger sample sizes to increase the generalizability, and link client problems with interventions to provide a better description of care as described below.

Table 5-1 Studies That Describe Client Problems

Authors	Sample	Setting	Purpose	Design	Findings
Mundt (1988)	212 maternal-child clients	Maternal-child clinic of a county health department	Describe and document public health nursing services.	Descriptive	The majority of clients received health promotion interventions rather than sick care.
Reilly, Grier, & Blomquist (1992)	1064 clients age 18 and older	Nurse-managed clinic that served the homeless	Describe the living arrangements, clinic visit patterns, and health problems of clients by age and gender.	Descriptive	*Genito-urinary function** problems were frequently noted as problems for younger women. Living arrangements and visit patterns varied by age and gender.
Rose (1993)	11 HIV-positive women age 18 and older	Community agency	Explore the health concerns of women with HIV/AIDS.	Descriptive	The study identified 15 of the most common problems for HIV-positive women.
Hays & Willborn (1996)	237 home care clients	Large Midwestern home care agency	Explore differences between clients who received only registered nurse care and those who received RN care and HHA care.	Descriptive, correlational	Clients in the RN-only group had a mean of 7.48 problems, and the RN and HHA group had 8.67 problems. The groups shared the top three most frequent problems, but the HHA and RN group had *Personal care* as a unique problem.

Jacobson & Eckstrom (1997)	20 veterans	Homeless shelter	Assess the health care needs of homeless shelter residents and focus attention on sustaining interventions.	Descriptive	Most common problems were *Income*, *Residence*, *Social contact*, *Mental health*, *Dentition*, *Substance use*, and *Health care supervision*. Authors suggested interventions for each problem.
Kane & Mahony (1997)	145 drug-exposed infants	Home care	Describe the most common nursing judgments and their outcomes.	Descriptive	*Caretaking/parenting* was the most frequent client problem. Outcomes chosen for the study were not sensitive enough to evaluate nursing practice.
Sampson & Doran (1998)	20 adult patients who had CABG surgery	Tertiary medical center in the Midwest	Describe the health needs of CABG patients at the time of hospital discharge.	Descriptive	At discharge 42% to 54% scored basic or minimal *Knowledge* related to *Sexuality*, *Pain*, *Nutrition*, *Physical activity*, and *Substance use*. Patients who experienced lingering symptoms related four additional problems.

*Now separated into two problems: *Urinary function* and *Reproductive function*.
CABG, *Coronary artery bypass graft; HHA*, home health aide; *RN*, registered nurse.

Studies That Describe Clinical Practice

Seven studies demonstrate the value of standardized nursing documentation in describing clinical practice (Table 5-2). The structured data provided information and knowledge about the needs of particular types of clients and insight into the interventions of health care providers.

Bowles (2000a) used the Omaha System to content analyze and code the hospital records of 30 older adults hospitalized with cardiac conditions. Patients who experienced procedures such as a cardiac catheterization or coronary bypass surgery had a higher incidence of anxiety. Of the surgical patients, 90% had needs related to *Pain* and 60% to 80% had needs related to *Respiration*. The *Neuro-musculo-skeletal function* signs and symptoms of weakness, gait impairment, and decreased ability to perform activities of daily living provided information to discharge planners about problems that could impede recovery and prompt postdischarge referrals to physical therapy. Of 3951 interventions for the problem *Circulation,* 79% were *Surveillance.* Based on this study, a new concept called "discharge planning" was recommended to capture the needs of patients as they are discharged from acute care. Discharge planning was most frequently linked with *Teaching, Guidance, and Counseling* (49%). Bowles (1999; 2000a) suggested that a problem list generated during acute care can be used to improve communication across settings to home care as patients with unmet needs are transferred to another level of care.

In the Naylor, Bowles, and Brooten (2000) study of hospitalized patients with nine common medical and surgical conditions, medical patients had more comorbid conditions and decreased functional status than surgical patients. Medical patients also had more problems in the *Health-related Behaviors Domain*, reflecting issues such as polypharmacy as they coped with multiple health conditions. Surgical patient problems were more acute, with needs related to *Pain, Sleep and rest patterns, Nutrition, and Bowel function.* If practitioners understand these problems, they can identify appropriate resources for patients after hospital discharge and can focus and improve care. The average number of interventions for the surgical (n=187) and medical (n=140) groups was similar ($p = 0.49$) with *Surveillance* the most frequent, accounting for 66% of the interventions. This study included a description of the most frequent targets by intervention category for medical and surgical patients, a result not seen in other studies.

Clark and colleagues (Clark et al., 2001; Christensen, 2003) tested the Omaha System in Wales, United Kingdom, in a health visitor service caring for older adults and families with child protection problems. The Omaha System worked well to describe differences in the types of problems documented, the accuracy of documentation, the satisfaction of nurses with the System, and the measurement of client progress. Similar to other studies, *Surveillance* was the most common intervention, with *Treatments and Procedures* used the least. Future work includes plans to use the Omaha System with larger samples to aggregate caseload profiles and needs assessment. The authors state that the Omaha System has great potential for use in computerized documentation systems in the United Kingdom and will be valuable in supporting the audit process.

An abstract by Sakai (2002), translated from Japanese, summarized a study that analyzed the nursing records of 100 elderly home care clients and used the Omaha System to identify differences in nursing practice between early and late stage home care. Early stage was defined as the first month of home care and late stage after one month of home care. Significant differences were found in the types of problems during early versus late-stage home care, with *Communication with community resources, Caretaking/parenting*, and *Personal care* being most frequent in the early phase and *Physical activity* more com-

Table 5-2 Studies That Describe Clinical Practice

Authors	Sample	Setting	Purpose	Design	Findings
Bowles (2000a)	30 patients hospitalized for common cardiac conditions	Large academic medical center	Describe the patient problems and nursing interventions performed for hospitalized patients.	Descriptive	25 problems were identified, most from the *Physiological Domain*. Most frequent (68%) intervention was *Surveillance*.
Naylor, Bowles, & Brooten (2000)	30 randomly selected hospitalized patient records written by APNs	Large academic medical center	Examine the transitional care problems of hospitalized elders and the links between the problems and interventions used by APNs.	Descriptive	Medical patients' problems differed from surgical patients', with no significant differences in the number or types of interventions between the two groups.
Clark et al. (2001)	205 older adults and families with child protection problems	Health visitor service in Wales, United Kingdom	Describe the client problems encountered and interventions prescribed by health visitors.	Descriptive, retrospective	Different types of problems were revealed at different times in families. Client outcomes changed over time.
Sakai (2002)	100 elderly home care clients	Home care	Identify differences in nursing practice between early and late-stage phases of home care.	Descriptive	Significant differences were found between types of problems in the two time periods.
Schoneman (2002)	1506 clients, infants to 95 years	Three urban community nursing centers	Describe the nature of surveillance as a nursing intervention.	Descriptive	*Surveillance* comprised 27% of all interventions for 68.5% of the clients. Older female clients received significantly more *Surveillance*.

Continued

CHAPTER 5

Table 5-2 Studies That Describe Clinical Practice—cont'd

Authors	Sample	Setting	Purpose	Design	Findings
Brooten et al. (2002, 2003)	333 intervention group subjects of various age groups and diagnoses	Transitional care interaction logs of APN/patient/ provider encounters in acute care, home care, and outpatient settings	Describe problems and interventions in five clinical trials and begin to link problems and interventions with time, number of contacts, outcomes, and costs.	Descriptive	Significant differences ere noted across study groups in numbers and types of problems. *Surveillance* was the most frequent intervention across all groups.
Neff, et al. (2003)	781 vulnerable persons without health insurance or with low incomes	Academic community-based nurse-managed center	Examine the characteristics of clients, their primary health problems, and the most frequently used nursing interventions.	Descriptive, retrospective	Most frequent problems were in the *Environmental* and *Health-related Behaviors Domains*. The most frequent intervention was *Surveillance*.

APN, Advanced practice nurse.

mon in late-stage home care. Intervention frequencies were the same in both phases, with *Surveillance* the most frequent followed by *Teaching, Guidance, and Counseling*. Significant improvements in outcomes were more frequently seen in the early phase as compared to the later phase. This study supports the placement of more intense visits in the first month of home care, to treat and resolve more problems, and indicates the need for health-restorative or preventive activities such as physical therapy to ward off problems with *Physical activity*.

Schoneman (2002) focused on the intervention *Surveillance* for a large sample of clients receiving care in nursing centers. Study findings suggest that older, female clients and those with the problems *Circulation* and *Nutrition* receive the most *Surveillance,* and that conditions related to health promotion, disease prevention, and monitoring of risk factors required the most *Surveillance*. During a 12-month period, 27,898 interventions were provided; *Surveillance* accounted for 27% of them. *Surveillance* was provided most frequently for problems in the *Physiological Domain. Surveillance* for teens focused on *Interpersonal relationship, Vision,* and *Nutrition*, while 20- to 39-year-olds received *Surveillance* regarding *Nutrition, Pregnancy,* or *Postpartum*. These findings demonstrated the individualized approach achieved through nursing centers and affirmed that the interventions performed were in response to the most common health needs of the nursing center population.

A well-established program of research by Brooten et al. (2002) used the Omaha System to describe patients' problems and advanced practice nurse interventions by group. A resulting profile of advanced practice nurse care linked patient problems and advanced practice nurse interventions with costs, outcomes, practitioner time, and resources consumed (Brooten et al., 2003; Brooten et al., 2004; Marek et al., 2004). This study is an example of the types of studies that are needed to move Omaha System research forward. It included a large, diverse sample and all the important components of a full analysis of care, problems, interventions, outcomes, and costs. Omaha System Box 5-1 describes how this research team used the Omaha System to describe the transitional care that advanced practice nurses provided to diverse client groups when they were discharged from the hospital to their homes.

Neff and colleagues (2003) described the practice in their academic community-based nurse-managed center using Omaha System data. The description of client problems and nurse interventions resulted in practice changes at the center. Using data from the Omaha System, center staff developed new initiatives to meet needs related to weight reduction and circulatory concerns. They also were able to see where they needed to improve their services and increased their focus on health screening. This article is an excellent example of how to apply knowledge gained from Omaha System data to improve practice.

The seven studies that describe clinical practice are all descriptive studies that link client problems with nursing interventions. The studies add to the body of knowledge about specialized nursing care and illustrate the importance of *Surveillance* as a critical skill. *Surveillance* was the most frequent intervention across all studies, demonstrating that skillful physical assessment is critical to achieving high quality clinical care. These studies also demonstrate the value of the Omaha System to differentiate among client groups and patterns of care.

Further study in this area could explore the relationships among intervention frequencies or client outcomes and levels of nurse education, nurse autonomy, or time. Exploration of the patterns of care that lead to positive outcomes is also important for the development of evidence-based practice guidelines. Because these studies addressed only nursing care, a gap exists in the knowledge about how nursing practice differs from

OMAHA SYSTEM BOX 5-1

Omaha System Experiences in Research: Exploring Advanced Practice Nursing/Transitional Care

Dorothy Brooten, RN, PhD, FAAN
Professor
School of Nursing
Florida International University
North Miami, Florida

Interaction logs were created during a series of five randomized clinical trials that tested the effects of a model of advanced practice nurse (APN) transitional care on patient outcomes and health care costs. These 333 logs, which captured the process of APN care, were almost verbatim recordings of discussions and interactions between patients and the APN who provided care during hospital and home visits and telephone calls. Patient groups included very low birth-weight infants, women with high risk pregnancies, women with abdominal hysterectomies, women with unplanned cesarean births, and elders with cardiac conditions.

Content analysis was completed on the logs using the Omaha System. The smallest phrase or sentence represented a unit. Analysis of the units yielded over 150,000 patient problems and over 150,000 APN interventions. Patient problems were consistent with the health problems of the specific patient group. *Surveillance* was the most frequent APN intervention across all five patient groups, followed by *Teaching, Guidance, and Counseling* for four of five groups, then followed by *Case Management.* With all five patient groups *Treatments and Procedures* accounted for less than 1% of APN functions. Initial outcomes and cost analysis indicated that patient groups with greater amounts of APN time had greater health care cost savings and more positive patient outcomes. Ongoing analysis and research are focused on developing profiles of patient problems and the APN interventions that consume the most APN time. In addition, profiles of probiems associated with poor patient outcomes and high health care costs are being developed.

medical, physical therapy, or social work practice. Comparison studies are needed to compare the problems identified and interventions chosen by the various disciplines and their relationships to client outcomes.

Studies That Describe Client Outcomes

The measurement of client outcomes is critical in today's health care environment because consumers, third party payers, administrators, and practitioners expect cost effectiveness, high quality care, and accountability. The next group of four studies addresses an emerging area of research that demonstrates how the Problem Rating Scale for Outcomes can be used to meet the increased demand for outcome measures (Table 5-3). The Scale is useful for outcomes measurement and analysis because its Likert-type format quantifies changes in *Knowledge, Behavior,* and *Status* of client problems over time.

Because agencies need valid and reliable instruments to measure client outcomes, McGourthy's (1999) research is very apt. This pilot study compared the Outcome and Assessment Information Set (OASIS) (Shaughnessy, Crisler, & Schlenker, 1998; Centers for Medicare and Medicaid Services, 2003), which is routinely collected in home care, to the outcomes measured by the Problem Rating Scale for Outcomes. Omaha System Box 3-2 also addresses the OASIS and the Omaha System. A retrospective review of 10 client

Table 5-3 Studies that Describe Client Outcomes

Authors	Sample	Setting	Purpose	Design	Findings
McGourthy (1999)	10 Medicare-eligible clients with COPD	Home care	Evaluate the usefulness of the Omaha System and OASIS to measure outcomes data in home care.	Descriptive	The Omaha System provided more outcomes data than OASIS because it includes a rating of *Knowledge* and *Behavior* for each problem.
Resick (1999)	138 older adult client records	Two nurse-managed wellness centers	Develop and test a chart audit tool adapted from the Omaha System and Focus Charting.	Methodological instrument development	The study established face and content validity of terms and definitions. Interrater reliability was 81%.
Anderko, Uscian, & Robertson (1999)	45 clients with *Medication regimen*, 61 victims of domestic violence, 82 community college students	Nurse-managed health center	Identify client outcomes associated with a differentiated nursing model at the individual, family, and aggregate levels.	Longitudinal, quasi-experimental, one group pretest posttest	A differentiated practice model positively impacted client outcomes in all groups.
Slack & McEwen (1999)	54 clients, 98% female and Hispanic	Community health center and alternative high school in a rural town	Describe multidisciplinary case management with an underserved minority population.	Quasi-experimental one group pretest posttest	The study demonstrated a significant improvement in outcomes ratings for all measures.
O'Brien-Pallas et al. (2002)	366 home care clients	Not-for-profit regional home visiting nurse service	Determine the amount of variation in client outcomes explained by multiple variables.	Correlational, predictive	Medical and nursing diagnoses explained large variations in outcomes. Clients cared for by nurses with baccalaureate degrees were more likely to improve.

COPD, Chronic obstructive pulmonary disease; *OASIS,* Outcome and Assessment Information Set.

CHAPTER 5

OMAHA SYSTEM BOX 5-2

Omaha System Experiences in Research: Documenting Outcomes in Nurse-Managed Wellness Centers

Maureen E. Leonardo, RN, CRNP, BC, MN
Associate Professor
Manager, Nurse-Managed Wellness Centers
School of Nursing
Duquesne University
Pittsburgh, Pennsylvania
Lenore K. Resick, RN, CRNP, BC, MSN
Associate Professor
Director, Nurse-Managed Wellness Centers
School of Nursing
Duquesne University
Pittsburgh, Pennsylvania
Tsui-Yao Nydia Chien, RN, MSN
Former Research Assistant
School of Nursing
Duquesne University
Pittsburgh, Pennsylvania

Our two nurse-managed Wellness Centers, located in senior apartment buildings, offer service and learning opportunities for nursing, pharmacy, and health science students as well as practice sites for faculty and opportunities for research. We wanted to implement a documentation system that was capable of reflecting wellness and health promotion activities in our settings and could easily be used and understood by multidisciplinary students. We chose and implemented the Omaha System to record client assessment, processes of care, and client outcomes data, a task that required considerable work. In contrast, many documentation systems used in similar settings are based on a medical rather than a multidisciplinary model.

Our team addressed several challenges after the documentation system was implemented. As the work volume increased and time for documentation became more limited, it was difficult to document the pertinent information in an efficient way, especially for new Omaha System student users. We developed a user-friendly, quick-reference Record Charting Guide that depicted the Omaha System and sample forms. The Guide became an effective teaching resource.

Our greatest challenge involved data abstraction and analysis. Our manual system was inadequate for conducting quality improvement reviews and obtaining data for outcomes measurement. We needed improved tracking methods for our first major source of funding, a 1-year resource grant from the Pennsylvania Department of Health, and the ability to demonstrate that we could increase our client services and improve our clients' outcomes. Through a team effort involving our Wellness Center practitioners, a colleague with informatics expertise, and our research assistants, we are completing the next steps successfully. Practitioners will continue to use a manual record and will complete a log based on the Omaha System. Research assistants will enter data from the logs into a spreadsheet database and analyze our data using statistical analysis software. Our goal is to receive continued research funding so that we can compare an individual's health and wellness status across time, benchmark aggregate data, and generate meaningful information and knowledge.

records measured shortness of breath and medication management, suggesting that the Rating Scale is more comprehensive than the OASIS for measuring client outcomes because it includes a measure of client *Knowledge* and *Behavior* while the OASIS is limited to the measurement of symptoms. Although this study is an interesting start, some limitations necessitate more rigorous, comprehensive, and systematic analysis for full understanding of how the Problem Rating Scale for Outcomes compares to the OASIS. These limitations include a small sample size and the fact that language in the documentation did not match the tools. The investigator had to make judgments about the ratings, and another independent researcher did not validate the ratings. Gaskell & McGourthy (2002) support further research in this area. They question the reliability and validity of the OASIS to accurately portray client condition and measure outcomes.

Resick (1999) developed and tested a retrospective chart audit tool for nurses, pharmacists, and other health science practitioners who were using a manual version of the Omaha System in two nurse-managed wellness centers. The purpose was to identify the problems, multidisciplinary interventions, and outcomes of care. Study findings suggested that the tool had adequate reliability (81%). Useful information emerged, including a comparison of the types of problems at the two sites. Practitioners at the first center identified more *Actual* problems than practitioners at the second center; 89% of the problems at the second center were modified by *Health Promotion*. This information could be useful for staffing and education. It also demonstrated that practitioners in the first center evaluated client *Behavior* as an outcome only 8% of the time, valuable information for quality improvement. In Omaha System Box 5-2, these practitioners describe the challenges involved in developing their wellness center documentation system using the Omaha System. They continue to use the Omaha System in their centers, perfect their implementation, and expand their research (Leonardo et al., 2004).

Anderko, Uscian, and Robertson (1999) illustrated that the dyad of the Problem Classification Scheme and the Problem Rating Scale for Outcomes enabled practitioners and researchers to measure outcomes specific to each problem label. Their study examined the outcomes of differentiated practice by measuring client outcomes of care provided at the individual, family, and aggregate levels. The nurse-managed clinic employed three types of nurses, those prepared at the master's, baccalaureate, and associate degree levels. A before-after design indicated that 100% of the clients being treated for sexually transmitted diseases improved in their *Knowledge,* 95% demonstrated improved *Behavior,* and 95% were symptom-free (*Status*). The report provided a full description of the measurements and the positive outcomes achieved for a variety of client groups, including victims of domestic violence and college students at risk for sexually transmitted diseases.

Slack and McEwen (1999) used the Omaha System to document and evaluate the impact of interdisciplinary case management. Effect size is the degree to which a phenomenon is present in a population and is usually described in a range of small (0.2), moderate (0.5), or large (0.8) (Burns & Grove, 2001). In this study, the effect sizes ranged from 0.4 to 1.5, moderate to very large, and referred to the amount of improvement in *Knowledge, Behavior,* and *Status* for 54 clients. The effect size was consistently largest for the *Knowledge* outcome and smallest for *Status*, especially for the problems in the *Psychosocial Domain*. Study results suggest the intervention *Case Management* had the least effect on problems in the *Environmental Domain*. The authors, while recognizing some study limitations, offered insights into the use of Omaha System data for program evaluation and quality improvement activities.

O'Brien-Pallas and colleagues (2002) explained the variation in client outcomes related to client complexity, the organization, and the environment of the nursing work force. This broad examination of the factors that influence client outcomes showed that the greater the number of nursing diagnoses, the less clients improved in *Knowledge* and *Behavior*. Clients with problems with coping and stress had poorer *Knowledge* and *Status* outcomes, and clients cared for by nurses with a baccalaureate degree achieved significantly improved *Knowledge* and *Behavior*. A strength of this study is that the investigators used the SF-36 collected by an independent rater, in addition to the Problem Rating Scale for Outcomes, to decrease the risk of practitioner bias and add validity to the outcome measures. The findings from the SF-36 correlated strongly with the Omaha System outcomes. NOTE: The SF-36 is a commonly used reliable and valid measure of quality of life, health status, and functioning (Ware & Sherbourne, 1992).

The previous five studies demonstrate how the Problem Rating Scale for Outcomes can be used to evaluate the effectiveness of care. Except for the O'Brien-Pallas (O'Brien-Pallas et al., 2002) study with 366 clients, in general there were small sample sizes ranging from 10 to 138 clients. The studies included a variety of ages, client conditions, ethnic groups, and variables. Further, all except one of these studies had the practitioners who were caring for the clients rate their own client's progress, risking the introduction of bias. Two more rigorous approaches are (1) to independently use another instrument to correlate with and therefore validate the outcomes ratings (O'Brien-Pallas et al., 2002) or (2) introduce an independent rater to interview the client and rate their outcomes. Omaha System Box 5-3 describes how a research team used the Problem Rating Scale for Outcomes in this way to objectively evaluate diet, activity, and medication adherence for patients living with heart failure.

Studies That Explain Health Care Resource Utilization

Studies that explain health care resource utilization are needed to increase understanding of what influences resource expenditures. The seven studies in Table 5-4 suggest that knowledge gained from such research can guide administrators, practitioners, and policy makers to make more informed decisions about care delivery.

Pasquale (1987) began the work in this area with a pilot study that used the Omaha System to classify 50 components of the plan of care and explain resource consumption (defined as number of visits and hours of service). Plan of care was divided into two categories: assessments/education and procedures. Assessments explained a large percentage of the variance in nursing visits that ranged from 61% to 87% depending on age cohort. In comparison, 65% of the variance in total resource consumption was explained by procedures, assessments, functional status, and living arrangements. This study was an early example of how the components of the Omaha System could be used to predict and explain resource consumption.

Hays (1992) conducted a study that examined the relationship between client problems, nursing intensity, and resource consumption. Findings demonstrated the influence that client problems have on the number of direct hours of nursing care provided. The study explained the greatest amount of variation in nursing hours consumed (26%) according to the presence or absence of all *Health Promotion, Potential*, and *Actual* problem modifiers. This is an important finding, indicating that *Health Promotion* and *Potential* problems require nursing time. Further variations in hours consumed were explained by *Actual* problems alone (21%) and the total number of nursing diagnoses (16%). This calls for further research into the weight or intensity of each nursing diagnosis and its corresponding intervention, since the total number of diagnoses influenced resource consumption less than the presence or absence of types of interventions.

OMAHA SYSTEM BOX 5-3

Omaha System Research:
Measuring Patient Adherence With the Problem Rating Scale for Outcomes

Mary D. Naylor, RN, PhD, FAAN, FAHA
Marian S. Ware Professor in Gerontology
School of Nursing
University of Pennsylvania
Philadelphia, Pennsylvania

Since 1989 our multidisciplinary research team has been testing a model of discharge planning and home follow-up implemented by advanced practice nurses (APNs) with high risk, older adults who are making the transition from hospital to home. To date, findings from three randomized clinical trials funded by the National Institute for Nursing Research (NR02095-01, NR02095-04, and NR04315) consistently demonstrate the effectiveness of advanced practice nurses in improving patient outcomes and decreasing health care costs. The advanced practice nurses work closely with patients and their caregivers to increase knowledge, self-management skills, and overall adherence to the treatment regimens.

In our third clinical trial, we focused exclusively on elders with heart failure. The Problem Rating Scale for Outcomes was selected to measure adherence to *Nutrition*, *Physical activity*, and *Medication regimen*. Improvements in *Knowledge* and *Behavior* and decreased symptoms were operationally defined as positive indications of patient adherence. Research assistants, master's students in nursing, were trained to use probe questions to ask patients about their diet, activity, and medications and to rate their responses using the Problem Rating Scale for Outcomes. For example, the patient was asked to name two foods that are high in sodium or to describe how often they walk. The use of research assistants to collect data, rather than the nurse who was caring for the patient, increased the objectivity and enabled data collection from control group patients. Cronbach's alpha reliabilities ranged from 0.75 to 0.85 for six data collection points over 1 year, indicating adequate internal consistency. Work is under way to examine the use of a summary score (obtained by adding all of the outcomes scores together; possible range 9-45) to reflect overall adherence for diet, physical activity, or medication management. Ongoing work is assessing the relationships between patient adherence and health and cost outcomes.

Building on the Pasquale (1987) and Hays (1992) studies, Helberg, (1993, 1994) established that a multivariable concept referred to as "nursing dependency" is an important variable to consider in utilization research. In the 1993 Helberg study, nursing dependency accounted for 24.5% of the total 27% variance in the number of nursing problems encountered. Nursing dependency included the client's performance of activities of daily living and instrumental activities of daily living. The correlation of nursing dependency to Omaha System problems indicated the adequacy of the Omaha System to capture functional status deficits experienced by many home care clients. These functional status deficits were often the barrier to client recovery and, therefore, important to recognize and treat.

Helberg's follow-up study (1994) demonstrated that nursing dependency was a significant predictor of home health care resource utilization. Clients with more problems and nursing care activities, and with decreased functional status and family coping, required more home care visits and longer time in home care. This important study suggested that the concept of nursing dependency be included in future studies that examine factors

Table 5-4 Studies That Explain Health Care Resource Utilization

Authors	Sample	Setting	Purpose	Design	Findings
Pasquale (1987)	100 home care clients	Home care	Define factors that affect home health care resource consumption.	Correlational, predictive	Assessments explained large amounts of variance in all age cohorts.
Hays (1992)	237 discharged home care clients	Large Midwestern home care agency	Explore the relationship between nursing care requirements and resource consumption.	Correlational, predictive	Types of client problems explained various amounts of resource consumption.
Helberg (1993)	438 home care clients	Metropolitan home care agency	Determine the influences of sociodemographic, medical, and nursing dependency factors on the number of client problems and amount of nursing care.	Correlational, predictive	Nursing dependency accounted for 24.5% of the variance in client problems.
Helberg (1994)	236 home care clients age 65 and older	Metropolitan home care agency	Explore the influence of nursing dependency over and above sociodemographic and medical factors on the number of home care visits and length of home care service.	Correlational, predictive	Nursing dependency explained a significant amount of the variance in number of visits and length of home care beyond sociodemographic and medical factors.
Keyzer (1994)	241 home care clients	Home care agencies located in Australia	Name and code nursing activities; create a data management system.	Descriptive	Staff experienced little difficulty using the Omaha System. Health care groups were formed from client problems.
Coenen, Marek, & Lundeen (1996)	331 clients of all ages who received primary health services	Community nursing center	Examine the usefulness of client problems (nursing diagnoses) in explaining utilization of primary health care services.	Correlational, predictive	22 of the 40 client problems were significantly correlated with clinic visits. Seven problems accounted for 45% of the variance.
Marek (1996)	317 home care clients	Home care	Identify client characteristics that explain variation in utilization and outcomes of home care.	Correlational, predictive	Client problems (nursing diagnoses) were the only significant predictor for every utilization measure.

related to the number of client problems and home care resource utilization. These studies demonstrated the value of clinical documentation using the Omaha System to retrieve information about the problems clients experience beyond their medical diagnosis alone. For example, the problems of *Nutrition, Medication regimen,* and *Physical activity* are much more descriptive of clients' needs than a medical diagnosis of congestive heart failure.

Keyzer (1994) applied the Omaha System in Australian home care agencies. There was a direct correlation between complexity of care (number of problems), demands for care, the client's dependency on nursing service, and the time taken to complete an episode of home care. In a second article from this study, Keyzer (1996) described how the Omaha System was used in agencies to link the demand for care to the cost per episode of home care. Study findings led to categorization of nursing care into health care groups: direct, face-to-face nurse-client interactions; indirect nursing work, including administrative tasks that supported the medical staff or the organization; and other work, including domestic work in the client's home. Indirect nursing work that supported the medical staff and the organization was more prevalent than work that supported the care of the client. Some nursing interventions created dependency and inhibited the client's self-care ability. The ability to analyze and categorize nursing care based on Omaha System data can assist agencies to increase their efficiency as they plan quality assurance activities, measure effectiveness, and restructure.

Coenen, Marek, and Lundeen (1996) expanded the work of Hays (1992) and Helberg (1993; 1994) by exploring the relationship among demographic variables, client problems, and clinic utilization. Similar to Helberg (1994), client problems were a significant predictor of utilization, explaining 45% of the variance in numbers of visits. *Medication regimen* was the strongest predictor of utilization, reflecting the importance of client teaching and management of medication administration.

Published results by Marek (1996) revealed the power of client problems in predicting resource utilization. Client problems (nursing diagnoses), measured by the Problem Classification Scheme, were the only client characteristics that were consistently significant predictors for all measures of utilization. Those measures included number of visits, number of registered nurse visits, intensity of visits, hours of care, registered nurse hours of care, length of home care episode, and number of nursing interventions.

The previous seven studies show that the research in resource utilization has increased knowledge regarding specific types of problems as predictors of resource utilization. This is an important area in utilization research because it will identify clients who have high risk, high cost problems and need specialized interventions, and possibly prevent poor and costly outcomes. Future utilization research could explore the associations among Omaha System problems and outcome ratings with the likelihood of recertification for another episode of home care. Such research might enable agencies to build a profile of clients who need more home care services and to avoid the costly mistake of discharging clients too soon. Gaps also exist in knowledge about the relationship between individual types of client problems, nursing interventions, and nursing time. These studies may provide knowledge for developing and testing alternative ways of providing care or directing educational programming to focus on areas where it is needed most. This area of research should also expand to other clinical sites. The majority of these seven studies were completed in home care.

Studies That Advance Classification Research

Seven studies have been completed that advance knowledge in classification research (Table 5-5). Using a variety of methodologies, investigators explored the adequacy and

Table 5-5 Studies that Advance Classification Research

Authors	Sample	Setting	Purpose	Design	Findings
Zielstorff et al. (1993)	NANDA-International nursing diagnoses and Problem Classification and Intervention Schemes	Laboratory of Computer Science of Massachusetts General Hospital and Harvard Medical School	Evaluate whether the NLM Metathesaurus includes terminology relevant to clinical nursing practice.	Nontraditional, concept matching, descriptive	Initial match of nursing terms and the Metathesaurus was 12%; it increased to 32% when the terms were separated into concepts.
Hoskins (1997)	NANDA-International nursing diagnoses, HHCC diagnoses, and Omaha System problems	ANA Committee	Link terms having the same or similar meanings from the three languages.	Nontraditional, concept matching, descriptive	Concepts were linked into 60 diagnostic health concepts.
Bakken et al. (2002)	Problem Classification Scheme, NANDA-International Taxonomy I, SNOMED CT®, ISO, and CEN models	Not applicable	Evaluate the usefulness of CEN and ISO as terminology models for integrating nursing diagnosis concepts into SNOMED CT.	Nontraditional, concept matching, descriptive	It was possible to describe the Problem Classification Scheme using the CEN and ISO models and to anticipate that the Problem Classification Scheme could be integrated into SNOMED CT.
Hyun & Park (2002)	974 terms from NANDA-International, the Omaha System, HHCC, and NIC	Not applicable	Evaluate the inclusiveness and expressiveness of ICNP® terms with four nursing terminologies.	Nontraditional, concept matching, descriptive	The ICNP described 72.7% of the Problem Classification Scheme and 71.4% of the Intervention Scheme.

Bakken et al. (2000)	1039 nursing activity terms from from 300 patients hospitalized with an AIDS-related condition	Large, urban, academic medical center	Evaluate the adequacy and utility of a proposed type definition for nursing activity concepts.	Nontraditional, concept matching, descriptive	All three elements of the type definition were present 63.5% of the time.
Zielstorff et al. (1998)	396 terms from three nursing diagnosis and problem nomenclatures	Not applicable	Link the problem or diagnosis terms from NANDA-International, Omaha System, and HHCC.	Nontraditional, concept matching, descriptive	21 concepts accounting for 63 terms were the same or similar across all three nomenclatures.
Bowles (2000b)	30 cardiac patient records	Large, urban, academic medical center	Evaluate the utility of Omaha System in acute care.	Nontraditional, concept matching, descriptive	97% of Omaha System terms matched with acute care terms. Three acute care problems could not be coded.

ANA, American Nurses Association; *CEN,* European Committee for Standardization; *HHCC,* Home Health Care Classification; *ICNP,* International Classification of Nursing Practice; *ISO,* International Organization for Standardization; *NIC,* Nursing Interventions Classification; *NLM,* National Library of Medicine; *SNOMED CT,* Systematized Nomenclature of Medicine Clinical Terms.

utility of the Omaha System in relation to taxonomic principles, reference terminologies, other standardized languages, and various care settings.

A body of work is ongoing to compare and contrast the standardized languages and apply that knowledge toward the development of a reference terminology for health care. For example, the Unified Medical Language System (UMLS) of the National Library of Medicine is a project designed to facilitate the retrieval of machine-readable information from literature, clinical records, databases, and medical knowledge bases. Although most of the research with the Unified Medical Language System has been done with medical terminology, Zielstorff et al. (1993) tested the Unified Medical Language System with two nursing terminologies: NANDA-International's nursing diagnoses and the Omaha System's Problem Classification and Intervention Schemes. This study was important because it evaluated the extent to which nursing terms are included in the Metathesaurus, a source vocabulary originally designed for indexing medical terms. Automated scanning and manual sorting resulted in few exact matches, suggesting that the Metathesaurus contained insufficient nursing terminology. The authors suggest searching for each nursing term based on its definition and semantic type and requested guidelines from the National Library of Medicine on how to link terms to the Metathesaurus to increase consistency. Further work is needed on this important research area to improve the representation of nursing terms in the Unified Medical Language System.

Hoskins (1997) first reported about American Nurses Association Committee activities to link the nursing diagnoses and problem terms from three terminologies: NANDA-International, Home Health Care Classification, and Omaha System. The purpose was to identify terms having the same or similar meanings so that comparisons could be made. The diagnoses and problems were sorted under 60 basic concepts to enable the mapping and comparison of terms in a tree diagram.

As efforts proceeded to develop a reference terminology for health care, Bakken and colleagues (2002) evaluated the usefulness of the models developed by the Comité Europeén de Normalisation (European Committee for Standardization [CEN]) and the International Organization for Standardization (ISO) Categorical Structure for Nursing Diagnoses for integrating nursing diagnosis concepts into the Systematized Nomenclature of Medicine Clinical Terms (SNOMED CT®). Study findings demonstrated the ability to dissect NANDA-International's nursing diagnoses and the Omaha System's problem terms and link them 100% of the time with the semantic categories *focus, bearer,* and *judgment* of the CEN and ISO models. SNOMED CT contained all but one of the semantic links needed to model the Problem Classification Scheme. This study was a beginning attempt to test the usefulness of the two models for integrating the Omaha System into SNOMED CT. Future research is needed to explore the performance of the models with other vocabularies that will lead to revisions and improvements. In Omaha System Box 5-4 the ongoing work to link the Omaha System with SNOMED CT is described.

Hyun and Park (2002) contributed to knowledge development related to reference terminologies. Their research evaluated the inclusiveness of the International Classification of Nursing Practice (ICNP®) by matching and linking terms from NANDA-International, the Omaha System, the Home Health Care Classification, and the Nursing Interventions Classification. The International Classification of Nursing Practice described 87.5% of NANDA-International's diagnoses, 89.7% of the Home Health Care Classification's diagnoses, and 72.7% of the Omaha System's Problem Classification Scheme. The authors reported using 44 Omaha System problem terms, because they used the 1992 version and included four instances of "other." With this approach, they increased the total available terms from 40 distinct terms to 44 with the four "other" terms not being unique. If

OMAHA SYSTEM BOX 5-4

Omaha System Experiences in Research: Reviewing the Omaha System and SNOMED CT®

Debra J. Konicek, RN, MSN, BC
Terminology Manager, Nursing
SNOMED International
Northfield, Illinois

SNOMED CT (SNOMED Clinical Terms) is a comprehensive clinical reference terminology, containing over 350,000 concepts, that provides a common language designed to consistently capture, share, and aggregate health care data across clinical specialties and sites of care. The terminology combines the content and structure of two existing efforts: the robust strength of the College of American Pathologists' SNOMED RT® and the richness of the United Kingdom's National Health Service Clinical Terms Version 3, formerly known as the Read Codes.

In September 2000, representatives of the College of American Pathologists and the Omaha System agreed to integrate Omaha System concepts within SNOMED CT. This relationship converges Omaha System terms and definitions with similar concepts from other standardized languages recognized by the American Nurses Association within the SNOMED CT framework.

The reference terminology model used for the SNOMED efforts is consistent with the model developed by the Nursing Vocabulary Summit Group that originated at Vanderbilt University. The Summit Group meets annually to develop strategies for resolving standardized vocabulary issues and to increase collaboration among nursing vocabulary developers, multidisciplinary model experts, and vendors. The Summit Group's model was proposed and accepted as a draft standard by the International Organization for Standardization. The model provides the foundation for "defining" nursing concepts from a variety of sources in such a way as to make each concept unique and computer-readable.

As work progresses, electronic client records that employ SNOMED CT as the underlying reference terminology and that use the Omaha System as the standardized classification for point-of-care documentation will be able to share data across multidisciplinary health care information systems, regardless of the software vendor application. Although some research limitations exist, the potential for conducting large database studies nationally and internationally increases dramatically with the release of SNOMED CT in 2004 and thereafter.

the four "other" terms were removed, the degree of match would rise. The Omaha System target terms from the Intervention Scheme were matched at a rate of 71.4%. Study findings suggest the International Classification of Nursing Practice has a good start in capturing the terms within the major nursing terminologies; however, it has some distance to go to reach full inclusion. To fully evaluate the inclusion of the Omaha System Intervention Scheme, researchers should examine each combination of intervention categories and targets. This study considered only the 63 targets of the 1992 Omaha System when matching intervention terms. For example, the category *Teaching, Guidance, and Counseling* with the target *dressing change/wound care* is very different from the category *Treatments and Procedures* with the target *dressing change/wound care.* A full evaluation could potentially include 252 intervention terms.

The Hyun and Park (2002) study provides sound methodological advice and a list of terms as recommended additions to future versions of the International Classification of Nursing Practice. Replication of this work with the modifications described above would be valuable. This type of research is needed to continually test and improve upon existing classification systems or aid in the development of new systems. Omaha System Box 5-5 summarizes the development of the International Classification of Nursing Practice (Wake et al., 1993; Coenen et al., 2001; ICN, 2001) and the links between it and the Omaha System.

In classification research, type definitions state the essential properties or attributes of a concept. For nursing, the type definition for nursing activities or interventions includes three components: activity focus, delivery mode, and recipient. These components are necessary to create the formal concept representations needed to manage and manipulate clinical nursing information. Bakken et al. (2000) evaluated the adequacy and utility

OMAHA SYSTEM BOX 5-5

Omaha System Experiences in Research:
Exploring the International Classification for Nursing Practice and the Omaha System

Amy M. Coenen, RN, PhD, FAAN
Director, International Classification for Nursing Practice
International Council of Nurses
Geneva, Switzerland
Associate Professor, College of Nursing
Marquette University
Milwaukee, Wisconsin

The International Classification for Nursing Practice (ICNP)® is a project of the International Council of Nursing and is defined as a classification of nursing phenomena (diagnoses, problems), nursing actions, and nursing outcomes that describes nursing practice. It is a combinatorial terminology for nursing practice and provides a unifying framework into which local language and existing nursing classifications and terminologies can be linked to enable comparison of nursing data across organizations, across sectors within health care systems, and among countries.

The International Classification for Nursing Practice was intended to build on and unify the existing work in nursing classifications such as the Omaha System, rather than create something that would not be complementary to existing work. While early nursing terminology work primarily occurred in isolation and resulted in some duplicative efforts, more recent activities demonstrate a move toward collaboration and convergence not only within the discipline of nursing, but with multidisciplinary standards initiatives.

One of the first steps in the development of the International Classification for Nursing Practice was to collect and compare all the nursing concepts in existing nursing terminologies, including the Omaha System. The Classification is intended to be more comprehensive than national or specialty nursing terminologies.

Research has shown that the International Classification for Nursing Practice–Beta Version is able to represent many of the Omaha System concepts. Further research in this area will influence the ongoing development of the Classification and could potentially advance the use of the Omaha System internationally as a catalogue or subset for community-oriented nursing services.

As a unifying framework, the goal of the International Classification for Nursing Practice is to provide mapping capabilities from one classification to another and among local terminologies. In addition to promoting comparable nursing data, the International Classification for Nursing Practice is intended to facilitate comparison of nursing data with data from other health disciplines. Ongoing collaboration among nursing and health care terminology developers will advance the opportunities to describe, compare, and evaluate nursing practice internationally.

of this definition for the nursing intervention concepts found in the Omaha System and the Home Health Care Classification. The Omaha System intervention categories were equivalent to delivery mode and Omaha System targets were equivalent to activity focus; therefore the terms were present for 100% of the interventions. Recipient was coded as explicit, implicit, or ambiguous and was present 63% of the time. In addition, the researchers determined whether the intervention terms could reliably be decomposed into the three components. An interrater reliability of 100% was achieved for the activity focus and delivery mode, but fell to 68.9% for recipient with disagreement regarding whether the recipient was implicit or ambiguous. The results of this study indicate the importance of accurate and full use of the Omaha System for documentation. The Omaha System links problems to the recipient of care (client) through a series of coding options or modifiers that are individual, family, and community. Therefore, if used properly, the recipient of interventions should always be documented and never ambiguous.

Concerned about continuity of care and searching for a vocabulary that might work across care settings, Zielstorff and colleagues (1998) compared the problems or nursing diagnoses of the Omaha System, the Home Health Care Classification, and NANDA-International. Study findings revealed that only 16% of the terms were the same or similar across all three vocabularies, with 91 terms being unique to the nomenclature in which they originated. The majority (79%) of the unique terms came from the Omaha System. Most of the terms were related to others as a broader or narrower version of the same term in another nomenclature, rather than as an exact match. The Omaha System terms were the broadest of all the nomenclatures. The linking was difficult because of differences in the conceptual frameworks and structures and inconsistencies in definitions and levels of abstraction among the three nomenclatures. This information is useful when making revisions and improvements in the systems.

Bowles (2000b) evaluated the capacity of the Omaha System to code the terms used by nurses in acute care. In future studies, researchers could apply the findings to demonstrate that the Omaha System can facilitate the communication of client problems discovered and treated in the acute care setting to practitioners in community settings in a standard, consistent manner. As health care systems adopt electronic health record systems, it is of paramount importance that the flow of information from one setting to another be consistent and seamless. Bowles (2000b) found that the Omaha System was broader than most of the acute care terms, enabling coding of 97% of the hospital terms into 65% of the Problem Classification Scheme's problems, as well as all of the Intervention Scheme's categories and 86% of the targets. Problems related to the health care environment, discharge planning, and fever of unknown origin could not be coded, requiring the use of the "other" category. Study findings indicate beginning knowledge about how the Omaha System might perform across settings in an electronic health record. Level of abstraction, semantic clarity, and relevance were also evaluated, providing valuable information for updating the Omaha System. Close examination of the signs and symptoms related to the discharge planning problem indicated that a problem could be coded by using existing Omaha System terms and a new problem was not needed. For example, patients who did not know how to take their medications would receive discharge teaching as part of the discharge planning process. The problem associated with that sign and symptom and the teaching is *Medication regimen*. The addition of the new target *continuity of care* will be very helpful to document many of the interventions related to discharge planning and to the transition from hospital to home or other transitions. Further research is needed to more fully evaluate the system with a broader acute care population, because this study was limited to older adults with cardiac problems.

Seven studies have been completed to test the Omaha System and evaluate the match with NANDA-International, Home Health Care Classification, Unified Medical Language System, SNOMED CT, and International Classification of Nursing Practice. As reference terminologies evolve and updates are made to the Omaha System, further research is needed to continue to evaluate the fit of the Omaha System within the context of a larger reference terminology. Current and future technological developments offer the potential to use reference terminologies across care settings and internationally. Therefore further testing of the utility of the Omaha System is necessary to ensure adequate content coverage and cultural sensitivity.

Studies That Involve Students

As described in Chapter 4, the use of the Omaha System in educational settings with faculty and students is growing rapidly, providing the opportunity for faculty and students to get involved in Omaha System research (Table 5-6).

Gilbey (1990) used the Omaha System to evaluate the types of client problems and the outcomes of care at a health-screening clinic where student nurses provided care. Client problems detected at the initial visits were rated using the Problem Rating Scale for Outcomes, and change was measured over a period of 1 to 3 years. The primary nursing intervention was *Teaching, Guidance, and Counseling,* with the main goals of increased client health-promoting behaviors and self-care ability. At the time of the return visit, 70% of client problems were resolved or somewhat relieved and 30% remained the same. Problems in the *Health-related Behaviors Domain* were the most common, but client success for this type of problem was the least. *Health-related Behavior* problems included poor *Nutrition* or overweight, lack of *Physical activity*, and *Substance use*. Only 20% of the overweight problems were resolved or improved, and men and women were equally unsuccessful. Study results clearly demonstrated where the students' interventions were the most effective and where they were not, helping students see where modifications in the plans of care were needed.

Burns-Vandenberg and Jones (1999) evaluated the match between the client problems and interventions identified and completed by students, and those commonly found in the postpartum literature. Using the Omaha System as their assessment guide, students identified more problems in all four domains than recommended in the literature, and their interventions far exceeded the literature as well. Study findings illustrate the diversity of problems that may occur during the postpartum period and the scope of the Omaha System in guiding a thorough assessment.

A study reported by Connolly and Elfrink (2002) described a profile of clients with serious mental illness and the outcomes of the care provided by baccalaureate student nurses. As described in Chapter 4 and related publications (Connolly, Huynh, & Gorney-Moreno, 1999; Connolly & Novak, 2000), San Jose State University nursing and other students have been using the Nightingale Tracker® since 1997 to document client care and electronically transfer information to their instructors. Study findings suggest that physical health concerns of mentally ill clients are as common as emotional concerns, indicating the importance of providing primary care services in addition to traditional mental health care. Findings prompted the faculty to review the curriculum to determine the adequacy of primary care content, and the numbers and quality of referrals increased. Students also benefited by using the Omaha System and Nightingale Tracker in that they developed confidence and skills in using information technology and increased their documentation efficiency.

Table 5-6 Studies That Involve Students

Authors	Sample	Setting	Purpose	Design	Findings
Gilbey (1990)	56 clients who attend a health clinic	Community-based health clinic	Evaluate the effect of attendance at a screening clinic on client problems and health behaviors.	Quasi-experimental, pretest posttest	32% of client problems were resolved, 38% somewhat corrected, and 30% were the same at follow-up visit.
Burns-Vandenberg & Jones (1999)	11 maternal-child assessments	Home visits	Evaluate whether problems and interventions documented by student nurses were consistent with those in the literature.	Descriptive, retrospective	Student nurses found more problems than were found in the literature. Interventions far exceeded those recommended in the literature.
Connolly & Elfrink (2002)	30 clients with serious mental illnesses; included 480 episodes of care over 15 weeks	Six nurse-managed health centers	Describe a profile of clients with serious mental illness and the outcomes of the care provided by student nurses.	Descriptive, retrospective	Clients had multiple physical and mental health problems, indicating the importance of primary health care for the mentally ill.
Kaiser et al. (2002)	205 adult clients ages 18-96	Primary and secondary preventive, community-based case management practice for families	Examine family health problems and intensity of need for care and their relationship to each other.	Descriptive, correlational	Families had an average of four problems. *Environmental Domain* problems correlated significantly with intensity of need for care.
Barton, Clark, & Baramee (2004)	27 refugee and immigrant families	Public health outreach faculty practice	Describe the problems, interventions, and outcomes of practice.	Descriptive	Common problems and interventions were identified, and outcomes improved statistically from admission to discharge.

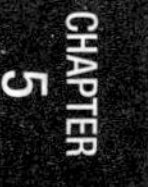

The growing interest in evidence-based practice prompted Kaiser and colleagues (2002) to examine family health problems and intensity of care, and their relationship to each other. Using the Problem Classification Scheme, the investigators retrospectively labeled client problems from the clinical records generated by five cohorts of student nurses. Intensity of care was also scored at the time of service and retrospectively reviewed by the investigator. All of the most common family health problems were in the *Environmental Domain*. *Income* was a problem for half of the clients and one-third had problems with *Residence* and *Neighborhood/workplace safety*. The total number of family problems was significantly correlated with intensity of need for care ($r = 0.586$, $p < 0.001$), and in 74% of the cases there was agreement between the numbers of problems and the intensity of need scores. However, that left 26% of clients where the use of both measures provided a conflicting view of their needs. The authors provided reliability scores for the coding of the Omaha System problems, but did not address reliability measures for how the intensity of need scores were assigned. The intensity of need scores were higher in this study than in other published studies and, according to the authors, may be related to the setting, the type of clients, or the student nurses who did the scoring (Kaiser et al., 2002). Further research is needed in this interesting area. Little is known about the relationship between the number and types of Omaha System problems and the intensity of nursing care. Using the Omaha System and an intensity of care measure prospectively and providing rigorous checks of reliability could strengthen this area of research.

Barton, Clark, and Baramee (2004) used the Omaha System as a tool for student nurses to document their public health experience. Twenty-seven cases were analyzed from the care of refugee and immigrant families in the Denver area. An average of six problems per family was documented across all domains. The authors reported that the data correlated well with findings from other research, where race and ethnicity were the greatest predictors of client health. Higher levels of diabetes in the Hispanic population coincided with the problems, *Health care supervision* and *Nutrition*. *Case Management* and *Teaching, Guidance, and Counseling* were common intervention categories. The University of Colorado team has published related articles (Moritz & Barton, 2001; Barton et al., 2003a; Barton et al., 2003b).

Conducting Omaha System research with students is a convenient way to introduce the use of standardized data in practice. Routinely exposing students to standardized terminologies will produce graduates who value the ability to describe and evaluate their practice. They will learn about the strengths and weaknesses of the terminologies and be informed users of electronic health records. This may help to ensure the presence and quality of nursing data elements available in electronic health records because the more informed, next generation of nurses will know and demand what they want and need in those systems.

Report on the Community Nursing Organization Project

Shorter hospitalizations and the need for more posthospitalization services were results of the 1987 Omnibus Budget Reconciliation Act that introduced diagnostic-related groups and a new reimbursement process to acute care settings. Soon after, the Health Care Financing Administration, now referred to as the Centers for Medicare and Medicaid Services, funded a Community Nursing Organization demonstration project to test a nurse-managed and capitated model for reimbursing Medicare services in community settings. Four nationally dispersed sites participated and provided case management services, home health care, durable medical equipment, medical supplies, outpatient services, prosthetics, and ambulance services. The sites chose the Omaha System as their method of assessment and documentation. Schraeder et al. (1996) described the clinical operations at Carle Clinic in Urbana, Illinois. Storfjell, Mitchell, and Daly (1997) reported on the Visiting Nurse Service in New York City. Omaha System data demonstrated that preventive education and screening were frequently used with problems from the *Psychosocial Domain*. Tracking sociodemographic and health characteristics of clients allowed caseload management, monitoring of quality and costs, and increased efficiency. The Carondelet site in Tucson, Arizona, used the Omaha System to identify and rate *Actual* and *Potential* health problems and *Health Promotion* needs. Ratings of common problems at 6-month intervals showed a consistent trend toward stable or improved *Knowledge* and *Behavior* over time, with no difference by socioeconomic or cultural groups (Lamb and Zazworsky, 1997). The Community Nurse Organization project enrolled more than 11,000 clients. Interested researchers should consider the Omaha System data held by the four sites as a rich source for future studies.

Unpublished Master's Theses and Doctoral Dissertations

A search of the digital dissertations database produced five citations of theses or doctoral dissertations that used the Omaha System to describe care. Four additional ones were found through personal communication. These studies have not been formally peer-reviewed and published. Two of the studies listed sample sizes over 500, and three others did not list the sample size in the abstract. Eight studies were descriptive and took place in a variety of settings, including an elementary school (Kahn, 1997), hospital to home care (Coward, 1998), home care (Swan, 1997), community nursing centers (Coenen, 1993; Kreuser, 1998), public health (Monsen, 2002), a cardiovascular/thoracic outpatient clinic in Thailand (Sangwattanarat, 2002), and 28 home care agencies in Taiwan (Du, 2003). The ninth study used a GALEN approach with its GRAIL representation language to link the Omaha System, Nursing Interventions Classification, and Home Health Care Classification interventions. The purpose was to compare concepts and levels of abstraction in the three terminologies, and their ability to represent nursing care (Hardiker, 2001).

AREAS FOR FUTURE RESEARCH

Since 1975, knowledge generated from Omaha System research has led to a description of client problems and clinical practice; an understanding of the relationship among client problems, care interventions, and client outcomes; predictions about health care resource utilization; and advances in the science of classification. However, although much has been learned, careful review of these studies reveals significant gaps where future research is needed.

The sample size of studies to date varies from 10 subjects to over 1500, with most samples including less than 100 subjects. With the increase in automation and the availability of large databases, future research should include larger samples that will increase the statistical power and generalizability of the results. Most of the studies published to date take place in home care, public health, community-oriented clinics or nursing centers, or the hospital, in descending order of frequency. The majority of studies focused on adults or, more commonly, older adults, with few studying the needs and outcomes of infants, children, adolescents, or families. Future research must address the 2004 revisions to the Omaha System. For example, the new problem *Communicable/infectious condition* may be used by various organizations with individual, family, or community modifiers. Few organizations have used the modifier *Community,* so diverse studies that address population-focused concerns are very important.

BOX 5-1 Areas for Future Research

1. What effect does the use of the Omaha System as an assessment, care planning, and documentation tool have on client outcomes and cost?
2. How does the use of the Omaha System affect documentation time and quality?
3. What effect does the Omaha System have on continuity of care when used to communicate client information across care settings?
4. What is the relationship among cost of care, types of client problems, and interventions?
5. Does the Problem Classification Scheme provide the terminology necessary to describe problems experienced by critically ill clients?
6. Is the granularity of the Omaha System terms adequate to avoid the loss of detail in clinical documentation?
7. Are the new Omaha System (Appendix A) problems and targets useful in and across a variety of situations?
8. How well do the Problem Classification Scheme, Intervention Scheme, and Problem Rating Scale for Outcomes capture data when using the new modifier *Community?*
9. How do practitioners in a variety of settings rate the usefulness of the various classification systems and terminologies?
10. What is the effect of specific clusters of Omaha System interventions and targets on client outcomes?
11. How does the reliability of the Problem Rating Scale for Outcomes compare when rated by a third party and by the nurse caring for the client?
12. What are the most common needs of infants, children, adolescents, and families, and what interventions are most commonly used for these groups?
13. Which Omaha System problems or outcomes ratings are associated with the need to recertify for another episode of home care?
14. How does the Omaha System facilitate communication across disciplines such as physical therapy, nursing, social work, and medicine?
15. What are the language and cultural strengths and limitations of the Omaha System when used internationally?

The most common research design was descriptive and based on retrospective data analyses. A few studies were of correlational design, describing the relationships among the components of the Omaha System and predicting the level of health resource utilization based on the problems identified or nursing care provided. Less common was quasi-experimental design using one group pretest posttest measurements, and no studies were of true randomized controlled experimental design. There has been steady production of published Omaha System research since 1996, averaging four to five studies per year.

Future research should include the more rigorous design of randomized controlled experiments to answer important research questions. In order to promote the acceptance and use of electronic health records, more studies are needed on the benefits of standardized language and its effects on nursing practice, client outcomes, and costs. There is also a need for more international research on the Omaha System to address how well the system captures differences in language and culture. Box 5-1 suggests some examples of potential research questions to address gaps in knowledge.

SUMMARY

The increasing adoption of the Omaha System in practice and educational settings, and subsequent research, will provide knowledge useful to address these unanswered questions and more. Practitioners are encouraged to use the Omaha System to document care, making it all the more convenient when called upon to provide measurable, accurate outcomes of their work. Educators are encouraged to expand the use of the Omaha System with their students and to publish their experiences. Researchers and others who publish are encouraged to use the term Omaha System in the title or to provide Omaha System as a keyword, thereby increasing the ability to retrieve the work. This chapter has shown how the science generated from Omaha System research has developed over time and how bits of data become information and knowledge that can be used to describe client needs, improve care, justify reimbursement, and plan resources. With the growth in electronic health records and databases, it is an exciting time for Omaha System users and researchers. Data collection can be streamlined to be more efficient and accurate than in the past, with the opportunity to do more rigorous prospective studies and choose methods to make Omaha System research a seamless link to quality improvement.

REFERENCES

Anderko, L., Uscian, M., & Robertson, J. F. (1999, June). Improving client outcomes through differentiated practice: A rural nursing center model. *Public Health Nursing, 16*(3):168-175.

Bakken, S., Cashen, M.S., Mendonca, E.A., O'Brien, A., & Zieniewicz, J. (2000, January/February). Representing nursing activities within a concept-oriented terminological system: Evaluation of a type definition. *Journal of the American Medical Informatics Association, 7*(1):81-90.

Bakken, S., Warren, J. J., Lundberg, C., Casey, A., Correia, C., Konicek, D., & Zingo, C. (2002, December). An evaluation of the usefulness of two terminology models for integrating nursing diagnosis concepts into SNOMED clinical terms. *International Journal of Medical Informatics, 68*(1-3):71-77.

Barton, A.J., Baramee, J., Sowers, D., & Robertson, KJ. (2003b, December). Articulating the value-added dimension of nurse practitioner care. *Nurse Practitioner, 28*(12):34-40.

Barton, A.J., Clark, L., & Baramee, J. (2004, April). Tracking outcomes in community-based care. *Home Health Care Management and Practice, 16*(3):171-176.

Barton, A.J., Gilbert, L., Erickson, V., Baramee, J., Sowers, D., & Robertson, K.J. (2003a, May/June). A guide to assist nurse practitioners with standardized nursing language. *CIN: Computers, Informatics, Nursing, 21*(3):128-133.

Bowles, K.H. (1999, Winter). The Omaha System: Bridging hospital and home care. *On-line Journal of Nursing Informatics, 3*(1)7-11. Retrieved March 8, 2004 from the Internet: http://www.eaa-knowledge.com/ojni/ni/dm/ojni.html.

Bowles, K.H. (2000a, April). Patient problems and nurse interventions during acute care and discharge planning. *Journal of Cardiovascular Nursing, 14*(3):29-41.

Bowles, K.H. (2000b, April). Application of the Omaha System in acute care. *Research in Nursing & Health, 23*(2):93-105.

Brooten, D., Naylor, M.D., York, R., Brown, L. P., Hazard Munro, B., Hollingsworth, A. O., Cohen, S. M., Finkler, S., Deatrick, J., & Youngblut, J. M. (2002, Fourth Quarter). Lessons learned from testing the quality cost model of advanced practice nursing (APN) transitional care. *Journal of Nursing Scholarship, 34*(4):369-375.

Brooten, D., Youngblut, J.M., Deatrick, J., Naylor, M., & York, R. (2003, First Quarter). Patient problems, advanced practice nurse (APN) interventions, time and contacts across five patient groups. *Journal of Nursing Scholarship, 35*(1):73-79.

Brooten, D., Youngblut, J.M., Kutcher, J., & Bobo, C. (2004, January/February). Quality and the nursing workforce: APNs, patient outcomes, and health care costs. *Nursing Outlook, 52*(1):45-52.

Burns, N. & Grove, S.K. (2001). *The Practice of Nursing Research. Conduct, Critique & Utilization.* Philadelphia, Saunders.

Burns-Vandenberg, J. & Jones, E. (1999, Fall). Evaluating postpartum home visits by student nurses. *Journal of Undergraduate Nursing Scholarship, 1*(1):1-5.

Centers for Medicare and Medicaid Services. (2003). *Conditions of Participation: Home Health Agencies.* Retrieved September 1, 2003 from the Internet: http://www.cms.hhs.gov/.

Christensen, J. (2003). A language for health visiting. In Clark, J. (Ed.), *Naming Nursing: Proceedings of the First ACENDIO Ireland/UK Conference* (pp. 241-248). Bern, Switzerland, Hans Huber.

Clark, J., Christensen, J., Mooney, G., Davies, P., Edwards, J., Fitchett, L., Spowart, B., & Thomas, P. (2001, March). New methods of documenting health-visiting practice. *Community Practitioner, 74*(3):108-112.

Coenen, A. M. (1993). Case management at a community nursing center. (Unpublished Doctoral dissertation, University of Wisconsin-Milwaukee, Milwaukee, Wisconsin). Dissertation Abstracts International, 55/05, 1800.

Coenen, A. M., Marin, H. F., Park, H-A., & Bakken, S. (2001, May/June). Collaborative efforts for representing nursing concepts for computer-based systems: International perspectives. *Journal of American Medical Informatics Association, 8*(3):202-211.

Coenen, A., Marek, K.D., & Lundeen, S. P. (1996, October). Using nursing diagnoses to explain utilization in a community nursing center. *Research in Nursing & Health, 19*(5):441-445.

Coenen, A., McNeil, B., Bakken, S., Bickford, C., & Warren, J. (2001, November/December). Toward comparable nursing data: American Nurses Association criteria for data sets, classifications systems, and nomenclatures. *Computers in Nursing, 19*(6):240-246.

Connolly, P. M. & Elfrink, V. L. (2002, August). Using information technology in community-based psychiatric nursing education: The SJSU/NT Project. *Home Health Care Management and Practice, 14*(5):344-352.

Connolly, P.M. & Novak, J.M. (2000, December). Teaching collaboration: A demonstration model. *Journal of American Psychiatric Nurses Association, 6*(6): 183-190

Coward, P.M. (1998). Use of standardized nursing language in home care referral. (Unpublished Doctoral dissertation, Case Western Reserve University, Cleveland, Ohio). UMI No. 9835505.

Du, C.M-S. (2003). Evaluation of the quality of home care nursing in Taiwan. School of Public Health. (Unpublished doctoral dissertation, University of South Carolina, Columbia, South Carolina).

Gaskell, S.M. & McGourthy, R. (2002, May/June). Is OASIS data a mirage? *The Remington Report, 10*(3):16-18.

Gilbey, V. (1990, Fall). Screening and counselling clinic evaluation project. *The Canadian Journal of Nursing Research, 22*(3):23-38

Hardiker, N.R. (2001). A logical ontology for nursing interventions. (Unpublished doctoral dissertation, University of Manchester, Manchester, England, United Kingdom).

Hays, B. J. (1992, May/June). Nursing care requirements and resource consumption in home health care. *Nursing Research, 41*(3):138-143.

Hays, B. J. & Willborn, E.H. (1996, February). Characteristics of clients who receive home health aide service. *Public Health Nursing, 13*(1):58-64.

Helberg, J.L. (1993, October). Factors influencing home care nursing problems and nursing care. *Research in Nursing & Health, 16*(5):363-370.

Helberg, J.L. (1994, April). Use of home care nursing resources by the elderly. *Public Health Nursing 11*(2): 104-112.

Hoskins, L.M. (1997). Linking nursing diagnoses across the NANDA, Home Health Care, and Omaha Classification Systems. In Rantz, M.J. & LeMone, P. (Eds.), *Classification of Nursing Diagnoses: Proceedings of the Twelfth Conference, North American Diagnosis Association* (pp. 8-12). Glendale, CA, Cinahl Information Systems.

Hyun, S. & Park, H.A. (2002, June). Cross-mapping the ICNP with NANDA, HHCC, Omaha System and NIC for unified nursing language system development. *International Nursing Review, 49*(2):99-110.

International Council of Nurses. (2001). *International Classification for Nursing Practice–Beta 2 Version.* Geneva, International Council of Nurses.

Jacobson, J. M. & Eckstrom, D.L. (1997, February). Assessing homeless veterans using the Omaha Assessment Tool in a nontraditional home care setting. *Home Care Provider, 2*(1):22-29.

Kahn, R. (1997). The numbers and types of interventions developed and employed for a population of ADHD students by an advanced nurse practitioner in a middle-sized urban school district in Michigan Title I Health Program during the 1995-1996 school year. (Unpublished master's thesis, Michigan State University, Lansing, Michigan). UMI # 1386869.

Kaiser, K.L, Hays, B.J., Cho, W.J., & Agrawal, S. (2002, Spring). Examining health problems and intensity of need for care in family-focused community and public health nursing. *Journal of Community Health Nursing, 19*(1):17-32.

Kane, A.T. & Mahony, D.L. (1997, December). Issues in the integration of standardized nursing language for populations: A study of drug-exposed infants' records. *Public Health Nursing, 14*(6):346-352.

Keyzer, D.M. (1994, January). Nurse management systems in the context of district nursing: The case of rural Australia. *Journal of Nursing Management, 2*(1):9-14.

Keyzer, K. (1996, May-June). Patient classified systems and rural district nurses in South West Victoria: Two studies in the process and cost of nursing services. *Informatics in Healthcare – Australia, 5*(2):48-51.

Kreuser, N.J. (1998). Access to primary health care: The nature of health problems and utilization for a vulnerable community nursing center population. (Unpublished Doctoral dissertation, University of Wisconsin-Milwaukee, Milwaukee, Wisconsin). UMI No. 9908204.

Lamb, G.S. & Zazworsky, D. (1997, March). The Carondelet model. *Nursing Management, 28*(3):27-28.

Leonardo, M.E., Resick, L.K., Bingman, C.A., & Strotmeyer, S. (2004, April). The alternatives for wellness centers: Drown in data or develop a reasonable electronic documentation system. *Home Health Care Management and Practice, 16*(3):177-184.

Marek, K.D. (1996, June). Nursing diagnosis and home care nursing utilization. *Public Health Nursing, 13*(30):195-200.

Marek, K.D., Jenkins, M.L., Stringer, M., Brooten, D., & Alexander, G.L. (2004, April). Classifying perinatal advanced practice data with the Omaha System. *Home Health Management and Practice, 16*(3):214-221.

Martin, K.S., Norris, J., & Leak, G.K. (1998, January/March). Psychometric analysis of the Problem Rating Scale for Outcomes. *Outcomes Management for Nursing Practice, 3*(1):20-25.

Martin, K.S. & Scheet, N.J. (1992). *The Omaha System: Applications for Community Health Nursing.* Philadelphia, Saunders.

Martin, K.S., Scheet, N.J., & Stegman, M.R. (1993, December). Home health clients: Characteristics, outcomes of care, and nursing interventions. *American Journal of Public Health, 83*(12):1730-1734.

McGourthy, R.J. (1999, February). Omaha and OASIS: A comparative study of outcomes in patients with chronic obstructive pulmonary disease. *Home Care Provider, 4*(1):21-25.

Monsen, K.A. (2002). Using the Omaha System to describe outcomes of clients receiving public health nurse home visiting services. (Unpublished master's thesis, University of Minnesota, Minneapolis, Minnesota).

Moritz, P. & Barton, A.J. (2001, July/August). Linking remote practice to research: Technology in action. *Nursing and Health Care Perspectives, 22*(4):189-193.

Mundt, M.H. (1988, Spring). An analysis of nurse recording in family health clinics of a county health department. *Journal of Community Health Nursing, 5*(1):3-10.

Naylor, M.D., Bowles, K.H., & Brooten, D. (2000, March/April). Patient problems and advanced practice nurse interventions during transitional care. *Public Health Nursing, 17*(2):94-102.

Neff, D.F., Mahama, N., Mohar, D.R.H., & Kinion, E. (2003, April/June). Nursing care delivery at an academic community-based nurse-managed center. *Outcomes Management, 7*(2):84-88.

O'Brien-Pallas, L.L., Irvine, D.D., Murray, M., Cockerill, R., Sidania, S., Laurie-Shaw, B., & Lochhaas-Gerlach, J. (2002, January-February). Evaluation of a client care delivery model, Part 2: Variability in client outcomes in community home nursing. *Nursing Economic$, 20*(1):13-21, 36.

Pasquale, D.K. (1987, Winter). A basis for prospective payment in home care. *IMAGE: Journal of Nursing Scholarship, 19*(4):186-191.

Reilly, F.E., Grier, M.R., & Blomquist, K. (1992, Summer). Living arrangements, visit patterns, and health problems in a nurse-managed clinic for the homeless. *Journal of Community Health Nursing, 9*(2):111-121.

Resick, L.K. (1999, August). Challenges in measuring outcomes in two community-based nurse-managed wellness clinics: The development of a chart auditing tool. *Home Health Care Management and Practice, 11*(5):52-59.

Rose, M.A. (1993, July-September). Health concerns of women with HIV/AIDS. *Journal of the Association of Nurses in AIDS Care, 4*(3):39-45.

Sakai, M. (2002). Home care nursing practice during the first month of care and a later month: Comparison of nursing problems, interventions and outcomes. *Journal of St. Luke's Society for Nursing Research, 6*(1):1-8.

Sampson, B.K., & Doran, K.A. (1998, May/June) Health needs of coronary artery bypass graft surgery patients at discharge. *Dimensions of Critical Care Nursing, 17*(3):158-168.

Sangwattanarat, W. (2002). Health related problems and home care needs among the elderly after coronary artery bypass grafting. (Unpublished master's thesis, Chiang Mai University, Chiang Mai, Thailand).

Schoneman, D. (2002, Spring). Surveillance as a nursing intervention: Use in community nursing centers. *Journal of Community Health Nursing, 19*(1):33-47.

Schraeder, C., Shelton, P., Britt, T., & Buttitta, K. (1996, Summer). Case management in a capitated system: The Community Nursing Organization. *Journal of Case Management, 5*(2):58-64.

Shaughnessy, P.W., Crisler, K.S., & Schlenker, R.E. (1998, February). Outcome-based quality improvement in the information age. *Home Health Care Management and Practice, 10*(2):11-19.

Slack, M.K., & McEwen, M.M. (1999, October). The impact of interdisciplinary case management on client outcomes. *Family Community Health, 22*(3):30-48.

Storfjell, J. L., Mitchell, R., & Daly, G. M. (1997, October). Nurse-managed healthcare: New York's Community Nursing Organization. *The Journal of Nursing Administration, 27*(10):21-27.

Swan, A.R. (1997). Outcome measurement in home care. (Unpublished doctoral dissertation, Rush University, Chicago, Illinois).

Wake, M.M., Murphy, M., Affara, F.A., Lang, N.M., Clark, J., Mortensen, R. (1993, May-June). Toward an international classification for nursing practice: A literature review and survey. *International Nursing Review,* 40(3):77-80.

Ware, J.E. Jr & Sherbourne, C.D. (1992, June). The MOS 36-item short form health survey (SF-36): Conceptual framework and item selection. *Medical Care, 30*(6):473-483.

Zielstorff, R.D., Cimino, C., Barnett, G.O., Hassan, L., & Blewett, D.R. (1993). Representation of nursing terminology in the UMLS Metathesaurus: A pilot study. In Frisse, M.E. (Ed.), *Proceedings of the 16th Annual Symposium on Computer Applications in Medical Care* (pp. 392-396). New York, McGraw Hill.

Zielstorff, R.D., Tronni, C., Basque, J., Reeves Griffin, L., & Welebob, E.M. (1998, Fourth Quarter). Mapping nursing diagnosis nomenclatures for coordinated care. *IMAGE: Journal of Nursing Scholarship, 30*(4):369-373.

6

USE OF INFORMATION TECHNOLOGY WITH THE OMAHA SYSTEM

Karen S. Martin

Only recently have comprehensive clinical information systems been developed that are based on the Omaha System and are capable of operating compatibly with other management information systems. Such systems were a primary goal of the Visiting Nurse Association of Omaha administrators when they initiated pioneering research early in the 1970s. From the onset, the Omaha System was designed to be an integrated practice and documentation system, and a method to standardize, record, and report client data and information within a computerized or manual management information system. The Omaha System was intended to be used by practitioners at the point-of-care as a "front end" or interface terminology. For a few years in the early 1980s, the Visiting Nurse Association of Omaha developed and sold software. Soon other groups began to create software for their own use. In the 1990s, companies started designing software based on the Omaha System and making it commercially available for agencies, public health departments, community-oriented clinics and nurse-managed centers, and schools of nursing. The number and type of software applications continues to expand rapidly.

DEVELOPMENTS

The explosive global developments and adoption of information technology such as computers, telecommunications, and networks is nothing less than amazing. It was 38 years before radio had 50 million listeners in the United States, 13 years before television had an equal number of viewers, and just 4 years until the Internet had that many users (Bridis, 1998). The Internet was launched in 1991; there were 300 million Internet users worldwide in 2000, and one billion are expected by 2005. The most frequent Internet visitors live in the United States and Canada, whereas people in Europe and Japan are more likely to use Web-enabled wireless devices (Stone, 2000). According to a 2002 report (U.S. Department of Commerce), more than half of United States residents are on-line. Internet use is closely associated with age. Children and young adults are the most frequent Internet users globally; 90% of children who live in the United States and are between the ages of 5 and 17 years now use computers. Many who are computer-literate do not view technology as important for its own sake, but as a tool or a means to an end. Many children and young adults are not intimidated by the speed with which technology changes or its short half-life and readily accept that they must be continuous learners.

That leaders continue to be referred to as pioneers reflects the reluctance of the health care industry to fully embrace automation (Martin & Scheet, 1992a and 1992b; Elfrink, 1996; Carty, 2000; Nightingale Tracker Clinical Field Test Nurse Team, 2000; Du, 2003; Martin, 2004). The skepticism involving computers, standardization, problem-oriented medical records, and the continuum of data, knowledge, information, and wisdom were described in Chapter 1 along with references. Few nurses, physicians, or other practitioners understood the need for standardization and the potential of clinical informatics and technology until the 1990s. Exceptions included those who began referring to themselves as "informaticists," the authors of *Next-Generation Nursing Information Systems* (Zielstorff, Hudgings, & Grobe, 1993), and Dame June Clark (1997) who said, "In the future, nursing will be defined, managed, and controlled by the information about it that is held in computerised information systems." The groundswell of multidisciplinary health care practitioners and institutions willing to share information or knowledge did not begin until the start of the current century. Although still few in number, nurses and members of other health care disciplines are becoming more vocal about the need for and the characteristics of adequate clinical information systems. They are leading the shift from a data-driven model to one that is practice and knowledge-driven (Tidd, 1998; Turley, 2002; Androwich et al., 2003; Clark, 2003; Thede, 2003; Wang et al., 2003).

Consumers of all ages access the Internet and make use of telehealth and other information technology advances to obtain health-related information and become partners in the health care communication loop. Frequently, consumers who are Internet-savvy motivate practitioners to develop skills and to recognize and evaluate authenticated and inaccurate Web sites. Approximately 80% of adult Internet users in the United States have searched for health topics on-line. This makes looking for health information the third most popular on-line activity, after using e-mail and investigating a product or service before buying it (Pew Internet and American Life Report, 2003). An expanding segment of the public is also becoming informed about the need for electronic health records and issues of standardized terminology, privacy, confidentiality, and reduction of errors (Landro, 2002; Landro, 2003). Considerable public attention has been focused on medication errors in the United States and the potential benefits of automation (Institute of Medicine, 2000; Institute of Medicine, 2004). Consumer demands for accurate, timely, and complete health-related information will only increase.

Although critics remain, the capability of information technology to collect, sort, document, classify, analyze, retrieve, and communicate client data is critical to providing effective health services, describing the outcomes of those services, and being reimbursed in a timely and efficient manner (Martin, 1982; Martin & Scheet, 1985; Crews et al., 1986; Jonkergouw, 1991; Bowles, 1997; Bender, 1998; Koch, 1998; Tidd, 1998; Mallard, 2000; Coenen et al., 2001; Elfrink et al., 2001; American Nurses Association, 2002; Humphrey, 2002a and 2002b; Sawyer et al., 2002; Martin, Baisch, & Bell-Calvin, 2003; Journal of Biomedical Informatics, 2003; O'Carroll, et al., 2003; Thede, 2003; Martin, 2004; Nelson, 2004; Sienkiewicz, 2004). Historically, the security and privacy of clients' records have been of such concern that some practitioners attempt to resist automation because of confidentiality. In the United States, the regulations for Health Insurance Portability and Accountability Act of 1996 (HIPAA) have added even more complexity to privacy and security issues (Centers for Medicare and Medicaid, 2003). At the same time, the federal government is encouraging providers to use electronic health records as an important strategy for promoting health care safety, quality, and efficiency (U.S. Department of Health and Human Services, 2003). It is likely that federal reimbursement regulations and legislation will mandate the keeping of electronic health records in the near future (Johnson, 2003).

In another development to encourage United States providers to implement electronic health records, the U.S. Department of Health and Human Services asked the Institute of Medicine to build on previous committee efforts and form the Committee on Data Standards for Patient Safety. This committee identified eight core functions that records should facilitate: health information and data, result management, order management, decision support, electronic communication and connectivity, patient support, administrative processes, and reporting (Institute of Medicine, 2003b). Efforts are continuing with additional committees and publications that urge adoption of information technology to improve work environments and increase client safety (Institute of Medicine, 2004). National organizations that focus on technology such as Health Level Seven (HL7), Healthcare Information and Management Systems Society (HIMSS), Systematized Nomenclature of Medicine (SNOMED) and the American Medical Informatics Association, as well as those who represent providers, such as the American Nurses Association and the American Medical Association, are endorsing the Institute of Medicine efforts and the adoption of electronic records. Open forums were scheduled throughout the United States as a strategy to publicize the efforts and gain more professional and public support. The national organizations plan to work together to define functional requirements of electronic health records as a necessary developmental step.

Individuals and groups in the United States and globally suggest that terminologies such as the Omaha System need to be included in technology to support comprehensive, on-line relational or object-oriented database models, to establish interrater reliability, and to compare data (Hettinger & Brazile, 1992; Carty, 2000; Elfrink et al., 2001; Englebardt & Nelson, 2002; Monsen & Martin, 2002a and 2002b; Clark, 2003; Thede, 2003; Omaha System Web site, 2004). While data sets, classification systems, and nomenclatures can be used without information technology, they cannot thrive without it. Because of the driving forces already mentioned, large data sets, often abstracted from client records, are now available. These data sets require adequate hardware, software, data managers, and researchers to mine the data, merge clinical information with other financial and statistical information, and create knowledge to improve care. The need for such research is described in Chapter 5.

Companies that develop and sell automated clinical information software entered the market relatively recently. While some software designed for service and academic settings was available commercially during the 1980s, the number and types available increased dramatically during the 1990s and since. The market has been volatile, with companies emerging, merging, separating, thriving, or failing, partly because the health care information industry is so new, but also because the extended technology industry and global economics have been volatile and less than financially stable.

Androwich et al. (2003) clearly summarized the past, present, and future of information technology. The authors referred to a major conceptual shift and a striking contrast between the Institute of Medicine's 1991 and 2001 recommendations involving clinical information systems (Institute of Medicine, 1991; Institute of Medicine, 2001). The 1991 recommendations suggested a very ambitious, comprehensive approach to clinical information systems and described the ideal computerized record that should be adopted as a standard. Computerization was viewed almost as a "silver bullet" that was capable of eliminating all organizational problems. The 1991 recommendations have been implemented in variable rather than consistent ways because of enormous complexity, cost, and technology factors. In contrast, the 2001 recommendations focus on information technology as a means rather than an end, and the necessity for health care delivery to be touched by the revolution that has been transforming the rest of society. The focus is on the need for health care that is safe, effective, client-centered, timely, efficient, and equitable, *and* that can be supported by appropriately designed clinical and administrative information systems. The shift between the Institute of Medicine's two reports confirms the original Omaha System goal: not to capture data for data's sake, but to use data as information and knowledge to improve care. Figure 6-1 is a flow chart designed to graphically depict that shift, the relationship among the concepts, and the critical importance of clinical knowledge (Androwich, et al., 2003). Related flow charts, conceptualizations, and models are described in Chapter 1.

Education

Many universities started the transition to technology slowly, beginning with accounting and word processing functions and staff who were comfortable with quantitative data and equipment. Frequently, universities developed systems and resources before educators or students were involved. Not surprisingly, students often had more computer skills than educators and exerted pressure for change. Many academic settings require new students to own or rent a computer and have basic computer skills and an email account, offer

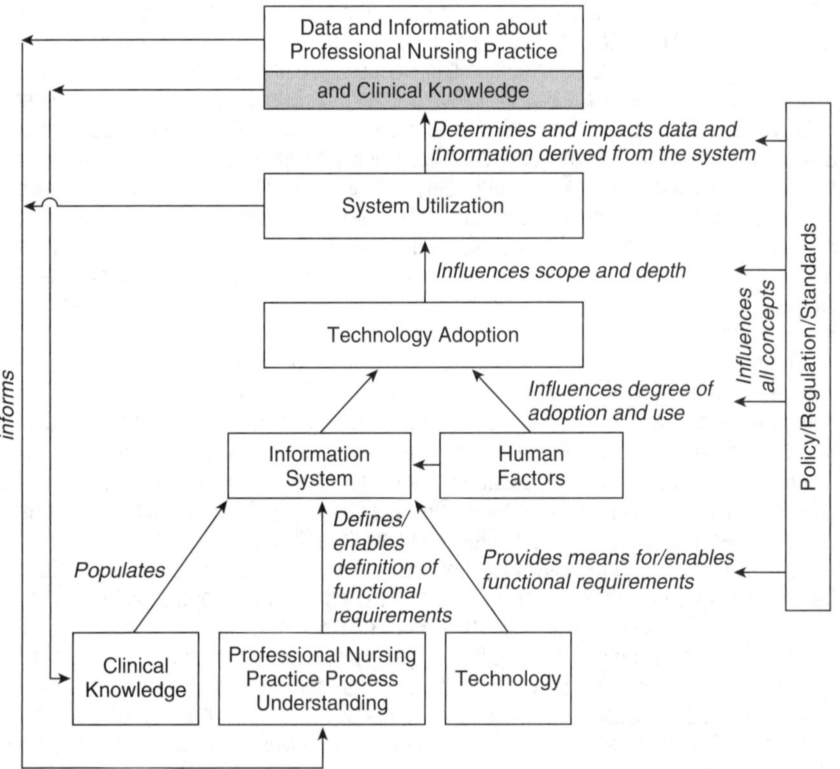

Figure 6-1 Organizing Framework for Clinical Information Systems: Clinical Knowledge as Critical Factor.

(From Androwich, I.M., Bickford, C.J., Button, P.S., Hunter, K.M., Murphy, J., & Sensmeier, J. [2003]. *Clinical Information Systems: A Framework for Reaching the Vision.* Washington, DC, American Nurses Publishing.)

extensive computer laboratories and media, provide sophisticated simulations and technology in health science buildings, offer on-line courses, and require data-based research. However, few universities have implemented a comprehensive information technology plan; typically, wide variations exist among departments (Katz, 1999; Turley, 2002). Often, top administrators and board members do not view technology as an asset. Because information technology is very expensive and universities face ever increasing economic strain and competition from new sources that are providing on-line educational opportunities, the relationship between higher education and information technology has been described as a dance with the devil (Katz, 1999).

Even if the university environment is positive, health care educators and researchers, including nursing faculty, face challenges in becoming technology leaders. Some must complete a significant learning curve and attitude changes. All are limited by time, money, and resources as described in Chapter 4 and in other publications (Connolly, Huynh, & Gorney-Moreno, 1999; Nightingale Tracker Clinical Field Test Nurse Team, 2000; Thomas, Coppola, & Feldman, 2001; Connolly & Elfrink, 2002; Wilson, 2002; Clark, 2003; Wilson & Roy, 2003). The university may be equipped adequately for students, educators, and researchers to use technology in campus buildings, but not have the infrastructure for networking off-site, securing client data, or recovering lost data. Although some health care educators develop sufficient programming, equipment, infrastructure, and maintenance skills, most need a team approach that combines their skills with those of competent, available technical support staff. Only then can faculty teach students to organize new knowledge, integrate it into existing knowledge structures, and apply their knowledge to solve information-related problems (Turley, 2002).

It is important for today's health care students to be introduced to terminologies and the value of clinical data and information technology. Thomas, Coppola, & Feldman (2001) summarized major challenges they faced when introducing the Nightingale Tracker® technology to students in an academic setting as well as smaller, equally critical, but often not anticipated, challenges. While still in an educational setting, students need to observe expert practitioners successfully using terminologies such as the Omaha System and computerized devices to make sound clinical decisions, document care, and analyze data. The more students develop related knowledge and skills, the better prepared they will be for the transition to the workforce. Omaha System Box 6-1 relates the story of a student who successfully transitioned to the role of an employee.

Practice

Accounting and word processing staff members were often the first employees to adopt information technology in health care organizations, the pattern just described for universities. In contrast to universities, a large percentage of employees in practice settings use client records each day. Until recently, those records were manual and had little structure or standardization, similar to the records to which multidisciplinary practitioners were introduced as students. Often, practitioners were skeptical about technology, quantitative data, and standardization; they viewed automation as a low priority, and even suggested that automation interfered with their ability to provide quality care, although Florence Nightingale implemented quantitative methods successfully in the 1800s (Geraci, 1997; Larrabee, 1999; Elfrink, 2001; Monsen & Martin, 2002a; Handly et al., 2003).

While administrators and managers have traditionally been as skeptical as practitioners, their attitudes are slowly changing. Williams (2002) reported that most administrators viewed information technology as a necessary evil required for billing rather than a strategic asset to improve the speed and efficiency of operations, decrease cost, and encour-

CHAPTER 6

OMAHA SYSTEM BOX 6-1

Omaha System Experiences with Information Technology: Welcoming Technology

My-Phuong T. Huynh, RN, BSN
Registered Nurse II
Kaiser Permanente Hospital
Santa Clara, California

Before I started using the Omaha System and the Nightingale Tracker® during my undergraduate nursing program at San Jose State University, I had basic computer experience, as did most of my classmates. Learning to operate the Tracker was relatively easy and offered unique opportunities to merge technology and nursing practice in contrast to manual documentation at other clinical sites, and to participate in research. The Omaha System was standardized and more applicable to our community health course than the previous nursing diagnosis terminology I had learned. It helped me formulate better care plans for my clients. I especially loved carrying the little reference book to our clinical sites!

I appreciated using the Tracker as a communication device with my instructors. It facilitated discussion, decreased the "us versus them" attitude, especially when we, the students, could understand and use the Tracker better than our instructors! Sometimes it was easier and faster to communicate with the instructors while using the Tracker than it was in person. We had fun, and our instructors consistently encouraged us to develop our skills and be successful. I had several very special opportunities, particularly special because I am a shy person. I coauthored a publication while I was still in my undergraduate program and spoke at several conferences.

I am a more competent and confident nurse because of my experiences using the Omaha System and Tracker. Yes, it was frustrating at times. I had to repeat some of my work when technology failed, it was not easy to be patient, and the long-term benefits were a blur at the time. However, the benefits are now clear. In the hospital where I work, we have automated medication distribution and documentation. Some nurses had difficulty with this during orientation, but it was an easy transition for me. It is wonderful that nursing schools are preparing students for what I like to call "the real nursing world." Welcome, technology!

age growth. More than 700 health care administrators in the United States and 28 other countries completed a survey about electronic health records. They reported that lack of adequate funds was their primary barrier (64%), and that lack of support by physicians (37%) and inability to find an affordable system (32%) were also serious barriers (Medical Records Institute, 2003).

Automation permeates acute care practice more than it does community practice in the United States. According to the 287 respondents of an acute care-oriented survey done in 2003, the top priority currently and during the next several years is to increase client safety and decrease provider errors (Healthcare Information and Management System Society, 2003b). Other high priorities include upgrading their clinical systems, implementing clinical applications and sharing information throughout their health care systems, and initiating a computerized client record. Client records were reported by 20% of the respondents to be computerized. Many acute care practitioners use point-of-care technology. However, acute care software may be limited to entry of physician or pharmacy orders or medication management, scheduling, client education, and other specific functions. Often, because of the new software that is available and packages that are already installed, acute care settings purchase more software that cannot be integrated and does not provide health care professionals, especially nurses, with a unified method to track client care or analyze clinical data throughout the institution. This is in contrast to purchasing one large clinical information system that is integrated into an even larger management information system (Case, Mowry, & Welebob, 2002; Sensmeier, 2002; Solovy, 2002).

Estimates indicate that no more than 15% to 20% of home care practitioners in the United States use point-of-care technology. The percentage is even lower for those employed in public health and other community settings (Koch, 1998; Reichley, 2001; Williams, 2002; Monsen & Kerr, 2004). Contrast these statistics with the Omaha System adopters depicted in Table 1-3 and described in Chapter 1. Williams expects the use of electronic health records to increase dramatically and states that "it is virtually impossible to develop a scenario for the future of health care that does not have home care and technology as central elements" (p. 7, 2002). Many administrators and managers have concluded that they cannot afford to delay automation. Others will reach that conclusion soon, especially if reimbursement and legislative mandates continue to increase at a dramatic rate (Johnson, 2003; U. S. Department of Health and Human Services, 2003).

Technology Standards

Standards rarely if ever precede the development of innovations. Information technology innovations clearly preceded standards that made it possible to store and compare data among health care providers and sites (Katz, 1999; Bakken, 2000; Turley, 2002; Healthcare Information and Management Systems Society, 2003a). Those who used early versions of word processing software recall their frustration and inability to send information from one computer or system to another. The development of standards eliminated those problems and increased interoperability. Currently, standardization efforts are occurring at several levels. Local, regional, and national provider organizations must establish standards involving their wiring plans, guidelines for adding and replacing software and computers, data management, backup and storage plans, and other highly technical system aspects.

Various groups have established complex and technical industry standards nationally and globally. Many of these groups are voluntary rather than governmental. For example, the Internet consortium developed and adopted the extensible markup language (XML) that is a standard in products from all major database developers. This technology allows materials to be accessed by previously incompatible personal computers, handheld devices, and Web-enabled telephones (Turley, 2002). Examples of diverse organizations involved with developing and coordinating health care standards are the National Committee on Vital and Health Statistics (NCVHS), Systematized Nomenclature of Medicine (SNOMED), the Healthcare Information and Management Systems Society (HIMSS), the International Organization for Standardization (ISO), Comité Européen de Normalisation (European Committee for Standardization)(CEN/TC), Logical Observation Identifiers, Names, and Codes (LOINC), Vanderbilt Nursing Terminology Summit Group, Health Level Seven (HL7), the Institute of Electrical and Electronic Engineers (IEEE), the American National Standards Institute (ANSI), and the American Society for Testing and Materials (ASTM).

As described in Chapter 1, many of these organizations are promoting the development of information and terminology models that have the potential for increasing the comparability (interoperability) of data, including terminologies such as the Omaha System

(Humphreys, McCray, & Cheh, 1997; Hwang, Cimino, & Bakken, 2003). In the United States, the National Library of Medicine has negotiated contracts with SNOMED CT®, LOINC, and HL7 on behalf of federal health care agencies. The three codes sets will be part of the Metathesaurus and serve as the standards for providers as they link and exchange clinical data. In time these contracts could dramatically change practitioners and providers' access to clinical data and the ability to track and analyze those data.

IMPLEMENTATION: CURRENT PERSPECTIVES

Since the initial development of the Omaha System early in the 1970s, some myths or assumptions have circulated among service organizations, schools, and software vendors. These myths must be clarified or refuted (Box 6-1). While the myths and the implementation information that follow are intended to apply to practice, education, and research, the issues that are emphasized originate in the practice setting. However, educators and researchers

BOX 6-1 Myths and Responses Frequently Associated With the Omaha System and Clinical Information Systems

- Myth 1: Automation is easy.
  Response: It is not easy, fast, or painless.
- Myth 2: It is reasonable to develop software by programming manual forms because administrators, managers, or educators are strongly attached to them or because vendors say that it is a good idea.
  Response: Few users will be satisfied with the completed software and its extensive limitations.
- Myth 3: You can save money by developing your own software.
  Response: Do not try unless your requirements are very simple and an Access, Excel, or similar database meets your needs. The organization that believes this approach can decrease its costs will be unpleasantly surprised, practitioners will be angry, and managers will not have the reports they expected.
- Myth 4: Electronic health records are basically the same, so it doesn't matter which system we purchase.
  Response: Not true. In addition to becoming very well informed about all aspects of the software, you need to obtain accurate information about the vendor's orientation and implementation process, the reports that will be available, their track record of service and responsiveness, the cost of and the way they handle upgrades, and how their software integrates with other software. See suggestions in Chapter 3 and *do your homework*.
- Myth 5: Vendors, systems analysts, and programmers know more about what information systems users need than users do. Few administrators, managers, or educators are informatics experts.
  Response: If you plan to purchase a system, you must become informed beyond the novice level, identify your short- and long-terms goals, and establish a multidisciplinary project team with members who have proficient and expert information technology skills.
- Myth 6: It is fine to develop software that includes some of the Omaha System problems, interventions, and ratings and even combine the Omaha System with other, similar, standardized vocabularies.
  Response: It is not fine. The entire published version of the Omaha System must be available to practitioners to maintain integrity and standardization, for practitioners to use it consistently and accurately, for the resulting data to be reliable and valid, and for the opportunity to have useful reports.

Continued

BOX 6-1 Myths and Responses Frequently Associated With the Omaha System and Clinical Information Systems—cont'd

- Myth 7: A "big bang approach" is a good way to implement an automated clinical information system. Provide practitioners or managers with little preparatory information, provide orientation, and tell them they will start using software immediately.*
  Response: This is a very dangerous approach and has resulted in low morale, resignations, and near mutiny in some organizations. If end users (practitioners) do not support a clinical information system, they are likely to find ways to undermine or even destroy your action plans.
- Myth 8: Detailed narrative records ("novels") are preferable when involved with the legal system or court.
  Response: Not true unless you are trying to hide data. Concise, structured, legible documentation that is accurate and consistent is preferable and can lead to comparable data, information, knowledge, and wisdom.
- Myth 9: Electronic health records drive practice.
  Response: They should not. They should enhance and modify practice in a positive way. Computers do not know more than good practitioners, and practitioners must always remember that.
- Myth 10: The more reports your information system generates, the better.
  Response: More is not necessarily better. Having a few reports that you know are accurate and complete is much better than having dozens of reports that include errors and omissions. Especially during early stages, identify which few Omaha System problems, interventions, or outcomes reports will provide the information to practitioners, managers, and administrators that has the potential to improve client care, decrease costs, or increase the opportunity to communicate with others within or outside the organization. Focus collective efforts on the steps to collect, enter, analyze, and communicate needed data for several reports before expanding. Remember the audience when selecting and sharing reports.
- Myth 11: Expect to experience a rapid time and cost savings.
  Response: Using computerized records takes more time initially. Studies do not support marked decrease in practitioner documentation time even after 6 to 18 months. If the information system is implemented and used successfully by the entire team, communication improves dramatically; documentation is legible, timely, and less likely to be lost; practitioners document improved clinical decision making and outcomes of care; managers and administrators have access to accurate and consistent clinical data that they never had before; and certain support staff requirements decrease.

*Anderson, L.K. & Stafford, C.J. (2002, January/February). *The "big bang" implementation: Not for the faint of heart.* Computers in Nursing, 20(1):14-22.

CHAPTER 6

should become well informed about these issues. Educators must prepare graduates to function successfully, and researchers have to conduct their studies successfully.

The process of converting a manual record to an automated clinical information system is one of the most complex, costly, and challenging changes a health care organization can undertake. The necessity of using a realistic and comprehensive action plan for planning, orientation, implementation, evaluation, and refinement cannot be overstated (see Box 6-4 later in the chapter) (Martin & Scheet, 1992a; Standish Group International, Inc., 1999; Mallard, 2000; Anderson & Stafford, 2002; Englebardt & Nelson, 2002; Monsen & Martin, 2002a.) Too often, administrators and board members want the process to cost less and be completed quickly, whereas employees want it to be easy and not interfere with their other responsibilities. The conversion will never be easy and will cause a strain throughout the organization. It requires that many employees change work patterns, maintain a positive attitude, and resolve predicted and unpredicted difficulties that continue to occur for months or even years. Too often, practitioners and managers underestimate the culture or habits associated with using and reviewing manual records, and the new attitudes and behaviors that are necessary to complete the transition to automated records. Holding focus groups with representatives of a health care organization is a strategy to identify needed steps of the implementation plan and to revise them, and to reduce anxiety and resistance, especially among experienced practitioners. In addition to encouraging the use of focus groups, Stricklin et al. (2000) suggested that the four critical success factors for implementation were technology skills, support in the workplace, client interaction, and integration of the technology into daily practice.

No two organizations will have identical experiences when they begin to use Omaha System software, any more than they would when implementing any other major change. It is reasonable to expect that organizations identify both advantages and disadvantages of use that vary considerably over time (Box 6-2).

Larrabee (1999) applied Benner's (1984) five-stage novice to expert framework to nurses and laptops in home care agencies (Box 6-3). Although all of Larrabee's details do not apply to other users, the model establishes useful expectations for practitioners, managers, administrators, and software vendors that can be individualized to a specific setting. In addition, if an organization establishes a series of stages at the beginning of the implementation process, practitioners can be acknowledged and rewarded when they advance to the next stage. The previous chapters of this book and other publications offer more suggestions for implementation (Geraci, 1997; Baldwin, 1998; Bender, 1998; Tidd, 1998; Larrabee et al., 2001; Handly et al., 2003; O'Carroll, et al., 2003; Thede, 2003; Rosebaugh, 2004).

Omaha System Boxes 6-2 and 6-3 are designed to describe the perspectives of a practitioner and a manager or administrator, respectively. Note that the practitioner has a negative attitude, especially initially, whereas the director has a positive attitude; in reality, people are not that predictable. The practitioner's perspective is intended to be lighthearted, does not reflect 11 consecutive days in the "Omaha System" diary, and was developed specifically for this book in contrast to other Omaha System Boxes throughout the book that report authors' actual experiences. The attitudes and behaviors in Omaha System Box 6-2 are typical of those expressed by many when they face major changes such as automation and use of the Omaha System. In contrast, the author of Omaha System Box 6-3 is a director who understands the necessity of timely and accurate performance and productivity reports, and anticipates using the Omaha System and other clinical data for benchmarking.

A team approach and sense of ownership are essential characteristics demonstrated by health care organizations that implement technology successfully. It is important to develop champions who are practitioners and managers and support positive reactions to change. The extent of change process that occurs when the Omaha System and an automated information system are implemented is usually in direct proportion to a number of factors, many of which are described in Omaha System Box 6-4 and in Chapter 3. Omaha System Box 6-4 encourages the reader to apply a building block approach to identify the steps needed for successful implementation; it reflects the box author's previous publications (Westra & Raup, 1995; Westra, 1996; Westra, Martin, & Swan, 1996; Westra & Solomon, 1999). It should not come as a surprise that some practitioners need praise for learning very basic computer skills. Although the dramatic increase in adoption of e-mail and the Internet were described at the beginning of this chapter, many individuals, groups,

BOX 6-2 Potential Advantages and Disadvantages of Using Omaha System Software

ADVANTAGES

- Continual access to information from multiple locations
- Easier to track mobile clients
- Improved coordination of care
- More accurate, consistent, and legible documentation
- Standardized structure for entering assessments, care plans, and interventions that can be customized for specific client populations
- Visible links and congruence among problems, interventions, and ratings (also visible if absent)
- Increased potential to note data trends that suggest level of risk and need for prioritization
- Improved access to data so that quality improvement is a reality, not just an exercise
- Capability of measuring outcomes of care that can be used for diverse internal and external reports
- Streamlined office processes for tracking client data
- Improved communication between clients, families, office personnel, practitioners, managers, and external personnel
- Increased sense of connectedness
- Provides a better supervisory tool for managers
- Improved timeliness for physicians' orders, the OASIS, and other mandatory activities
- Improved documentation for third party payers, surveyors, auditors, accreditors, or legal action
- Improved billing cycles
- Increased practitioner field time and decreased office time
- Increased sense of professionalism

DISADVANTAGES

- Realization that software is not perfect and does not fit organization's entire wish list
- Learning curve required for practitioners to develop competence (varies dramatically)
- Requires ongoing support and monitoring for correct use of the Omaha System
- Requires continuing support from software vendor
- Requires ongoing system management support from organization's information technology staff
- Requires alternative plan if device or system fails
- Increased tension and negative reactions to change by employees, clients, referral sources, and third party payers; it is hard to change a technophobic's belief system
- Initial and ongoing costs

Adapted from Struk, C. (2002, December). Frequently asked questions about computer technology for clinicians. *Home Healthcare Nurse, 20*(12):811-813.

CHAPTER 6

and areas in the United States and the world do not have access to technology and are not computer-literate. Successful implementation requires an action plan that meets diverse users' needs and skill levels when they prepare for automation, introduce practitioners to the Omaha System and software, and manage the change to automation. While the content and schedule of action plans have to be tailored for specific sites, general themes must be included in all successful plans. Box 6-4 summarizes the planning, orientation, and implementation experiences of the Marion County Health Department (Indianapolis, Indiana) and provides valuable tips for each phase (Handly et al., 2003).

BOX 6-3 Model for Implementing a Clinical Information System in a Home Care Agency Based on Benner's Novice to Expert Theory

The novice stage: The orientation week plus 6 weeks. Competency is based on participation and assimilation. Productivity is measured by the addition of one client per week. *Interpretive goal:* Nurse will be able to verbalize needs and seek assistance.
The advanced beginner stage: 6 weeks to 6 months. Competency is measured in increasing productivity to at least 4 clients a day. *Interpretive goal:* Nurse will feel comfortable with laptop and ask appropriate questions.
The competent stage: 6 months to 1 year. Competency is measured by productivity of 6 clients in 8 hours, per department policy. All documentation will be complete and timely. *Interpretive goal:* Nurse will be able to utilize laptop to plan care and participates in users' group meetings.
The proficient stage: After 1 year. Competency is measured by the nurse's complete integration of the laptop into practice. Nurse serves as a preceptor to new laptop users. Nurse participates in agency activities to refine system. *Interpretive goal:* Nurse will be able to state preference for laptop to paper.
The expert stage: Based on demonstrated ability. At this point, the nurse is at the highest level of understanding of both the laptop clinical documentation system and its components. *Interpretive goal:* Nurse will be able to teach new laptop users, mentor them, troubleshoot for the agency, and serve as a facilitator for discussion on the upgrading and changing of the system.

From Larrabee, S.B. (1999, August). Benner's Novice to Expert Nursing Theory applied to the implementation of laptops in the home care setting. *Home Health Care Management and Practice*, *11*(4):41-47.

Practical, useful, and very current information about purchasing and implementing clinical information systems is not readily available in the literature. Few articles are written and published by administrators, managers, practitioners, educators, students, and software vendors that describe their actual experiences, lessons learned, and suggestions for newer adopters (Connolly, Huynh, & Gorney-Moreno, 1999; Pearce, Castleman, & Elfrink, 1999; Westra & Solomon, 1999; Hockenjos & Wharton, 2001; Larrabee et al., 2001; Souther, 2001; Tressa & Barber, 2001; Monsen & Martin, 2002a and 2002b; Sloan & Delahoussaye, 2003; Rosebaugh, 2004). Reference librarians at colleges or even local libraries may help identify relevant publications or regular features in other publications. In addition to implementation literature, leaders of the organization or agency and members of the project team are likely to benefit from reading publications about change, chaos, force, field, diffusion, and related theories (Lewin, 1951; Polanyi, 1967; Rogers, 1995; Woods & Grant, 1995; Geraci, 1997; Connolly, Huynh, & Gorney-Moreno, 1999; Hilz, 2000; Slotnick & Shershneva, 2002; Bozak, 2003). Many practitioners are frustrated, frightened, and stressed by the changes related to an automated clinical information system.

Consider obtaining information from additional sources. Conferences that include software exhibits and demonstrations, consultants, contact with staff members of national organizations, word of mouth, and visits to other users are listed in Chapter 3 as valuable resources. Software vendors can provide information about the advantages and costs of specific software and hardware, assistance with a budget and cost justification for board members or others who must approve a purchase, and details about the necessary steps and schedule, especially if they offer an implementation guide. Use a search engine to identify current Web sites, listservs, and information that is available on the Internet to the

OMAHA SYSTEM BOX 6-2

Omaha System Experiences with Information Technology: Peeking into My Diary

Kimberly W. Field, RN, MSN
Tuberculosis Program Coordinator
Washington State Department of Health
Olympia, Washington

Day 1: O = Omaha System, they said. WHY do we need a new record? Ours worked swell for 11 years. Does it matter that no one else can read my notes?
Day 2: M = Molly said she worked somewhere that used the Omaha System and that we CAN do it. She promised to help, especially if I have a bad day. Sure I will.
Day 3: A = Automation is the new buzz word. Good that I started using a PC years ago. Never dreamed that I'd use a computer at work.
Day 4: H = HOW will I squeeze this stuff in my too busy schedule? Was glad to hear—will have things to read and a workshop.
Day 5: A = Again, again, again. PRACTICE, PRACTICE, PRACTICE. Yuck.
Day 6: S = Statistics all over the office today. IF we learn to use this stuff, we can count client data. Don't they know I do a good job just by watching and listening to me? When DID my manager go on a shared visit with me? Can't remember.
Day 7: Y = YMCA!! Can you believe it? Karen Martin, the workshop leader, made us stand up and sing this weird Omaha System song to YMCA! She said she has done these workshops since 1978 and we have to get involved and laugh if we're going to learn. REALLY!
Day 8: S = Success!! Our manager put up a big sign today: SUCCESS!! Our new records are automated. Now we just have to do the rest.
Day 9: T = Trouble. My laptop crashed 2 days ago. Was it my fault? Funny thing is that I MISS that little box. HOW can I remember all these visits?
Day 10: E = Easy. I admitted a new client today and it was EASY—told Molly. Almost scary.
Day 11: M = My prize!! Had a drawing and I won a free lunch at Tiko's! Maybe this Omaha stuff isn't so bad after all!

P.S. Hope you chuckled when you read my Omaha System diary! You read a lot of pages to find it. Keep reading; you may find more chuckles! But then again, you may not!!

public, by subscription, or through membership. Some examples are California HealthCare Foundation's ihealthBeat; Stony Hill Publishing's Home Care Automation Report; Phoenix Health System's HIPAAlert, Home Care Information Technology Council; Healthcare Information and Management Systems Society (HIMSS), HealthLeaders, Inc.; National Library of Medicine; Nurses, Midwives, and Allied Professions/United Kingdom's National Electronic Library for Health; Association for Common European Nursing Diagnoses, Interventions, and Outcomes; British Computer Society nursing specialist group; Nursing Informatics Europe; vendors' Web sites; and the Omaha System Web site. Thoughtful questions, reports of automation successes, and descriptions of barriers are often shared on listservs such as those hosted by the Omaha System, the American Medical Informatics Association, and other membership organizations, rather than in the formal literature.

OMAHA SYSTEM BOX 6-3

Omaha System Experiences with Information Technology: Learning from the Past and Preparing for the Future

Julie Pahlen, RN, BS, PHN
Director
Roseau County Home Health Care
Roseau, Minnesota

Our small, rural hospital-based home care, hospice, and public health agency is state-licensed, Medicare-certified, and Joint Commission on Accreditation of Healthcare Organizations-accredited. In 1999 we recognized that automation was an essential method to increase productivity and become more efficient. When I compare our initial and current status, I think about:

1. The use of laptops was intimidating. Some nurses needed months to become comfortable and confident even though we encouraged them to play games. Recently we hired a new nurse who has extensive computer experience and a very different attitude. Her learning curve was dramatically different than our initial nurses.
2. Using the Outcome and Assessment Information Set (OASIS), required by our Medicare certification, would have been a nightmare without automation. We continue to improve our skills, but often are frustrated by OASIS questions and answers. Automation has been a definite benefit when we prepare for and experience accreditation site visits.
3. We have been fortunate to have good vendor and agency information technology support. Even so, I realize that I must be "tough" and continually insist on that support, fight for the right software and hardware updates, and maintain the vision. We experienced a major internal failure and lost a large amount of data; our decision not to go paperless was the only thing that kept that failure from being a disaster.
4. We have a number of goals. We want to continue our annual record audits, become more accurate and consistent Omaha System users, link our Omaha System and OASIS data, and use aggregate data to demonstrate trends and the effectiveness of our services.

We celebrated our progress as we moved from a ten-lane documentation highway, where nurses created their own documentation styles, to a six-lane highway; we believe we are approaching four lanes. We will not limit ourselves to only one or two lanes—our nurses and clients require more flexibility to reflect the quality of practice and the success of outcomes of care.

Sample Screen Images and Scannable Forms

Forms for manual records were included in the 1992 Omaha System text (Martin & Scheet, 1992a) to illustrate how diverse practice and educational settings developed and documented client data. Forms completed with case study data were placed throughout the application chapters; blank forms were included in the Appendixes so users could adopt them partially or totally.

Because of the incredible advances and implementation of information technology, screen images and scannable forms are included in this edition rather than forms for manual records. Figures 6-2 and 6-3 are excerpts of software designed by vendors to support the extensive and complex clinical information system requirements of diverse health care provider organizations. Figure 6-4 is used by a university-based nurse-managed center to support data entry and analysis.

OMAHA SYSTEM BOX 6-4

Omaha System Experiences with Information Technology: Implementing the Software

Bonnie L. Westra, RN, PhD

Vice President, Planning

CareFacts Information Systems, Inc.
St. Paul, Minnesota

The advantages of using a computerized documentation system are numerous. Redundant data entry can be greatly reduced. Automation provides cues and prompts practitioners to record consistently and to comply with regulatory requirements. During the nursing shortage, automation can be a recruitment tool for many employers.

There are important steps to successfully implementing a clinical information system. The first step is to involve practitioners in the initial decision making process. Choose a vendor who has experienced staff members to guide you through implementation. Once you select software, divide implementation into building blocks for orientation:

- Computer knowledge
- Typing skills
- Nursing/problem solving process
- Basic care planning knowledge
- Omaha System knowledge
- Introduction for moving through the software program

The world does not stop when you are implementing a new system, and your practitioners can expect to be very busy, if not overwhelmed. Therefore, it is vital to incorporate accountability and ensure that learning occurs. Each of the building blocks must include objectives, step-by-step guidelines, and competency testing to demonstrate accountability and build staff confidence so they know they mastered previous building blocks.

Practice time is required and can be improved in various ways. Have objectives that specify the intended outcomes of the practice sessions. Provide guidelines for what practitioners should practice, such as case studies. Supervise practice times so practitioners learn correctly the first time. Provide positive feedback for all achievements to increase morale and encourage success.

Learning is more successful if practitioners have fun and feel positive. Use humor; be playful, and share toys such as huggable bears or squeezable stress balls. Take pictures and post them to create a sense of camaraderie. Use visual aides, even as simple as hash marks on a board, to acknowledge every time someone does something right, has an important insight, or helps others. Be generous: give credit initially for the smallest accomplishment, such as demonstrating how to turn on a computer, getting into the program, or finding the right screen. An optimistic atmosphere makes transitioning to computers a successful adventure.

Readers need to remember that the screen images are limited examples of how the Omaha System appears in software applications. The figures are not intended to be a substitute for vitally important activities described in Chapter 3, such as visiting vendors' Web sites, talking to vendors, viewing computer demonstrations, and visiting customers where software is installed. In addition, the screen images and scannable forms will become outdated because the vendors update their software regularly.

The screen images in Figures 6-2 and 6-3 and the scannable forms in Figure 6-4 are from three different sources, as noted in the following paragraphs.

CHAPTER 6

BOX 6-4 Computerized Information Management Tips

The following tips are based on the experiences of the Marion County Health Department, Indianapolis, Indiana.

PLANNING

- Have a vision—believe that you can successfully achieve it.
- Evaluate current documentation for consistency, accuracy, and readability.
- Plan for multidisciplinary representatives to research and attend software demonstrations, and listen to their recommendations.
- Identify core values and needs—decide if a standardized vocabulary is an essential feature.
- Realize that no system will be perfect.
- Recognize that information technology staff involvement is critical because automation does not follow a natural course.
- Evaluate staff computer knowledge and skills, and look for ways to enhance them.
- Explore realistic costs and benefits of implementing and maintaining an automated system.
- Expect problems involving existing hardware and software compatibility regardless of what is purchased.
- Establish a small, multidisciplinary core team to share ownership of the project.

ORIENTATION

- Acknowledge that expert consultants are needed to provide orientation for staff.
- Develop a flexible schedule based on the consultants' recommendations for orienting staff.
- Encourage staff to *practice, practice,* and *practice.*
- Realize that staff need support and encouragement as they move toward computerized documentation.

IMPLEMENTATION

- Recognize that change is difficult—staff will resist.
- Understand that there will be varied and ongoing challenges.
- Address staff anxiety as soon as it develops.
- Keep a positive attitude; it is essential for success.
- Be prepared to have ongoing orientation for updates, new programs, and improvements within the system, as well as orientation for newly hired staff.
- Praise staff, celebrate achievements, and acknowledge progress toward goals.
- Continue primary staff responsibilities and services—automation should not consume one's professional life.
- Explore additional ways to expand the use of clinical information.

From Handly, M.J., Grubb, S.K., Keefe, N.A., & Martin, K.S. (2003, January). Essential activities for implementing a clinical information system in public health nursing. *Journal of Nursing Administration*, *33*(1):14-16.

Figure 6-2 is from CareFacts Information Systems, Inc. Customers include home care, hospice, public health, and other community providers in the United States. Contact information is Gateway Center, 2140 W. County Road C, St. Paul, Minnesota 55113; telephone: 651-636-3890; Web site: www.carefacts.com.

Figure 6-3 is from CHAMP Software, Inc. (the client name is fictitious). Customers include home care, public health, and other community providers in the United States.

Contact information is 115 E. Hickory Street, Suite 400, Mankato, Minnesota 56001; telephone: 507-388-4141; Web site: www.champsoftware.com.

Figure 6-4 is from the University of Colorado Health Sciences Center School of Nursing. The school purchased Teleform® technology, an optical character recognition system from Cardiff software, and developed a 1-page Omaha System summary form that can be scanned into the computer. The school's contact information is 4200 East Ninth Street, Denver, CO 80262; telephone: 303-315-7687; e-mail: amy.barton@uchsc.edu.

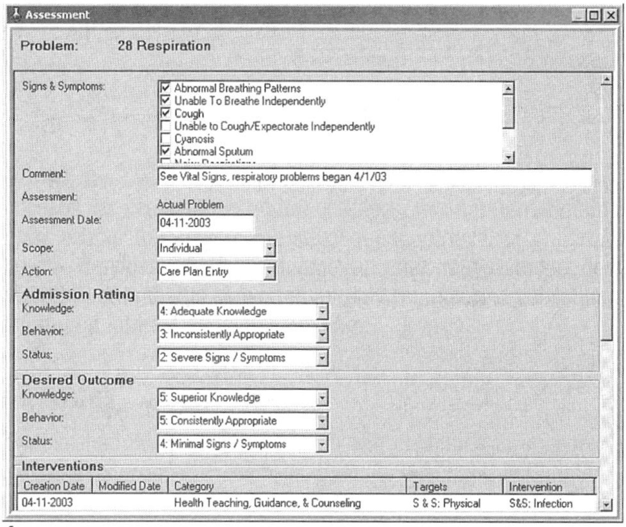

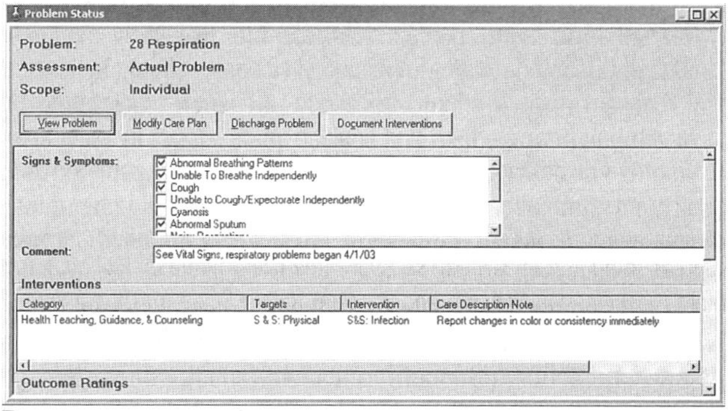

Figure 6-2 Screen images from CareFacts software. **A.** Illustrates use of the Problem Classification Scheme and the Problem Rating Scale for Outcomes. **B.** Illustrates use of the Problem Classification Scheme and the Intervention Scheme. **C.** Illustrates use of the Problem Classification Scheme and the Intervention Scheme.

(Courtesy CareFacts Information Systems, Inc., St. Paul, Minnesota. Contact information: Gateway Center, 2140 W. County Road C, St. Paul, Minnesota 55113; telephone: 651-636-3890; Web site: www.carefacts.com.)

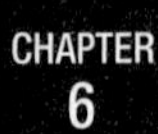

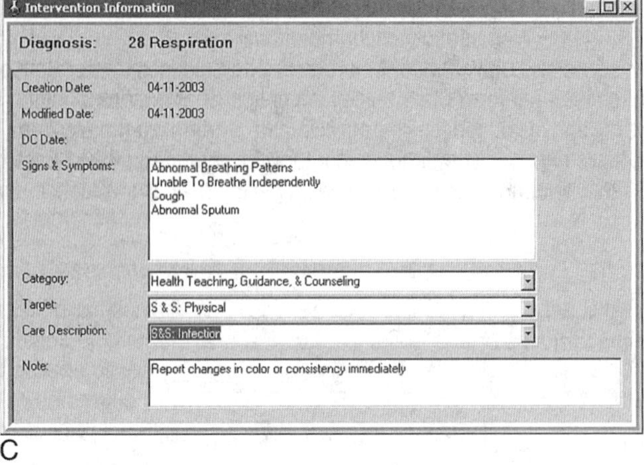

Figure 6-2, cont'd, Screen Images from CareFacts Software.

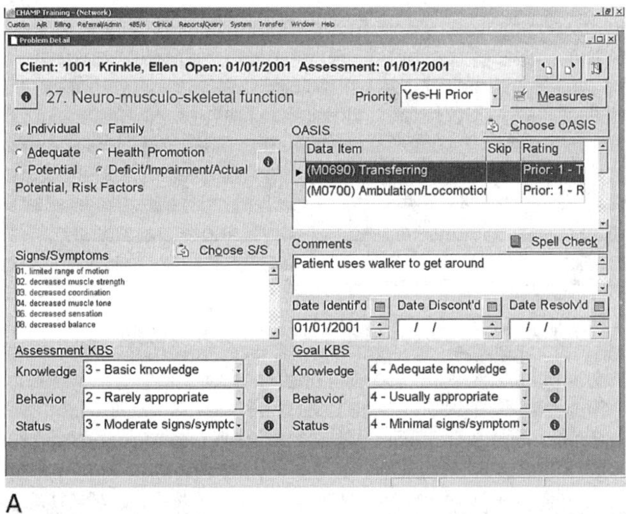

Figure 6-3 Screen images from CHAMP software (the client name is fictitious). **A,** Illustrates use of the Problem Classification Scheme and Problem Rating Scale for Outcomes.

Continued

Other vendors and groups are in various stages of developing diverse software applications based on the Omaha System. For example, Alternative Link developed ABC Codes to compare the economic and health outcomes of conventional, complementary, and alternative practices (http://www.alternativelink.com). The Omaha System is one of the classification systems included. Nurse practitioners are likely candidates to employ the ABC Codes for billing purposes. A team at FITNE in Athens, Ohio, developed and sold the Nightingale Tracker to many schools of nursing in the United States and in New Zealand (http://www.fitne.net/). Chapter 4 includes examples of student and educator adopters.

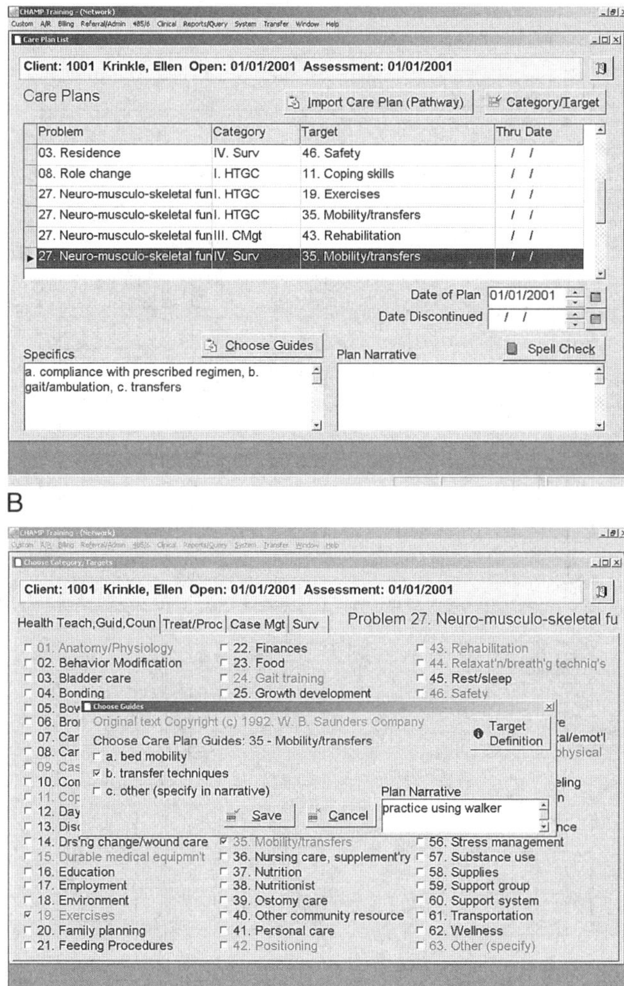

Figure 6-3, cont'd, **B,** Illustrates use of the Problem Classification Scheme and Intervention Scheme. **C,** Illustrates use of the Problem Classification Scheme and Intervention Scheme.
(Courtesy CHAMP Software, Inc., Mankato, Minnesota. Contact information: 115 E. Hickory Street, Suite 400, Mankato, Minnesota 56001; telephone: 507-388-4141; Web site: www.champsoftware.com.)

The New Zealand PDA initiative, KIWIN®, intended for use by students, is described in Omaha System Box 4-9. This software combines demographic data, New Zealand required data, and the Omaha System (Wilson & Roy, 2003).

IMPLEMENTATION: FUTURE PERSPECTIVES

Although most of the strategies in this chapter focus on implementation, work does not end when a clinical information system is installed and is functioning well. Time, energy, and

CHAPTER 6

15968

Case Management

Pt initial M. L. Age 23 Diagnosis

Gender ○ Male ● Female

Ethnicity ● Spanish origin/Hispanic ○ Non-Spanish/Non-Hispanic

Race ● White ○ Black ○ Asian/Pacific islander ○ American Indian/Eskimo ○ Other

Payer ○ Medicare ○ Medicaid ○ Other insurance ○ Self-pay ● Other

Problems	Modifiers	Signs & Symptoms	Intervention Categories	Intervention Targets	Outcomes	Adm	D/C
01	○ HP	0102	● Health Teaching	22	K	3	3
	○ P	04	○ Treatment				
	● A		● Case Manager	22	B	3	4
	○ Individual		○ Surveillance		S	3	4
	● Family						
06	○ HP	0102	● Health Teaching	1040	K	2	4
	○ P	0305	○ Treatment				
	● A		● Case Manager	40	B	2	3
	○ Individual		○ Surveillance		S	3	3
	● Family						
35	○ HP	0104	● Health Teaching	0237	K	1	3
	○ P	05	○ Treatment				
	● A		● Case Manager	2340	B	1	3
	○ Individual		○ Surveillance		S	2	3
	● Family						
	○ HP		○ Health Teaching		K		
	○ P		○ Treatment				
	○ A		○ Case Manager		B		
	○ Individual		○ Surveillance		S		
	○ Family						
	○ HP		○ Health Teaching		K		
	○ P		○ Treatment				
	○ A		○ Case Manager		B		
	○ Individual		○ Surveillance		S		
	○ Family						

Figure 6-4 One-page Omaha System summary form developed by the University of Colorado Health Sciences Center School of Nursing. The school purchased Teleform® technology, an optical character recognition system from Cardiff software, and developed a 1-page Omaha System summary form that can be scanned into the computer.

(Courtesy University of Colorado Health Sciences Center School of Nursing, Denver, Colorado. Contact information: 4200 East Ninth Street, Denver, Colorado 80262; telephone: 303-315-7687; e-mail: amy.barton@uchsc.edu).

money are essential to stay informed, maintain data and equipment, upgrade software and hardware, and convert clinical data to information and knowledge so it can be used for meaningful and accurate reports (Monsen & Martin, 2002a and 2002b; Monsen & Kerr, 2004). As noted by Westra in Omaha System Box 6-4, automation does not occur in a vacuum. Practitioners, managers, and administrators must continue to confront staffing, client, economic, and other challenges while they maintain an information technology vision.

The increasing sophistication of Omaha System users contributes to change. Organizations are starting to analyze and use their data, a definite step in the process of converting data to information (Monsen & Martin, 2002a; Monsen & Martin, 2002b; Monsen & Kerr, 2004). As they gain skills and use their data more frequently, they will ask for software modifications. For example, some users are now interested in documenting a "C" for caregiver when the *Knowledge* and/or *Behavior* rating is completed for the caregiver, rather than the client (i.e., K = 2/C; B = 3/C). The identity of the caregiver would be documented in free text.

The future is always unknown. Numerous authors and speakers offer educated guesses about anticipated practice, education, software, communications, and interface revolutions (Sibbald, 1995; Jenkins & Erdman, 1998; Katz, 1999; Carty, 2000; Elfrink, 2001; Institute of Medicine, 2001; Androwich et al., 2003; Institute of Medicine, 2003a; Institute of Medicine, 2003c; Pentland, 2003; Thede, 2003; Institute of Medicine, 2004). Tweed (2003) suggests that the most important advances will involve telehealth, point-of-care "palm-top" or handheld computing, digital imaging, microdiagnostics, wireless connectivity, Internet-based data access, and voice recognition. Wilhelm (2003) compares essential information technology investments and decisions to the ups and downs of riding a roller coaster. It is likely that organizations that purchase Omaha System software, as well as vendors who sell it, have memories that resemble those of roller coaster rides. Turley (2002) predicts changes that seem very plausible and present challenges to practitioners, educators, and researchers who use the Omaha System (Box 6-5). Strategic alliances that are created to facilitate standardized reporting, benchmarking, and quality improvement are expected to be part of the Omaha System's future. Such alliances would involve users' groups, researchers, and software vendors, as well as the partnerships described in Chapter 1.

Omaha System Boxes 6-5 and 6-6 are designed to offer additional predictions about the future. One message about the future is very clear in Box 6-5 and both of these Omaha

BOX 6-5 Future Informatics Trends

- Larger amounts of client information will be linked.
- Information will be able to be aggregated by several overlapping grouping cohorts: family, geography, workplace, genetics, risk factors, etc.
- Health care will become increasingly targeted to meet the needs of individuals; therapies will be based on one's genetics, lifestyle, preferences, etc.
- The amount of information will be overwhelming and will require computational assistance at all levels.
- The professions will either adapt to these changes in health care, or they will be replaced.
- Health care will be increasingly seen as knowledge work.
- Technology will pervade all aspects of health care.

From Turley, J.P. (2002). The future of health care informatics education. In Englebardt, S.P. & Nelson, R. (Eds.), *Health Care Informatics: An Interdisciplinary Approach* (pp. 479-503). St. Louis, Mosby.

System Boxes: dramatic and unyielding changes will occur. The changes will affect everyone: health care providers, administrators, managers, and organizations, as well as educators, students, and academic institutions. Providers, consumers, and payers will share information more freely and rapidly while protecting privacy and confidentiality. Preparing for change requires a positive attitude, willingness to be curious and be a continuous learner, serving as a teacher, and being patient (Tweed, 2003).

OMAHA SYSTEM BOX 6-5

Omaha System Experiences with Information Technology: Dreaming for the Future

Barbara A. Thomas, RN, MA, MS, FNP
Former Director, Learning Resource Center
Adjunct Professor of Nursing
Pace University
Pleasantville, New York

Jean F. Coppola, BS, MS, PhD
Adjunct, Technology Systems
Manager, Major Information Technology Initiatives
Pace University,
Pleasantville, New York

To dream is only human. . . .
To dream is merely natural. . . .
Author unknown

Learning about and obtaining FITNE Inc.'s Nightingale Tracker® was just the beginning; a beginning that we did not realize would have no real end. The journey started with our use of the Omaha System-based Tracker for our community health undergraduate nursing students and accelerated rapidly from a single-lane road to a multilane throughway! Our students quickly learned to use what they affectionately called their "Trackers," and carried them proudly in their brightly colored (lunch) bags. At the end of the semester, students returned their Trackers, immediately purchased their own personal digital assistants (PDAs) that were based on the Palm operating system, and found software applications on the Web that was free or very inexpensive to download.

Although not included in the Tracker, nursing students wanted a physical assessment application. FITNE had developed an early, unfinished prototype, and graciously allowed us to review the application. About the same time, a computer science professor started offering software engineering courses and instructed students to select real-world applications and work with "customers." Thus, the partnership between FITNE, Pace University, and the students changed the throughway to an expressway with interconnecting highways! As nursing students met with computer science students to test the application for usability, they wanted to push the program to its limits and planned for future flexibility. We hope to beta test our application in nursing schools, revise it, and make it available on a larger scale to improve data collection, planning, and quality services at the point of care.

The dream continues! We are communicating with an international team to migrate another program. Would it work well to put the Omaha System on a PDA? The answer is overwhelming – YES! Our vision includes new partnerships with a variety of organizations to develop yet to be determined computer applications for nursing programs of the future.

OMAHA SYSTEM BOX 6-6
Omaha System Experiences with Information Technology: Getting Ready for Change

David L. Rosebaugh, BS, MURP
CEO
CHAMP Software, Inc.
Mankato, Minnesota
Erin M. Young, BS, BA
Project Coordinator
CHAMP Software, Inc.
Mankato, Minnesota

Health care is changing at a rapid pace, but technology is changing much faster. Change is the one certainty of the future, and every practitioner, manager, administrator, institution, and agency must prepare. Noted futurist Arthur C. Clarke and Microsoft CEO Bill Gates have been quoted as saying that when it comes to technology, most people overestimate it in the short term and underestimate it in the long term.

Imagine the capabilities of today's tablet computer (a laptop computer designed to input data by writing on the screen with a stylus) reduced to a device the size of a legal pad that weighs less than 1 pound. Imagine using this device to read the daily newspaper, download electronic books, listen to college lectures in real-time, place a phone call with video, watch a movie or television show, or listen to music from any artist. Imagine being able to do it all from anywhere in the world, wireless. Imagine writing on the device or talking to it, and only as a last resort attaching a keyboard and pressing keys to input text. This is the dream of Microsoft's .NET platform, intended to share diverse data and information across diverse devices, anywhere.

Health care technology, increasingly referred to as *eHealth*, will experience dramatic changes in the near future. Some changes will be uniquely tailored to the cost-containment strategies required to deliver health care to an aging baby-boomer population. Increasingly, telehealth can enhance the efficiency and effectiveness of practitioners' visits. Other changes relate to advances in technology. Popularity of the personal digital assistants and tablets is expected to expand dramatically as they are transformed into new, multifunctional devices. Health services will be integrated via the Web through wireless devices. The ability to compare data and maintain sensitivity to differences in clients, target populations, providers, and terminologies will improve.

Where do you as a health care provider or student fit into this future? A posture of leaning forward to change, rather than rocking backward, is critical. Anticipate and embrace new technology developments, knowing that you are expected and required to share uniform data, while preserving privacy and security. The goal is better health care at lower cost. If you fully embrace this attitude, you will thrive.

SUMMARY

Change is the key word when considering information technology and health care. The amazing development and use of computers, telecommunications, and networks globally is changing the way people live and work. The pace is not expected to slow, but only to increase in speed. It is imperative that all health care providers become competent information technology users. They must collect, store, analyze, retrieve, and report client data and convert those data to information and knowledge as an important way to improve health care services and outcomes. They must develop partnerships with clients, families, and communities as they travel along the information superhighway.

REFERENCES

American Nurses Association. (2002). *Principles for Documentation.* PD-1. Washington, DC, American Nurses Publishing.

Anderson, L.K. & Stafford, C.J. (2002, January/February). The "big bang" implementation: Not for the faint of heart. *Computers in Nursing, 20*(1):14-22.

Androwich, I.M., Bickford, C.J., Button, P.S., Hunter, K.M., Murphy, J., & Sensmeier, J. (2003). *Clinical Information Systems: A Framework for Reaching the Vision.* Washington, DC, American Nurses Publishing.

Bakken, S. (2000). Standards for electronic health records and clinical decision support systems. In Carty, B. (Ed.), *Nursing Informatics Education for Practice* (pp. 179-203). New York, Springer.

Baldwin, D.R. (1998, February). Implementation of computerized documentation. *Home Health Care Management and Practice, 10*(2):43-51.

Bender, A. (1998, February). Management information systems: A required tool for survival. *Home Health Care Management and Practice, 10*(2):37-42.

Benner, P. (1984). *From Novice to Expert: Excellence and Power in Clinical Nursing Practice.* Menlo Park, California, Addison-Wesley.

Bowles, K.H. (1997, July/August). The barriers and benefits of nursing information systems. *Computers in Nursing, 15*(4):191-196.

Bozak, M.G. (2003, March/April). Using Lewin's Force Field Analysis in implementing a nursing information system. *CIN: Computers, Informatics, Nursing, 21*(2):80-85.

Bridis, T. (1998, April 16). Cyberspace is driving America's economy. *Pittsburgh Post Gazette, 71*(259):A-1.

Carty, B. (Ed.). (2000). *Nursing Informatics Education for Practice.* New York, Springer.

Case, J., Mowry, M., & Welebob, E. (2002, June). *The nursing shortage: Can technology help?* ihealthreports. California HealthCare Foundation. Retrieved March 20, 2004 from the Internet: http://www.chcf.org/documents/hospitals/NursingShortageTechnology.

Centers for Medicare and Medicaid Services. (2003). *Conditions of Participation: Home Health Agencies.* Retrieved September 1, 2003 from the Internet: http://www/cms.hhs.gov/ .

Clark, J. (1997, October). The elements of nursing are all but unknown. Inaugural Professional Lecture. University of Swansea, Swansea, Wales, United Kingdom.

Clark, J. (2003). *Naming Nursing: Proceedings of the First ACENDIO Ireland/UK Conference.* Bern, Switzerland, Hans Huber.

Coenen, A., McNeil, B., Bakken, S., Bickford, C., & Warren, J.J. (2001, November/December). Toward comparable nursing data: American Nurses Association criteria for data sets, classification systems, and nomenclatures. *Computers in Nursing, 19*(6):240-248.

Connolly, P.M. & Elfrink, V. (2002, August). Using information technology in community-based psychiatric nursing education: The SJSU/NT project. *Home Health Care Management and Practice, 14*(5):344-352.

Connolly, P.M., Huynh, M-P.T., & Gorney-Moreno, M.J. (1999, Winter). On the cutting edge or over the edge? Implementing the Nightingale Tracker. *On-line Journal of Nursing Informatics, 3*(1):20-30. Retrieved March 8, 2004 from the Internet: http://www.eaa-knowledge.com/ojni/ni/dm/ojni.html.

Crews, C., Connolly, K., Bruett, M., Whitted, P., & Beckwith, N. (1986, January-February). Computerized central intake: Streamlining community health-care admissions. *Nursing Economic$, 4*(1):31-36.

Du, C.M-S. (2003). Evaluation of the quality of home care nursing in Taiwan. (Unpublished doctoral dissertation. School of Public Health, University of South Carolina).

Elfrink, V. (1996, March/April). The information technology frontier: A call for pioneers. *Computers in Nursing, 14*(2):82-83, 88.

Elfrink, V. (2001, December). A look to the future: How emerging information technology will impact operations and practice. *Home Healthcare Nurse, 19*(12):751-757.

Elfrink, V., Bakken, S., Coenen, A., McNeil, B., & Bickford, C. (2001, February). Standardized nursing vocabularies: A foundation for quality care. *Seminars in Oncology Nursing, 17*(1):18-23.

Englebardt, S.P. & Nelson, R. (Eds.). (2002). *Health Care Informatics: An Interdisciplinary Approach.* St. Louis, Mosby.

Geraci, E.P. (1997, July/August). Computers in home care: Application of change theory. *Computers in Nursing, 15*(4):199-203.

Handly, M.J., Grubb, S.K., Keefe, N.A., & Martin, K.S. (2003, January). Essential activities for implementing a clinical information system in public health nursing. *Journal of Nursing Administration, 33*(1):14-16.

Healthcare Information and Management System Society. (2003a). *An Analysis of Health Information Standards Development Initiatives.* Retrieved September 8, 2003 from the Internet: http://www.himss.org/content/files.

Healthcare Information and Management System Society. (2003b). *Leadership Survey.* Retrieved November 3, 2003, from the Internet: http://www.himss.org/2003survey/.

Hettinger, B.J. & Brazile, R.P. (1992, May/June). A database design for community health data. *Computers in Nursing, 10*(3):109-115.

Hilz, L.M. (2000, November/December). The informatics nurse specialist as change agent: Application of Innovation-Diffusion Theory. *Computers in Nursing, 18*(6):272-281.

Hockenjos, G.J. & Wharton, A. (2001, December). Point-of-care training: Strategies for success. *Home Healthcare Nurse, 19*(12):766-773.

Humphrey, C.J. (2002a, October). The current status of home care nursing practice, Part 1. *Home Healthcare Nurse, 20*(10):677-684.

Humphrey, C.J. (2002b, November). The current status of home care nursing practice, Part 2. *Home Healthcare Nurse, 20*(11):741-747.

Humphreys, B.L., McCray, A.T., & Cheh, M.L. (1997, November/December). Evaluating the coverage of controlled health data terminologies: Report on the results of the NLM/AHCPR Large Scale Vocabulary Test. *Journal of the American Medical Informatics Association, 4*(6):484-500.

Hwang, J.-I., Cimino, J.J., & Bakken, S. (2003, July/August). Integrating nursing diagnostic concepts into the Medical Entities Dictionary using the ISO Reference Terminology Model for Nursing Diagnosis. *Journal of the American Medical Informatics Association, 10*(4):382-388.

Institute of Medicine. (1991). *The Computer-based Patient Record: An Essential Technology for Change.* Dick, R. and Steen, E. (Eds.). Washington, DC, National Academies Press.

Institute of Medicine. (2000). *To Err is Human: Building a Safer Health Care System.* Kohn, L.T., Corrigan, J.M., & Donaldson, M.S. (Eds.). Washington DC, National Academies Press.

Institute of Medicine. (2001). *Crossing the Quality Chasm.* Committee on Quality of Health Care in America. (Ed.). Washington, DC, National Academies Press.

Institute of Medicine. (2003a). *Health Professions Education: A Bridge to Quality.* Greiner, A.C. & Knebel, E. (Eds.). Washington, DC, National Academies Press.

Institute of Medicine. (2003b). *Key Capabilities of an Electronic Health Record System.* Retrieved November 3, 2003 from the Internet: http://www.nap.edu/catalog/1078.html?onpi_newsdoc073103.

Institute of Medicine. (2003c). *Who Will Keep the Public Healthy? Educating Public Health Professionals for the 21st Century.* Gebbie, K., Rosenstock, L. & Hernandez, L.M. (Eds.) Washington, DC, National Academies Press.

Institute of Medicine. (2004). *Keeping Patients Safe: Transforming the Work Environment of Nurses.* Page, A. (Ed.). Washington, DC, National Academies Press.

Jenkins, J. & Erdman, K. (1998, February). Web-based documentation systems. *Home Health Care Management and Practice, 10*(2):52-61.

Johnson, N. (2003, July 24). *National Health Information Infrastructure Act of 2003.* Retrieved November 3, 2003 from the Internet: http://www.house.gov/nancyjohnson/pr_nhii.htm.

Jonkergouw, P.H. (1991). Computerisation of the nursing process. In Hovenga, E.J.S., Hannah, K.J., McCormick, K.A., & Ronald, J.S. (Eds.), *Nursing Informatics '91: Proceedings of the Fourth International Conference* (pp. 457-463). New York, Springer.

Journal of Biomedical Informatics, 36(4/5). (2003, August/October). Entire iessue.

Katz, R.N. (1999). *Dancing with the Devil.* San Francisco, Jossey-Bass.

Koch, L.A. (1998, September). Eight essential steps for effective data collection and use. *Caring, XVII*(9):58-67.

Landro, L. (2002, August 15). Electronic medical records call for common language by doctors. *Wall Street Journal, CCXL*(33):D3.

Landro, L. (2003, July 1). Wired patients. *Wall Street Journal, CCXLII*(1):A10.

Larrabee, J.H., Boldreghini, S., Elder-Sorrells, K., Turner, Z.M., Wender, R.G., Hart, J.M., & Lenzi, P.S. (2001, March/April). Evaluation of documentation before and after implementation of a nursing information system in an acute care hospital. *Computers in Nursing, 19*(2):56-65.

Larrabee, S.B. (1999, August). Benner's Novice to Expert Nursing Theory applied to the implementation of laptops in the home care setting. *Home Health Care Management and Practice, 11*(4):41-47.

Lewin, K. (1951). *Field Theory in Social Science.* New York, Harper and Brothers.

Mallard, C.O. (2000). Nursing informatics in the home health care environment. In Carty, B. (Ed.). *Nursing Informatics Education for Practice* (pp. 252-270). New York, Springer.

Martin, K.S. (1982, November/December). A client classification system adaptable for computerization. *Nursing Outlook, 30*(9):515-517.

Martin, K.S. (2004, April). Your mission. *Home Health Care Management and Practice, 16*(3):170.

Martin, K.S., Baisch, M.J., & Bell-Calvin, J. (2003, January). Data mining produces gold. *Nursing Matters, 14*(1): 6-7.

Martin, K.S. & Scheet, N.J. (1985). The Omaha System: Implications for costing out nursing. In Shaffer, F.A. (Ed.), *Costing out Nursing: Pricing our Product* (pp. 197-206). New York, McGraw-Hill.

Martin, K.S. & Scheet, N.J. (1992a). *The Omaha System: Applications for Community Health Nursing.* Philadelphia, Saunders.

Martin, K.S. & Scheet, N.J. (1992b). *The Omaha System: A Pocket Guide for Community Health Nursing.* Philadelphia, Saunders.

Medical Records Institute. (2003). *MRI Fifth Annual Survey of HER Trends and Usage.* Retrieved November 3, 2003, from the Internet: http://www.medrecinst.com/resources/survey/results03/index.shtml.

Monsen, K.A. & Kerr, M.J. (2004, April). Mining quality documentation data for golden outcomes. *Home Health Care Management and Practice, 16*(3):192-199.

Monsen, K.A. & Martin, K.S. (2002a, April/June). Developing an outcomes management program in a public health department. *Outcomes Management, 6*(2):62-66.

Monsen, K.A. & Martin, K.S. (2002b, July/September). Using an outcomes management program in a public health department. *Outcomes Management, 6*(3):120-124.

Nelson, R.M. (2004, April). Measuring outcomes in home health care: Beyond the OASIS data set. *Home Health Care Management and Practice, 16*(3):200-205.

Nightingale Tracker Clinical Field Test Nurse Team. (2000, May/June). A comparison of teaching strategies for integrating information technology into clinical nursing education. *Nurse Educator, 25*(3):136-144.

O'Carroll, P.W., Yasnoff, W.A., Ward, M.E., Ripp, L.H., & Martin, E.L (Eds.). (2003). *Public Health Informatics and Information Systems.* New York, Springer.

Omaha System Web site. (2004). Retrieved March 8, 2004 from the Internet: http://www.omahasystem.org.

Pearce, K., Castleman, J., & Elfrink, V. (1999, June). One nurse's experience with technology. *Home Healthcare Nurse, 17*(6):361-372.

Pentland, A. (2003, March). Take two cell phones and call me in the morning: A glimpse into the future of health care technology. *Caring, XXII*(3):8-10.

Pew Internet and American Life Report. (2003, July 16). *Internet health resources.* Retrieved November 3, 2003 from the Internet: http://www.pewinternet.org/reports/toc.asp?Report=95.

Polanyi, M. (1967). *The Tacit Dimension.* London, Cox and Wyman.

Reichley, M. (2001, March/April). Reach for real-time data. *Success in Home Care, V*(2):18-25.

Rosebaugh, D.L. (2004, April). Getting ready for the software in your future. *Home Health Care Management and Practice, 16*(3):228-234.

Rogers, E.M. (1995). *Diffusion of Innovation*, 4th ed. New York, The Free Press.

Sawyer, L.M., Berkowitz, B., Haber, J.E., Larrabee, J.H., Marino, B.L., Martin, K.S., Mason, K.P., Mastal, M.F., Nilsson, M.W., Waldridge, S.E., & Walker, M.K. (2002, April/June). Expanding American Nurses Association quality indicators to community-based practices. *Outcomes Management, 6*(2):53-61.

Sensmeier, J. (2002). Advancing the state of data integration in healthcare. *Healthcare Information and Management Systems Society.* Retrieved November 26, 2003 from the Internet: http://www.himss.org/content/files/AdvDataIntegration.pdf.

Sibbald, B. (1995, March). 2020 vision of nursing. *The Canadian Nurse, 91*(3):33-36.

Sienkiewicz, J. (2004, June). The Quality Network Adverse-Event Benchmarking Project: A New Jersey perspective. *Home Health Care Management and Practice, 16*(4):280-285.

Sloan, H.L. & Delahoussaye, C.P. (2003, January/February). Clinical application of the Omaha System with the Nightingale Tracker. *Nurse Educator, 28*(1):15-17.

Slotnick, H.B. & Shershneva, M.B. (2002, Fall). Use of theory to interpret elements of change. *Journal of Continuing Education for Health Professionals*, *22*(4):197-204.

Solovy, A. (2002). Forward progress: Most wired survey and benchmark study. *Hospitals and Health Networks.* Retrieved November 3, 2003 from the Internet: http://www.hospitalconnect.com/hhnmostwired/archives/forward_prog.

Souther, E. (2001, March/April). Implementation of the electronic medical record: The team approach. *Computers in Nursing*, *19*(2):47-55.

Standish Group International, Inc. (1999). *Chaos: A recipe for success.* Retrieved August 4, 2003 from the Internet: http://pm2go.com/sample_research/PDFpages/chaos1998.pdf.

Stone, M. (2000, March 24). Study shows 300 Mil worldwide Internet users. *ACM TechNews*, *2*(34). Retrieved November 3, 2003, from the Internet: http://www-2.cs.cmu.edu.

Stricklin, M.L.V., Niles, S.A., Struk, C., & Jones, S. (2000, September). What nurses and managers expect from point of care technology. *Home Healthcare Nurse*, *18*(8):514-523.

Thede, L.Q. (2003). *Informatics and Nursing: Opportunities and Challenges*, 2nd ed. Philadelphia, Lippincott, Williams, and Wilkins.

Thomas, B.A., Coppola, J.F., & Feldman, H. (2001, Spring/Summer). Adopting handheld computers for community-based curriculum: Case study. *Journal of the New York State Nurses Association*, *32*(1):4-6.

Tidd, C.W. (1998, February). From data to information: Management tools for home health care clinical directors. *Home Health Care Management and Practice*, *10*(2):1-10.

Tressa, S.S. & Barber, D.A. (2001, September). Home care automation: An agency looks back. *Caring, XX*(9): 36-38.

Turley, J.P. (2002). The future of health care informatics education. In Englebardt, S.P. & Nelson, R. (Eds.), *Health Care Informatics: An Interdisciplinary Approach* (pp. 479-503). St. Louis, Mosby.

Tweed, S.C. (2003, October). Seven performance-accelerating technologies that will shape the future of home care. *Home Healthcare Nurse*, *21*(10):647-650.

U.S. Department of Commerce. (2002, February). *A nation on-line: How Americans are expanding their use of the Internet.* Retrieved November 3, 2003, from the Internet: http://www.ntia.doc.gov/ntiahome/dn/html/toc.htm.

U.S. Department of Health and Human Services. (2003, July 1). *HHS launches new efforts to promote paperless health care system.* Retrieved November 3, 2003, from the Internet: http://www.aspe.os.dhhs.gov/sp/nhii/News/NHIIJu11_03.htm.

Wang, S.J., Middleton, B., Prosser, L.A., Bardon, C.G., Spurr, C.D., Carchidi, P.J., Kittler, A.F., Goldszer, F.C., Fairchild, D.G., Sussman, A.J., Kuperman, G.J., & Bates, D.W. (2003, April). A cost-benefit analysis of electronic medical records in primary care. *The American Journal of Medicine, 114*(5):397-403.

Westra, B. (1996, November/December). Making the right choice: Computerizing clinical information. *The Remington Report*, *4*(6):32-35.

Westra, B.L., Martin, K.S., & Swan, A.R. (1996, August). Recognizing the need for standardized documentation and classifying patient needs. *Home Health Care Management and Practice*, *8*(5):24-31.

Westra, B.L. & Raup, G. (1995, August). Computerized charting: An essential tool for survival. *Caring*, *XIV*(8): 57-61.

Westra, B. & Solomon, D. (1999, Winter). The Omaha System: Bridging home care and technology. *On-line Journal of Nursing Informatics, 3*(1):12-14. Retrieved March 8, 2004, from the Internet: http://www.eaa-knowledge.com/ojni/ni/dm/ojni.html.

Wilhelm, L. (2003, March). Untangling home care's Gordion Knot. *Caring, XXII*(3):18-19.

Williams, T. (2002, May). Home care's changing technology perspective. *Home Care Automation Report*, *7*(5):4-7.

Wilson, S. (2002). Development of a personal digital assistant (PDA) as point-of-care technology in nursing education. *Journal of Mobile Informatics.* Retrieved November 3, 2003, from the Internet: http://www.pdacortex.com/pda_nursing_education.htm.

Wilson, S.K. & Roy, D. (2003). KIWIN: An automated documentation solution for nursing education. In Marin, H.D.F., Marques, E.P., Hovenga, E. & Goossen, W. (Eds.), *NI 2003: 8th International Conference in Nursing Informatics* (p. 707). Rio de Janeiro, Brazil, E-papers Servicos Editorials Ltd.

Woods, A. & Grant, T. (1995). *Reason in Revolt: Marxism and Modern Science.* London, Wellread.

Zielstorff, R.D., Hudgings, C.I., & Grobe, S.J. (1993). Next-Generation Nursing Information Systems: Essential Characteristics for Professional Practice. Washington, DC, American Nurses Publishing.

SECTION

II

User's Guide to the Omaha System

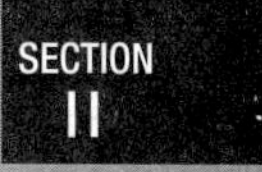

INTRODUCTION

The User's Guide is a reference designed for many purposes. It can help practitioners and students learn to use the Omaha System. During their introduction to the User's Guide, practitioners and students should also read Chapter 2, Appendix A, the Glossary, and receive an orientation to the Omaha System. Chapter 2 addresses the basic "what, why, when, and how" to facilitate understanding, and Appendix A includes the structure, terms, and definitions. Experienced practitioners and students should also use the User's Guide as a reference to complete their daily documentation accurately and consistently. Experienced users may benefit from reading the diverse case studies in Appendix B and the details about the revised Omaha System in Appendix E, since they need to change their recording patterns to reflect the revisions. Provider organization directors, managers, and quality improvement staff and faculty members should read the previously mentioned sections and become familiar with the rest of the book. Such reading will help them lead orientation discussions, teach use of clinical information software that includes the revised Omaha System, update their manual records, and modify their data analysis protocols so their organization's outcomes management program produces standardized, valid, and reliable information. For example, it is likely that user organizations will need to revise their agency documentation and quality improvement policies to reflect the addition of the modifier *Community* and retirement of the problem *Technical procedure.*

The User's Guide is organized according to the Omaha System's 42 problems and has three major sections: the Problem Classification Scheme, the Intervention Scheme, and the Problem Rating Scale for Outcomes.

Practitioners use the **Problem Classification Scheme** section for client assessment. It includes problem definitions, examples of problem modifiers *(Health Promotion, Potential, and Actual)*, signs/symptoms, and related medical diagnoses from the ICD-9-CM coding references. The modifier examples reflect three diverse themes and are intended to describe a small representative sample of individuals, families, and communities. If multidisciplinary users understand the concepts included in the examples, they will be able to replace details with those from their own clients and select the correct modifiers. The related medical diagnoses are suggestions for users to consider as they select codes for regulatory or reimbursement purposes. However, when submitting ICD-9 codes, users must refer to coding manuals and select more detailed, multidecimal choices. Furthermore, because many global organizations use ICD-10 codes, they will need to refer to those manuals.

Practitioners use the **Intervention Scheme** section when they develop a client care plan or document their activities. The suggested care planning/intervention guides are comprised of the categories, targets, and client-specific information statements. While the arrangement of targets and statements represents the most frequent practice patterns used by hundreds of multidisciplinary practitioners, users may follow guidelines and combine categories, targets, and information statements in many additional ways. Each selected target is accompanied by a list of "abc" statements, referred to as *client-specific information statements*, which are designed for use with individuals, families, and communities. Practitioners should select a small number of targets and statements to develop a care plan or document a single client encounter. For example, while only one or two generic support groups are mentioned in the case management sections, practitioners need to identify valuable resources available in their facility or community. Because the client-specific information statements are not a formal part of the Omaha System, they do not appear in Appendix A. After companies receive copyright permission from the publishing company, the statements are usually incorporated in software so users can quickly scan and select relevant information from a pick list.

Practitioners use the **Problem Rating Scale for Outcomes** to track client change over time. The examples for *Knowledge, Behavior,* and *Status* are focused and detailed, having three different themes for each problem that flow from most negative to most positive. The examples were developed as a template or conceptual bridge to help users apply the general meaning of a numeric rating to their own specific clients. This approach seems to help most new and experienced users; they are able to replace details such as "wets bed" with "has temper tantrum" or "walker" with "wheelchair." As noted for the problem modifier examples, users need to read the examples, practice adapting them to case studies, and discuss their conclusions with their colleagues. If organizations schedule practice and discussion opportunities initially and at periodic intervals, their practitioners' documentation entries will become more accurate and consistent, providing the necessary foundation for analyzing aggregate data and using an outcomes management program.

When the three components of the Omaha System are used to organize client records, the standardized terms of this Guide and some additional, limited narrative comments are needed for each component. A few details should be recorded to explain signs/symptoms, client-specific information, and ratings. For example, ratings are intended to reflect the *Knowledge, Behavior,* and *Status* of the individual for whom the problem was identified. Sometimes, as in the case of an infant's nutritional problem, the *Knowledge* specific to that problem does not apply to the infant but to the infant's caregiver. Documentation should reflect the caregiver's *Knowledge* and the infant's *Behavior* and *Status.* Users should note this exception in their documentation as described in Chapter 2.

In some organizations, practitioners developed pathways or program-specific examples, using the terms of the Omaha System and following the patterns of the User's Guide. Such involvement encourages practitioners to gain a sense of ownership and deeper understanding of the Omaha System. It also encourages them to include terms and details in the client-specific information statements designed for use with individuals, families, and communities that are easily understood and useful within their own organization. In addition, readers are encouraged to personalize their copy of the User's Guide by listing names, phone numbers, and addresses of frequently used contacts in the case management sections, or by establishing a computerized data base.

Environmental Domain

INCOME

Problem Classification Scheme

Definition. Money from wages, pensions, subsidies, interest, dividends, or other sources available for living and health care expenses.

Modifiers (select one):

Health Promotion

Example: employed individual wants guidance on budgeting and money management to prepare for retirement in 10 years.

Potential

Example: has newly diagnosed chronic illness; health insurance covers only the first year of treatment and medications.

Actual

Example: "partner fired from job last week" or "small pension is only source of income" suggest the sign/symptom *low/no income*.

SIGNS/SYMPTOMS OF ACTUAL (select those that apply)

- low/no income
- uninsured medical expenses
- difficulty with money management
- able to buy only necessities
- difficulty buying necessities
- other

Related Medical Diagnoses. V Codes Supplementary Classification of Factors Influencing Health Status and Contact with Health Services: Persons Encountering Health Services in Other Circumstances (V60-V68).

Intervention Scheme

Teaching, Guidance, and Counseling (suggested care planning/intervention guides)

behavior modification:

a. addictive behaviors
b. gambling
c. compulsive spending
d. other

finances:

a. crisis intervention/short-range planning
b. long-range planning/decision making
c. budgeting
d. community resources
e. family resources
f. other

other:

Treatments and Procedures (suggested care planning/intervention guides)

finances:

a. comprehensive analysis and action plan
b. other

other:

Case Management (suggested care planning/intervention guides)

finances:

a. community resources
b. pension/entitlement
c. governmental health/social service assistance
d. private social service agency
e. private insurance
f. health maintenance organization
g. Red Cross
h. charitable organizations
i. spiritual/faith communities
j. other

legal system:

a. public defender
b. attorney referral service
c. legal assistance
d. governmental child-adult protective services
e. guardian/conservator
f. financial support enforcement
g. law enforcement
h. other

social work/counseling care:

a. evaluation
b. schedule/provide services
c. coordination among providers
d. other

other:

Surveillance (suggested care planning/intervention guides)

finances:

a. income versus expenses
b. use of available resources
c. other

social work/counseling care:

a. receives care when scheduled
b. adequate/appropriate care
c. follows plan of care
d. other

other:

Problem Rating Scale for Outcomes

Knowledge

1-No knowledge
Example: cannot identify sources/amounts of expenses and income

2-Minimal knowledge
Example: identifies some sources/amounts of income and a few expenses

3-Basic knowledge
Example: identifies all sources/amounts of income and some expenses

4-Adequate knowledge
Example: identifies all sources/amounts of income and expenses
5-Superior knowledge
Example: understands current financial situation and can predict future needs

Behavior
1-Not appropriate behavior
Example: spends impulsively
2-Rarely appropriate behavior
Example: buys luxuries and some necessities, not interested in assistance programs
3-Inconsistently appropriate behavior
Example: buys necessities and few luxuries, is interested in idea of budget, does not use assistance programs
4-Usually appropriate behavior
Example: begins to develop, follow budget, applies for/uses some assistance programs
5-Consistently appropriate behavior
Example: follows budget consistently; has maximized income assistance resources

Status
1-Extreme signs/symptoms
Example: evicted from residence after not paying rent, no source of income or health care
2-Severe signs/symptoms
Example: in residence but utilities disconnected due to nonpayment, no source of income or health care
3-Moderate signs/symptoms
Example: has utilities but no consistent source of income or health care
4-Minimal signs/symptoms
Example: consistent income, decreasing debts, sometimes has source of health care
5-No signs/symptoms
Example: expenses do not exceed income, has consistent source of income and health care

SANITATION

Problem Classification Scheme

Definition. Environmental cleanliness and precautions against infection and disease.
Modifiers (select one):

Health Promotion
Example: expresses interest in proper food storage methods.
Potential
Example: many flies in area, and window screens need repair.
Actual
Example: the sign/symptom *inadequate food storage/disposal* is noted for "last night's meal on the kitchen table during this afternoon's visit." The sign/symptom *foul odor* is described by "dog excreta inside home," or "soiled diapers stored in open box and have strong odor."

SIGNS/SYMPTOMS OF ACTUAL (select those that apply)

- soiled living area
- inadequate food storage/disposal

- insects/rodents
- foul odor
- inadequate water supply
- inadequate sewage disposal
- inadequate laundry facilities
- allergens
- infectious/contaminating agents
- presence of mold
- excessive pets
- other

Related Medical Diagnoses. Infectious and Parasitic Diseases (001-139). Endocrine, Nutritional, and Metabolic Diseases, and Immunity Disorders (240-279). Diseases of the Nervous System and Sense Organs: Inflammatory Diseases of the Central Nervous System (320-326). Injury and Poisoning (800-999). V Codes Supplementary Classification of Factors Influencing Health Status and Contact with Health Services (V01-V83).

Intervention Scheme

Teaching, Guidance, and Counseling (suggested care planning/intervention guides)

environment:
a. relationship to disease
b. proper food handling
c. disposal of contaminated materials
d. allergy-proofing
e. pet management
f. other

infection precautions:
a. identify potential sources of infection
b. hand washing
c. disposal of soiled/contaminated materials
d. clean environment
e. other

safety:
a. sanitary disposal procedures
b. other

other:

Treatments and Procedures (suggested care planning/intervention guides)

environment:
a. disposal of contaminated materials
b. other

safety:
a. implement sanitary disposal procedures
b. other

specimen collection:
a. water
b. other

other:

Case Management (suggested care planning/intervention guides)

community outreach worker services:

a. evaluation
b. schedule/provide services
c. coordination among providers
d. other

environment:

a. public housing
b. health department
c. real estate agency
d. citizen complaint office
e. landlord
f. other

homemaking/housekeeping:

a. evaluation
b. schedule/provide services
c. coordination among providers
d. other

interpreter/translator services:

a. evaluation
b. schedule/provide services
c. coordination among providers
d. other

nursing care:

a. evaluation
b. schedule/provide services
c. coordination among providers
d. other

other community resources:

a. inspector/sanitarian
b. other

social work/counseling care:

a. evaluation
b. schedule/provide services
c. coordination among providers
d. other

other:

Surveillance (suggested care planning/intervention guides)

environment:

a. cleanliness
b. disposal of contaminated materials
c. other

nursing care:

a. receives care when scheduled
b. adequate/appropriate care
c. follows plan of care
d. other

safety:
a. uses sanitary disposal procedures
b. other
social work/counseling care:
a. receives care when scheduled
b. adequate/appropriate care
c. follows plan of care
d. other
other:

Problem Rating Scale for Outcomes

Knowledge

1-No knowledge
Example: does not understand relationship between excessive soil, insects/rodents, pets, contaminating agents, and health
2-Minimal knowledge
Example: understands some health hazards caused by excessive soil, insects/rodents, pets, and contaminating agents
3-Basic knowledge
Example: understands that excessive soil, insects/rodents, pets, and contaminating agents are hazardous to health but unable to identify methods to improve sanitation
4-Adequate knowledge
Example: understands some methods for eliminating insects/rodents and importance of proper sanitation
5-Superior knowledge
Example: knows appropriate methods, materials, and timing required for eliminating insects/rodents and maintaining proper sanitation

Behavior

1-Not appropriate behavior
Example: almost always disposes of soiled materials and refuse using unsafe procedures
2-Rarely appropriate behavior
Example: frequently disposes of soiled materials and refuse using unsafe procedures
3-Inconsistently appropriate behavior
Example: occasionally disposes of soiled materials and refuse using safe procedures
4-Usually appropriate behavior
Example: usually disposes of soiled materials and refuse using safe procedures
5-Consistently appropriate behavior
Example: consistently disposes of soiled materials and refuse using safe procedures

Status

1-Extreme signs/symptoms
Example: living area grossly unsanitary with garbage, excrement, insects/rodents, and excessive clutter
2-Severe signs/symptoms
Example: living area rarely clean; some insects/rodents and contaminants

3-Moderate signs/symptoms
Example: living area sometimes clean; some insects/rodents and contaminants
4-Minimal signs/symptoms
Example: living area clean most of time; few insects/rodents and contaminants
5-No signs/symptoms
Example: living area consistently clean; no insects/rodents and contaminants

RESIDENCE

Problem Classification Scheme

Definition. Living area.
Modifiers (select one):
Health Promotion
Example: middle-aged individual considers modifying the residence for future safety.
Potential
Example: uses electric space heater.
Actual
Example: "refrigerator located in front of door" and "many boxes and newspapers stored along walls" suggest the signs/symptoms *inadequate/obstructed exits/entries* and *cluttered living space.*

SIGNS/SYMPTOMS OF ACTUAL (select those that apply):

- structurally unsound
- inadequate heating/cooling
- steep/unsafe steps
- inadequate/obstructed exits/entries
- cluttered living space
- unsafe storage of dangerous objects/substances
- unsafe mats/throw rugs
- inadequate safety devices
- presence of lead-based paint
- unsafe appliances/equipment
- inadequate/crowded living space
- exposed wiring
- structural barriers
- homeless
- other

Related Medical Diagnoses. Injury and Poisoning (800-999). V Codes Supplementary Classification of Factors Influencing Health Status and Contact with Health Services (V01-V83). E Codes Supplementary Classification of External Causes of Injury and Poisoning (E800-E999).

Intervention Scheme

Teaching, Guidance, and Counseling (suggested care planning/intervention guides)
home:
a. long-range planning/decision making
b. community resources
c. crisis intervention/short-range planning
d. ramps

e. needed repairs
f. maintain adequate heating/cooling
g. modify for accessibility
h. other

legal system:

a. governmental child-adult protective services
b. health department
c. building permits/inspections
d. law enforcement
e. other

safety:

a. store/remove unsafe substance
b. remove mats/throw rugs
c. clear exits
d. fire prevention/safety
e. weather precautions
f. location/use of appliances/cleaning equipment
g. storage of weapons
h. other

other:

Treatments and Procedures (suggested care planning/intervention guides)

other:

Case Management (suggested care planning/intervention guides)

durable medical equipment:

a. bathroom safety devices
b. ramps
c. other

home:

a. community support systems
b. advocacy
c. public/governmental housing
d. organizations for elders
e. real estate agency
f. retirement home/assisted living
g. residential living
h. board and care homes
i. housing designed for functional limitations
j. landlord
k. other

legal system:

a. governmental child-adult protective services
b. health department
c. building permits/inspections
d. lawyer referral service
e. legal assistance
f. law enforcement
g. other

nursing care
a. evaluation
b. schedule/provide services
c. other
occupational therapy care:
a. evaluation
b. schedule/provide services
c. other
physical therapy care:
a. evaluation
b. schedule/provide services
c. other
other:

Surveillance (suggested care planning/intervention guides)
home:
a. state of repair
b. adequacy of space
c. accessibility
d. other
safety:
a. home safety assessment
b. location/use of hazards
c. location/use of appliances/equipment
d. other
other:

Problem Rating Scale for Outcomes

Knowledge
1-No knowledge
Example: unaware of hazards in living area
2-Minimal knowledge
Example: identifies some hazards in living area
3-Basic knowledge
Example: identifies hazards in living area but no solutions
4-Adequate knowledge
Example: identifies hazards in living area and a partial plan for correction
5-Superior knowledge
Example: identifies hazards in living area and solution

Behavior
1-Not appropriate behavior
Example: takes no action to improve unsafe and inaccessible bathroom
2-Rarely appropriate behavior
Example: arranges items in bathroom so accessible, but does not address safety hazards
3-Inconsistently appropriate behavior
Example: installs bathroom grab bars, but other safety hazards exist
4-Usually appropriate behavior
Example: installs walk-in shower and plans to address minimal safety concerns

5-Consistently appropriate behavior
Example: modifies bathroom structural and safety barriers or moves to adequate residence

Status
1-Extreme signs/symptoms
Example: home needs major repair, is dangerous for residents
2-Severe signs/symptoms
Example: home has extreme clutter and is crowded
3-Moderate signs/symptoms
Example: home has moderate clutter, some exits obstructed
4-Minimal signs/symptoms
Example: home has minimal clutter, no exits obstructed
5-No signs/symptoms
Example: home is functional, adequate size for number of residents

NEIGHBORHOOD/WORKPLACE SAFETY

Problem Classification Scheme

Definition. Freedom from illness, injury, or loss in the community or place of employment.

Modifiers (select one):
Health Promotion
Example: new parent requests advice regarding appropriate placement of playground for toddler.
Potential
Example: suspected illegal drug activity near residence.
Actual
Example: "a pack of dogs is roaming the neighborhood" near individual or family's home indicating the sign/symptom *uncontrolled/dangerous/infected animals.*
Signs/Symptoms of Actual (select those that apply):
- high crime rate
- high pollution level
- uncontrolled/dangerous/infected animals
- inadequate/unsafe play/exercise areas
- inadequate space/resources to foster health
- threats/reports of violence
- physical hazards
- vehicle/traffic hazards
- chemical hazards
- radiological hazards
- other

Related Medical Diagnoses. Infectious and Parasitic Diseases (001-139). Injury and Poisoning (800-999). V Codes Supplementary Classification of Factors Influencing Health Status and Contact with Health Services (V01-V83). E Codes Supplementary Classification of External Causes of Injury and Poisoning (E800-E999).

Intervention Scheme

Teaching, Guidance, and Counseling (suggested care planning/intervention guides)

environment:
a. health department
b. humane society
c. other

home:
a. landlord
b. real estate agency
c. other

other community resources:
a. neighborhood watch group
b. school parent-teacher organization
c. other

safety:
a. neighborhood watch group
b. law enforcement
c. avoid high-risk locations/times
d. other

other:

Treatments and Procedures (suggested care planning/intervention guides)

specimen collection:
a. radon
b. animals
c. other

other:

Case Management (suggested care planning/intervention guides)

environment:
a. law enforcement
b. health department
c. humane society
d. other

home:
a. landlord
b. other

safety:
a. neighborhood watch group
b. community safety organization
c. other

other:

Surveillance (suggested care planning/intervention guides)

environment:
a. reports of hazards
b. other

safety:
a. frequency of incidents
b. chemical reports
c. crime reports/locations
d. other
other:

Problem Rating Scale for Outcomes

Knowledge
1-No knowledge
Example: unaware of dangerous animals in neighborhood
2-Minimal knowledge
Example: some awareness of dangerous animals in neighborhood
3-Basic knowledge
Example: describes dangerous animals in neighborhood but no solutions
4-Adequate knowledge
Example: identifies partial plan for correcting dangerous animals in neighborhood
5-Superior knowledge
Example: identifies reasonable solutions for dangerous animals in neighborhood

Behavior
1-Not appropriate behavior
Example: only wears required protective gear when supervisors visit work site
2-Rarely appropriate behavior
Example: seldom wears protective gear at work site
3-Inconsistently appropriate behavior
Example: occasionally wears protective gear at work site
4-Usually appropriate behavior
Example: wears protective gear most of the time at work site
5-Consistently appropriate behavior
Example: wears protective gear consistently at work site

Status
1-Extreme signs/symptoms
Example: extremely unsafe neighborhood; with high crime rate
2-Severe signs/symptoms
Example: crime rate high but deceasing since neighborhood targeted for improvement
3-Moderate signs/symptoms
Example: moderate crime rate in neighborhood; few residents/landlords participating in organized efforts to decrease crime rate
4-Minimal signs/symptoms
Example: safety precautions (locks and lights) have decreased crime rate in neighborhood
5-No signs/symptoms
Example: low crime rate, active neighborhood watch group

Psychosocial Domain

COMMUNICATION WITH COMMUNITY RESOURCES

Problem Classification Scheme

Definition. Interaction between the individual/family/community and social service organizations, schools, and businesses in regard to services, information, and goods/supplies.

Modifiers (select one):

Health Promotion

Example: young adult wants to learn what services are available from local agencies.

Potential

Example: elderly man moved to the city from the farm recently.

Actual

Example: the signs/symptoms *unfamiliar with options/procedures for obtaining services* and *educational barrier* are appropriate for comments such as "I want to finish high school, but don't know how I can do it and take care of my baby."

SIGNS/SYMPTOMS OF ACTUAL (select those that apply):

- unfamiliar with options/procedures for obtaining services
- difficulty understanding roles/regulations of service providers
- unable to communicate concerns to provider
- dissatisfaction with services
- inadequate/unavailable resources
- language barrier
- cultural barrier
- educational barrier
- transportation barrier
- limited access to care/services/goods
- unable to use/has inadequate communication devices/equipment
- other

PSY

Related Medical Diagnoses. Mental Disorders (290-319). V Codes Supplementary Classification of Factors Influencing Health Status and Contact with Health Services (V01-V83).

Intervention Scheme

Teaching, Guidance, and Counseling (suggested care planning/intervention guides)

behavior modification:

a. new skills for new roles
b. recognize/change personal patterns
c. other

communication:

a. strategies to convey requests
b. procedures to obtain services
c. voices dissatisfaction with services
d. other

continuity of care:

a. description of available services
b. steps to increase continuity

c. other

day care/respite:

a. options
b. procedures to obtain services
c. benefits
d. other

durable medical equipment:

a. regular/adapted telephone
b. regular/adapted computer
c. telehealth monitor
d. lock/security/alert systems
e. wander/fall alert systems
f. safety devices such as grab bars
g. assistive devices such as reachers and long-handled shoe horns
h. ambulation equipment
i. toileting equipment
j. other

education:

a. options (traditional, special needs, correspondence, on-line)
b. procedures to obtain services
c. benefits
d. complete educational plan
e. other

employment:

a. options
b. procedures to obtain services
c. benefits
d. other

genetics:

a. family history
b. resources for testing/screening
c. other

interaction:

a. roles of service providers
b. coordination among providers
c. other

interpreter/translator services:

a. procedures to obtain services
b. other

legal system:

a. options
b. procedures to obtain services
c. benefits
d. other

other community resources:

a. eligibility requirements
b. resources for goods, services, and information
c. other

other:

Treatments and Procedures (suggested care planning/intervention guides)

other:

Case Management (suggested care planning/intervention guides)

community outreach worker services:
a. evaluation
b. schedule/provide services
c. coordination among providers
d. other

day care/respite:
a. programs for adults/elders
b. programs for children
c. other

durable medical equipment:
a. communicate with sources
b. other

education:
a. programs for adults/elders
b. programs for children
c. other

employment:
a. programs for adolescents/adults/elders
b. other

genetics:
a. evaluation
b. schedule services
c. other

interaction:
a. roles of service providers
b. coordination among providers
c. other

interpreter/translator services:
a. evaluation
b. schedule/provide services
c. client advocacy
d. coordination among providers
e. other

legal system:
a. public defender
b. attorney referral service
c. legal assistance
d. governmental child-adult protective services
e. guardian/conservator
f. financial support enforcement
g. law enforcement
h. other

nursing care:
a. evaluation
b. schedule/provide services

c. client advocacy
d. coordination among providers
e. other

occupational therapy care:
a. evaluation
b. schedule/provide services
c. client advocacy
d. coordination among providers
e. other

other community resources:
a. referral
b. coordination among providers
c. client advocacy
d. other

social work/counseling care:
a. evaluation
b. schedule/provide services
c. client advocacy
d. coordination among providers
e. other

other:

Surveillance (suggested care planning/intervention guides)

communication:
a. telehealth monitor findings
b. satisfactory communication
c. other

continuity of care:
a. adequate/appropriate services
b. coordination among providers
c. other

other community resources:
a. adequate/appropriate resources
b. other

other:

Problem Rating Scale for Outcomes

Knowledge

1-No knowledge
Example: immigrant group does not know about language classes

2-Minimal knowledge
Example: immigrant group knows location of language classes but not details

3-Basic knowledge
Example: immigrant group knows some details about language classes but not how to enroll or get there

4-Adequate knowledge
Example: immigrant group knows about language classes, how to enroll, and get there; details are not printed in group's language

5-Superior knowledge

Example: immigrant group knows about language classes; schedule and details are printed in group's language and distributed in their neighborhood

Behavior

1-Not appropriate behavior
Example: unwilling to use community resources
2-Rarely appropriate behavior
Example: will use service only if arranged by social worker
3-Inconsistently appropriate behavior
Example: communicates some problems appropriately to social worker
4-Usually appropriate behavior
Example: uses services appropriately most of the time
5-Consistently appropriate behavior
Example: communicates with social worker and providers, uses services

Status

1-Extreme signs/symptoms
Example: does not use needed transportation resources
2-Severe signs/symptoms
Example: using resources with great difficulty; refuses to ask for more information
3-Moderate signs/symptoms
Example: moderate difficulty using resources
4-Minimal signs/symptoms
Example: minimal difficulty using resources
5-No signs/symptoms
Example: appropriate use of resources

SOCIAL CONTACT

Problem Classification Scheme

Definition. Interaction between the individual/family/community and others outside the immediate living area.

Modifiers (select one):

Health Promotion
Example: parish nurse offers class about community resources to new area residents.
Potential
Example: does not drive car and has limited transportation options.
Actual
Example: statement, "new to community and has not made friends," suggests the sign/symptom *limited social contact*.

SIGNS/SYMPTOMS OF ACTUAL (select those that apply):

- limited social contact
- uses health care provider for social contact
- minimal outside stimulation/leisure time activities
- other

Related Medical Diagnoses. Mental Disorders (290-319). V Codes Supplementary Classification of Factors Influencing Health Status and Contact with Health Services: Persons Encountering Health Services in Other Circumstances (V60-V68).

Intervention Scheme

Teaching, Guidance, and Counseling (suggested care planning/intervention guides)

interaction:
a. family/friends
b. neighbors
c. volunteers
d. spiritual/faith communities
e. library
f. reliable Internet sites
g. leisure activities
h. crafts/hobbies
i. other

other community resources:
a. identify available resources
b. age/interest appropriate clubs/organizations
c. benefits
d. other

other:

Treatments and Procedures (suggested care planning/intervention guides)

other:

Case Management (suggested care planning/intervention guides)

day care/respite:
a. programs for adults/elders
b. programs for children
c. other

support group:
a. age/cultural/condition-specific groups for crafts, sports, faith communities, etc.
b. community-/facility-based services
c. reliable Internet sites
d. telephone information/reassurance
e. other

support system:
a. family/friends
b. spiritual/faith communities
c. schools
d. neighbors
e. work associates
f. other

other:

Surveillance (suggested care planning/intervention guides)

interaction:
a. adequate/appropriate
b. other

support group:
a. adequate/appropriate
b. other

support system:
a. adequate/appropriate
b. other
other:

Problem Rating Scale for Outcomes

Knowledge
1-No knowledge
Example: unaware of nearby group meal sites
2-Minimal knowledge
Example: does not understand relationship of limited social contact to nutrition and health problems
3-Basic knowledge
Example: expresses interest in information regarding meal sites
4-Adequate knowledge
Example: makes plans to attend meal sites 1-2 times a month
5-Superior knowledge
Example: makes plans to attend meal sites several times a week

Behavior
1-Not appropriate behavior
Example: refuses to leave home or allow others to come in
2-Rarely appropriate behavior
Example: allows only one nurse into home
3-Inconsistently appropriate behavior
Example: allows nurses and social workers into home with much prodding
4-Usually appropriate behavior
Example: leaves home occasionally to attend social activities
5-Consistently appropriate behavior
Example: actively involved in social activities

Status
1-Extreme signs/symptoms
Example: no social contacts
2-Severe signs/symptoms
Example: communicates with family or friends one time per week or less
3-Moderate signs/symptoms
Example: attends day care/elder center two times per week, otherwise alone
4-Minimal signs/symptoms
Example: attends day care/elder center five times per week; infrequent phone contact with family
5-No signs/symptoms
Example: attends day care/elder center five times per week; communicates with supportive network of family and friends frequently

ROLE CHANGE

Problem Classification Scheme

Definition. Additions to or removal of a set of expected behavioral characteristics.

Modifiers (select one):

Health Promotion

Example: individuals who are within 5 years of retirement are fully employed and are concerned that they participate only in employer-organized activities.

Potential

Example: in second trimester of unplanned pregnancy.

Actual

Example: the sign/symptom *involuntary role reversal* describes "independent member of a two-person family becomes dependent or vice versa."

SIGNS/SYMPTOMS OF ACTUAL (select those that apply):

- involuntary role reversal
- assumes new role
- loses previous role
- other

Related Medical Diagnoses. Mental Disorders (290-319). Complications of Pregnancy, Childbirth, and the Puerperium (630-677). Congenital Anomalies (740-759). V Codes Supplementary Classification of Factors Influencing Health Status and Contact with Health Services (V01-V83).

Intervention Scheme

Teaching, Guidance, and Counseling (suggested care planning/intervention guides)

behavior modification:

a. roles/responsibilities
b. recognize/change personal patterns
c. guided imagery
d. make choices to promote health
e. identify positive role models
f. other

coping skills:

a. time management
b. expected responses to role changes
c. role expectations
d. meditation
e. other

education:

a. complete educational plan
b. options
c. procedures to obtain services
d. other

support system:

a. active listening
b. emotional support
c. realistic expectations
d. other

other:

Treatments and Procedures (suggested care planning/intervention guides)

other:

Case Management (suggested care planning/intervention guides)

other community resources:
a. age/interest appropriate organizations
b. volunteer opportunities
c. other

social work/counseling care:
a. evaluation
b. schedule services
c. coordination among providers
d. other

support group:
a. age/cultural/condition-specific groups for new parents, job loss/change, etc.
b. community-/facility-based services
c. reliable Internet sites
d. telephone information/reassurance
e. other

support system:
a. family/friends
b. spiritual/faith communities
c. schools
d. neighbors
e. work associates
f. other

other:

Surveillance (suggested care planning/intervention guides)

coping skills:
a. adequate/appropriate
b. other

signs/symptoms—mental/emotional:
a. coping mechanisms
b. fear/anxiety
c. other

social work/counseling care:
a. receives care when scheduled
b. adequate/appropriate care
c. follows plan of care
d. other

stress management:
a. adequate/appropriate
b. other

other:

Problem Rating Scale for Outcomes

Knowledge

1-No knowledge
Example: lacks information about managing changed responsibilities

2-Minimal knowledge
Example: interested in relevant methods to manage changed responsibilities

3-Basic knowledge
Example: describes several methods of managing changed responsibilities but cannot personalize
4-Adequate knowledge
Example: sometimes/usually recognizes pertinent coping methods for changed responsibilities
5-Superior knowledge
Example: describes a relevant comprehensive system of managing changed responsibilities

Behavior
1-Not appropriate behavior
Example: does not care for new baby, not interested in returning to school
2-Rarely appropriate behavior
Example: infrequently helps with baby's care; indicates that it is "father's job"
3-Inconsistently appropriate behavior
Example: sometimes cares for baby, considering return to school
4-Usually appropriate behavior
Example: usually cares for baby, interested in returning to school
5-Consistently appropriate behavior
Example: provides total care for baby and household, and has applied for school

Status
1-Extreme signs/symptoms
Example: wellness center group members with newly diagnosed diabetes mellitus do not accept responsibilities for managing care
2-Severe signs/symptoms
Example: members accept new responsibilities occasionally with prodding
3-Moderate signs/symptoms
Example: members accept responsibilities with reminders
4-Minimal signs/symptoms
Example: members accept current responsibilities most of the time
5-No signs/symptoms
Example: members accept current responsibilities consistently

INTERPERSONAL RELATIONSHIP

Problem Classification Scheme

Definition. Associations or bonds between the individual/family/community and others.

Modifiers (select one):

Health Promotion
Example: school nurse and community outreach worker help plan community wide multicultural awareness celebration.

Potential
Example: history of serial relationships or three divorces.

Actual
Example: grandmother, mother, and children share home. The "grandmother and mother argue about child-rearing practices and discipline children differently" leading to

the signs/symptoms *incongruent values/goals/expectations/schedules* and *prolonged, unrelieved tension.*

Signs/Symptoms of Actual (select those that apply):

- difficulty establishing/maintaining relationships
- minimal shared activities
- incongruent values/goals/expectations/schedules
- inadequate interpersonal communication skills
- prolonged, unrelieved tension
- inappropriate suspicion/manipulation/control
- physically/emotionally abusive to partner
- difficulty problem solving without conflict
- other

Related Medical Diagnoses. Mental Disorders (290-319). V Codes Supplementary Classification of Factors Influencing Health Status and Contact with Health Services (V01-V83).

Intervention Scheme

Teaching, Guidance, and Counseling (suggested care planning/intervention guides)

anger management:
a. strategies
b. benefits
c. other

communication:
a. develop/improve skills
b. other

exercises:
a. local programs/facilities
b. suggested exercise program
c. balanced rest/activity
d. pacing activity
e. water/aquatics therapy
f. family activities
g. audiovisual materials, including videos
h. other

medical/dental care:
a. therapy to strengthen family support systems
b. other

relaxation/breathing techniques:
a. guided imagery
b. music
c. breathing techniques
d. yoga
e. progressive muscle relaxation
f. massage
g. other

stress management:
a. respite
b. meditation
c. other

support group:
a. benefits
b. realistic expectations
c. other
support system:
a. emotional support
b. active listening
c. realistic expectations
d. other
other:

Treatments and Procedures (suggested care planning/intervention guides)
other:

Case Management (suggested care planning/intervention guides)
social work/counseling care:
a. evaluation
b. schedule/provide services
c. coordination among providers
d. other
support group:
a. age/cultural/condition-specific groups for move/relocation, recent separation, etc.
b. community-/facility-based services
c. reliable Internet sites
d. telephone information/reassurance
e. other
support system:
a. family/friends
b. spiritual/faith communities
c. schools
d. neighbors
e. work associates
f. other
other:

Surveillance (suggested care planning/intervention guides)
anger management:
a. adequate/appropriate changes
b. other
interaction:
a. status of relationships
b. other
stress management:
a. coping ability
b. decreased tension/anxiety
c. other
other:

Problem Rating Scale for Outcomes

Knowledge

1-No knowledge
Example: cannot differentiate between positive and negative communication
2-Minimal knowledge
Example: expresses interest in learning better communication skills
3-Basic knowledge
Example: describes importance of positive communication, but not methods
4-Adequate knowledge
Example: describes some communication methods and when to use them
5-Superior knowledge
Example: knows various positive, open communication methods and when to use them

Behavior

1-Not appropriate behavior
Example: history of multiple short-term relationships with significant others
2-Rarely appropriate behavior
Example: slight decrease in number and increase in length of relationships with significant others
3-Inconsistently appropriate behavior
Example: greater decrease in number and increase in length of relationships with significant others
4-Usually appropriate behavior
Example: remains in 5-year, relatively positive relationship with a significant other
5-Consistently appropriate behavior
Example: remains in 10-year, positive relationship with a significant other

Status

1-Extreme signs/symptoms
Example: tense, volatile atmosphere
2-Severe signs/symptoms
Example: limited, brief communication and interaction, often tense
3-Moderate signs/symptoms
Example: some limited, polite communication and interaction
4-Minimal signs/symptoms
Example: some warm, usually polite, rarely tense communication and interaction
5-No signs/symptoms
Example: frequent, open communication and interaction

PSY

SPIRITUALITY

Problem Classification Scheme

Definition. Beliefs and practices that involve faith, religion, values, the spirit, and/or the soul.

Modifiers (select one):

Health Promotion

Example: Catholic parents are interested in learning about Japanese spiritual beliefs and practices because their son plans to marry a Japanese woman.

Potential

Example: scheduled for major surgery next month and wants to learn about relationships between health, positive spirituality, and the immune system.

Actual

Example: experiences stress caused by challenges to beliefs, values, or religious practices. Data suggest the sign/symptom *disrupted spiritual rituals,* as evidenced by "no longer attends religious services."

SIGNS/SYMPTOMS OF ACTUAL (select those that apply):

- expresses spiritual concerns
- disrupted spiritual rituals
- disrupted spiritual trust
- conflicting spiritual beliefs and medical/health care regimen
- other

Related Medical Diagnoses. V Codes Supplementary Classification of Factors Influencing Health Status and Contact with Health Services: Persons Encountering Health Services in Other Circumstances (V60-V68).

Intervention Scheme

Teaching, Guidance, and Counseling (suggested care planning/intervention guides)

end-of-life care:

a. recognition/acceptance
b. plans
c. no code (no resuscitation)
d. other

spiritual care:

a. allow expression of existential/faith preferences
b. offer active/passive prayer
c. other

other:

Treatments and Procedures (suggested care planning/intervention guides)

other:

Case Management (suggested care planning/intervention guides)

end-of-life care:

a. funeral home/morgue
b. memorial services
c. burial/cremation
d. other

spiritual care:

a. clergy or pastoral care
b. schedule/participate in rituals
c. other

support group:

a. age/cultural/condition-specific groups for separation, chronic/terminal illness, etc.
b. community-/facility-based services
c. reliable Internet sites

d. telephone information/reassurance
e. other

support system:

a. family/friends
b. spiritual/faith communities
c. schools
d. neighbors
e. work associates
f. other

other:

Surveillance (suggested care planning/intervention guides)

coping skills:

a. adequate/appropriate
b. other

spiritual care:

a. adequate/appropriate
b. other

other:

PSY

Problem Rating Scale for Outcomes

Knowledge

1-No knowledge

Example: does not know how to integrate spiritual rituals and current illness

2-Minimal knowledge

Example: concerned that prescribed treatments and medications may interfere with spiritual beliefs

3-Basic knowledge

Example: wants spiritual rituals but requests help making contacts

4-Adequate knowledge

Example: expects new partnership with health care providers to improve integration of care and spiritual rituals

5-Superior knowledge

Example: knows that treatment and medication plan are integrated with spiritual beliefs and rituals

Behavior

1-Not appropriate behavior

Example: spiritual practices prohibit use of health care

2-Rarely appropriate behavior

Example: spiritual practices conflict with health care needs; rarely uses health care

3-Inconsistently appropriate behavior

Example: spiritual practices do not conflict with health/self care

4-Usually appropriate behavior

Example: spiritual practices support health care/self care

5-Consistently appropriate behavior

Example: spiritual practices provide comfort and support and promote wellness behaviors

Status
1-Extreme signs/symptoms
Example: consistently anxious and distressed about spiritual faith or belief system
2-Severe signs/symptoms
Example: frequently anxious about spiritual faith or belief system
3-Moderate signs/symptoms
Example: sometimes questions spiritual faith or belief system
4-Minimal signs/symptoms
Example: usually comfortable with spiritual faith or belief system
5-No signs/symptoms
Example: comfortable with spiritual faith or belief system

GRIEF

Problem Classification Scheme

Definition. Suffering and distress associated with loss.

Modifiers (select one):

Health Promotion
Example: healthy young adult interested in classes on aging, death, and dying.

Potential
Example: employee anticipates losing job.

Actual
Example: a formerly employed young man whose foot was amputated 6 months ago "spends most of the day in a chair complaining about the unfriendly world" suggesting the sign/symptom *difficulty coping with grief responses.* Loss can be associated with death, chronic disease, divorce/separation, imprisonment, move, prolonged unemployment, or the inability to drive.

SIGNS/SYMPTOMS OF ACTUAL (select those that apply):
- fails to recognize stages of grief/process of healing
- difficulty coping with grief responses
- difficulty expressing grief responses
- conflicting stages of grief among individuals/families
- other

Related Medical Diagnoses. Neoplasms (140-239). Complications of Pregnancy, Childbirth, and the Puerperium (630-677). Congenital Anomalies (740-759). Symptoms, Signs, and Ill-Defined Conditions: Ill-Defined and Unknown Causes of Morbidity and Mortality (797-799). V Codes Supplementary Classification of Factors Influencing Health Status and Contact with Health Services (V01-V83). E Codes Supplementary Classification of External Causes of Injury and Poisoning (E800-E999).

Intervention Scheme

Teaching, Guidance, and Counseling (suggested care planning/intervention guides)

coping skills:
a. life review
b. share feelings

c. leisure activities
d. crafts/hobbies
e. volunteering
f. other

dietary management:
a. basic nutrition
b. eating patterns
c. supplemental vitamins and minerals
d. macrobiotics
e. other

end-of-life care:
a. recognition/acceptance
b. plans
c. no code (no resuscitation)
d. other

exercises:
a. local programs/facilities
b. suggested exercise program
c. balanced rest/activity
d. pacing activity
e. water/aquatics therapy
f. family activities
g. audiovisual materials including videos
h. other

relaxation/breathing techniques:
a. guided imagery
b. music
c. breathing techniques
d. yoga
e. progressive muscle relaxation
f. massage
g. other

rest/sleep:
a. benefits
b. regular patterns
c. strategies
d. other

signs/symptoms—mental/emotional:
a. expected stages of grief
b. concerns related to death/dying
c. other

other:

Treatments and Procedures (suggested care planning/intervention guides)

medical/dental care:
a. therapy
b. other

other:

Case Management (suggested care planning/intervention guides)

medical/dental care:
a. evaluation
b. schedule/provide services
c. coordination among providers
d. other

nursing care:
a. evaluation
b. schedule/provide services
c. coordination among providers
d. other

recreational therapy care:
a. evaluation
b. schedule/provide services
c. coordination among providers
d. other

social work/counseling care:
a. evaluation
b. schedule/provide services
c. coordination among providers
d. other

support group:
a. age/cultural/condition-specific groups for bereavement, move/relocation, etc.
b. community-/facility-based services
c. reliable Internet sites
d. telephone information/reassurance
e. other

support system:
a. family/friends
b. spiritual/faith communities
c. schools
d. neighbors
e. work associates
f. other

other:

Surveillance (suggested care planning/intervention guides)

signs/symptoms—mental/emotional:
a. coping mechanisms
b. behavioral changes
c. affect
d. other

signs/symptoms—physical:
a. sleep patterns
b. height
c. weight
d. vital signs/blood pressure
e. other

other:

Problem Rating Scale for Outcomes

Knowledge

1-No knowledge
Example: not aware of normal grief process
2-Minimal knowledge
Example: can state grief stages, does not relate information to self/others
3-Basic knowledge
Example: relates grief stages to others, not to self
4-Adequate knowledge
Example: usually able to relate own feelings to grief stages
5-Superior knowledge
Example: understands grief and relates to own feelings with acceptance and consistency

Behavior

1-Not appropriate behavior
Example: does not share feelings with family or providers, rejects offers of support
2-Rarely appropriate behavior
Example: rarely shares feelings with family or providers, indifferent to offers of support
3-Inconsistently appropriate behavior
Example: occasionally shares feelings with family or providers, responds positively to offers of support
4-Usually appropriate behavior
Example: usually shares feelings and occasionally seeks support
5-Consistently appropriate behavior
Example: shares feelings and seeks support appropriately

Status

1-Extreme signs/symptoms
Example: unable to perform basic activities, function independently, or cope with emotions
2-Severe signs/symptoms
Example: occasionally performs basic activities, but requires assurance and cannot resume employment
3-Moderate signs/symptoms
Example: performs basic activities, requires occasional assurance, copes with emotions some of the time, and is unsuccessful in resuming employment responsibilities
4-Minimal signs/symptoms
Example: functions independently, copes with emotions most of the time, and resumes partial employment
5-No signs/symptoms
Example: functions independently, copes with emotions consistently, and resumes gainful employment and normal activities

MENTAL HEALTH

Problem Classification Scheme

Definition. Development and use of mental/emotional abilities to adjust to life situations, interact with others, and engage in activities.

Modifiers (select one):

Health Promotion

Example: public health nurses conduct suicide awareness and prevention campaign in local secondary schools.

Potential

Example: family history of mental illness or dysfunction.

Actual

Example: reports "hearing messages or seeing people and objects regularly" denoting the sign/symptom *hallucinations/illusions*, or "doesn't care about anything anymore," suggesting the sign/symptom *loss of interest/involvement in activities/self-care*.

SIGNS/SYMPTOMS OF ACTUAL (select those that apply):

- sadness/hopelessness/decreased self-esteem
- apprehension/undefined fear
- loss of interest/involvement in activities/self-care
- narrowed to scattered attention/focus
- flat affect
- irritable/agitated/aggressive
- purposeless/compulsive activity
- difficulty managing stress
- difficulty managing anger
- somatic complaints/fatigue
- delusions
- hallucinations/illusions
- expresses suicidal/homicidal thoughts
- attempts suicide/homicide
- self-mutilation
- mood swings
- flash-backs
- other

Related Medical Diagnoses. Mental Disorders (290-319). Symptoms, Signs, and Ill-Defined Conditions (780-799). V Codes Supplementary Classification of Factors Influencing Health Status and Contact with Health Services (V01-V83). E Codes Supplementary Classification of External Causes of Injury and Poisoning (E800-E999).

Intervention Scheme

Teaching, Guidance, and Counseling (suggested care planning/intervention guides)

anger management:

a. strategies
b. benefits
c. other

communication:

a. steps to obtain services
b. other

coping skills:

a. adjustment to illness
b. crisis intervention
c. other

dietary management:
a. basic nutrition
b. eating patterns
c. supplemental vitamins and minerals
d. macrobiotics
e. other

laboratory findings:
a. interpretation of blood tests
b. other

medication action/side effects:
a. important to take as prescribed
b. purpose/benefits
c. changes to note and report in timely manner
d. need for timely laboratory tests
e. other

other community resources:
a. options
b. referral process
c. other

relaxation/breathing techniques:
a. guided imagery
b. music
c. breathing techniques
d. yoga
e. progressive muscle relaxation
f. massage
g. other

rest/sleep:
a. amount needed
b. planned rest
c. conducive environment
d. day/night schedule
e. other

signs/symptoms—mental/emotional:
a. affect
b. suicidal tendencies
c. depression
d. other

support group:
a. emotional support
b. active listening
c. others' experiences
d. other

support system:
a. benefits
b. strategies
c. other

other:

Treatments and Procedures (suggested care planning/intervention guides)

nursing care:
a. therapy
b. other

social work/counseling care:
a. therapy
b. other

specimen collection:
a. blood
b. other

other:

Case Management (suggested care planning/intervention guides)

continuity of care:
a. coordination among providers
b. other

day care/respite:
a. options
b. other

legal system:
a. governmental health/social service assistance
b. governmental child-adult protective services
c. courts
d. law enforcement
e. other

medical/dental care:
a. evaluation
b. schedule/provide services
c. coordination among providers
d. other

medication coordination/ordering:
a. obtains refills in timely manner
b. communicate with pharmacist/other providers
c. other

nursing care:
a. evaluation
b. schedule/provide services
c. coordination among providers
d. other

other community resources:
a. advocate for community services
b. mental health services
c. other

recreational therapy care:
a. evaluation
b. schedule/provide services
c. coordination among providers
d. other

support group:
a. age/cultural/condition-specific group for clients, family/caregivers, etc.
b. community-/facility-based services
c. reliable Internet sites
d. telephone information/reassurance
e. other

support system:
a. family/friends
b. spiritual/faith communities
c. schools
d. neighbors
e. work associates
f. other

other:

Surveillance (suggested care planning/intervention guides)

anger management:
a. adequate/appropriate
b. other

continuity of care:
a. coordination among providers
b. other

coping skills:
a. choices
b. adequate/appropriate
c. other

interaction:
a. adequate/appropriate with family/friends
b. adequate/appropriate at work/community
c. other

laboratory findings:
a. interpretation of blood tests
b. other

medication action/side effects:
a. takes as prescribed
b. notes and reports changes/side effects in timely manner
c. other

rest/sleep:
a. appropriate for age/condition
b. consistent patterns
c. other

signs/symptoms—mental/emotional:
a. frequency of symptoms
b. severity of symptoms
c. suicidal tendencies
d. disorganized speech/activity
e. other

other:

Problem Rating Scale for Outcomes

Knowledge

1-No knowledge

Example: not aware that symptoms are unusual or could be sign of mental illness

2-Minimal knowledge

Example: aware that symptoms are sign of disorder, but does not know treatment options or understand the impact of symptoms

3-Basic knowledge

Example: aware of symptoms, knows one treatment option and basic information about impact of illness on life

4-Adequate knowledge

Example: aware that symptoms are due to mental illness and impact mental illness has on life, knows various treatment options

5-Superior knowledge

Example: aware that symptoms are due to mental illness, knows lifestyle choices to decrease or prevent symptoms from returning, understands which symptoms suggest exacerbation, and knows treatment options

Behavior

1-Not appropriate behavior

Example: does not take medications, attend therapy, or see counselor/physician

2-Rarely appropriate behavior

Example: takes medications only when symptoms are severe, in hospital, or treatment is ordered by court; attends only initial therapy appointment; often uses ineffective self-treatment

3-Inconsistently appropriate behavior

Example: takes occasional "medication holidays"; attends therapy inconsistently; occasionally uses ineffective self-treatment

4-Usually appropriate behavior

Example: usually takes medications as prescribed; attends most therapy sessions; uses some healthy lifestyle changes to improve illness

5-Consistently appropriate behavior

Example: sees counselor/physician regularly and takes medications as prescribed

Status

1-Extreme signs/symptoms

Example: agitated, aggressive, depressed, frequent thoughts about suicide

2-Severe signs/symptoms

Example: talks about depression and other fears, does not express suicidal thoughts

3-Moderate signs/symptoms

Example: occasionally depressed, increased awareness of self and others needs

4-Minimal signs/symptoms

Example: increasingly engages in purposeful activity, has not expressed suicidal thoughts for 6 months

5-No signs/symptoms

Example: coping with daily stresses

SEXUALITY

Problem Classification Scheme

Definition. Attitudes, feelings, and behaviors related to intimacy and sexual activity.

Modifiers (select one):

Health Promotion

Example: school district requests relationship and sexuality education program for pre-teens.

Potential

Example: considering having unprotected sex.

Actual

Example: "complains of sexual needs being ignored by partner" suggesting the sign/symptom *difficulty expressing intimacy.*

Signs/Symptoms of Actual (select those that apply):

- difficulty recognizing consequences of sexual behavior
- difficulty expressing intimacy
- sexual identity confusion
- sexual value confusion
- dissatisfied with sexual relationships
- unsafe sexual practices
- sexual acting out/provocative behaviors/harassment
- sexual perpetration/assault
- other

PSY

Related Medical Diagnoses. Mental Disorders (290-319). Complications of Pregnancy, Childbirth, and the Puerperium (630-677). V Codes Supplementary Classification of Factors Influencing Health Status and Contact with Health Services (V01-V83).

Intervention Scheme

Teaching, Guidance, and Counseling (suggested care planning/intervention guides)

anatomy/physiology:

a. reproductive organs
b. reproductive cycle
c. other

behavior modification:

a. make choices to promote health
b. recognize/change personal patterns
c. safe sex
d. identify positive role models
e. guided imagery
f. other

communication:

a. skills
b. listening
c. other

growth/development care:

a. reasonable expectations
b. other

personal hygiene:
a. correct wiping
b. cleanliness
c. other

screening procedures:
a. self-screening
b. diagnostic tests including Papanicolaou test
c. other

signs/symptoms—physical:
a. evidence of disease/infection
b. other

wellness:
a. safe sex
b. comfort with own sexuality
c. consequences of sexual activity
d. other

other:

Treatments and Procedures (suggested care planning/intervention guides)

medical/dental care:
a. examination
b. treatment plan
c. other

nursing care:
a. examination
b. treatment plan
c. other

other:

Case Management (suggested care planning/intervention guides)

medical/dental care:
a. evaluation
b. schedule/provide services
c. coordination among providers
d. other

nursing care:
a. evaluation
b. schedule/provide services
c. coordination among providers
d. other

social work/counseling care:
a. evaluation
b. schedule/provide services
c. coordination among providers
d. other

support group:
a. age/cultural/condition-specific group for teens, singles, couples, etc.
b. community-/facility-based services
c. reliable Internet sites

d. telephone information/reassurance
e. other
other:

Surveillance (suggested care planning/intervention guides)
medical/dental care:
a. receives care when scheduled
b. adequate/appropriate
c. follows plan of care
d. other
nursing care:
a. receives care when scheduled
b. adequate/appropriate
c. follows plan of care
d. other
signs/symptoms—physical:
a. evidence of disease/infection
b. vital signs/blood pressure
c. other
social work/counseling care:
a. receives care when scheduled
b. adequate/appropriate
c. follows plan of care
d. other
wellness:
a. evidence of change
b. other
other:

Problem Rating Scale for Outcomes

Knowledge
1-No knowledge
Example: does not understand that own behavior is sexually inappropriate and leads to negative consequences
2-Minimal knowledge
Example: knows some examples of sexually inappropriate behavior, but does not relate to own behavior
3-Basic knowledge
Example: understands sexually inappropriate behavior and relates to own behavior, but does not understand the relationship between own behavior and negative consequences
4-Adequate knowledge
Example: understands what constitutes sexually inappropriate behavior and is beginning to relate own behavior to negative consequences
5-Superior knowledge
Example: relates own sexually inappropriate behavior to consequences and does not want to experience negative consequences

Behavior
1-Not appropriate behavior
Example: does not protect self; intimate with multiple partners

2-Rarely appropriate behavior
  Example: sometimes protects self; intimate with multiple partners
3-Inconsistently appropriate behavior
  Example: protects self; intimate with multiple partners
4-Usually appropriate behavior
  Example: has short-term monogamous relationship with partner who may be at risk
5-Consistently appropriate behavior
  Example: has long-term monogamous relationship with healthy partner

Status
1-Extreme signs/symptoms
  Example: unable to express sexual intimacy appropriately
2-Severe signs/symptoms
  Example: rarely expresses sexual intimacy appropriately
3-Moderate signs/symptoms
  Example: moderate difficulty in expressing sexual intimacy appropriately
4-Minimal signs/symptoms
  Example: minimal difficulty in expressing sexual intimacy appropriately
5-No signs/symptoms
  Example: expresses sexual intimacy comfortably and appropriately

CARETAKING/PARENTING

Problem Classification Scheme

Definition. Providing support, nurturance, stimulation, and physical care for dependent child or adult.

Modifiers (select one):

Health Promotion

Example: young woman who is not pregnant or a parent requests information about child care resources.

Potential

Example: grandparent comes to live with family that includes young children.

Actual

Example: the parent of three children and the daughter/caregiver of her 90-year old father exhibit the sign/symptom *dissatisfaction/difficulty with responsibilities* with the statement, "I can't take another day like this."

SIGNS/SYMPTOMS OF ACTUAL (select those that apply):

- difficulty providing physical care/safety
- difficulty providing emotional nurturance
- difficulty providing cognitive learning experiences and activities
- difficulty providing preventive and therapeutic health care
- expectations incongruent with stage of growth and development
- dissatisfaction/difficulty with responsibilities
- difficulty interpreting or responding to verbal/nonverbal communication
- neglectful
- abusive
- other

Related Medical Diagnoses. Mental Disorders (290-319). Complications of Pregnancy, Childbirth, and the Puerperium (630-677). V Codes Supplementary Classification of

Factors Influencing Health Status and Contact with Health Services (V01-V83). E Codes Supplementary Classification of External Causes of Injury and Poisoning (E800-E999).

Intervention Scheme

Teaching, Guidance, and Counseling (suggested care planning/intervention guides)

bonding/attachment:
a. activities to promote
b. responds to infant's cues
c. other

caretaking/parenting skills:
a. long-range planning/decision-making
b. support in-home care system
c. infant/child care
d. elder care
e. telephone reassurance
f. other

communication:
a. negotiate social systems
b. other

coping skills:
a. crisis intervention
b. stress reduction
c. planned time away
d. other

day care/respite:
a. selection criteria involving environment and staff
b. plan for regular day care
c. plan for emergency/alternative day care
d. other

dietary management:
a. nutritional requirements for age/physical condition
b. visual appeal
c. texture
d. quantity
e. calories
f. prevention of allergies
g. introduce/use new foods/liquids
h. other

discipline:
a. parent/caregiver's preferences/experiences
b. age/condition-appropriate measures
c. limit setting
d. clear expectations
e. reduce distractions/annoyances in environment
f. other

environment:
a. cleanliness
b. noise
c. lighting
d. other

feeding procedures:
a. appropriate methods for age/physical condition
b. formula preparation/storage
c. breast-feeding
d. schedule
e. burping
f. other

growth/development care:
a. maturation of child/adult
b. realistic expectations
c. other

infection precautions:
a. identify potential sources of infection
b. hand washing
c. disposal of tissues/pads/diapers
d. clean environment
e. avoid others with infections
f. keep skin dry
g. other

medical/dental care:
a. routine/preventive care
b. well-baby examinations
c. well-child/adult immunizations
d. appropriate care for symptoms
e. other

other community resources:
a. caretaking
b. other

personal hygiene:
a. skin care
b. hair/scalp care
c. bathing
d. mouth care
e. foot care
f. nail care
g. cord care
h. circumcision care
i. other

positioning:
a. hold to feed infant
b. back sleeping position for infant
c. stomach position for infant's supervised play
d. re-positioning to improve function and decrease pressure areas
e. other

rest/sleep:
a. amount needed
b. planned rest
c. conducive environment
d. day/night schedule
e. other

safety:
a. appropriate supervision
b. concerns for each stage of development/condition
c. drive car/operate hazardous outdoor equipment
d. electrical appliances
e. lock/security/alert systems
f. wander/fall alert systems
g. poison/medication control
h. appropriate furniture/placement
i. car seats/seat belts
j. other
sickness/injury care:
a. recognition/care of sick child/adult
b. temperature taking
c. routine/emergency care plans
d. other
stimulation/nurturance:
a. verbal
b. visual
c. tactile
d. day trips/outings
e. pet therapy
f. music/art/physical activity programs
g. games/play/toys
h. volunteers
i. other
support group:
a. options
b. realistic expectations
c. others' experiences
d. other
other:

Treatments and Procedures (suggested care planning/intervention guides)
other:

Case Management (suggested care planning/intervention guides)
caretaking/parenting skills:
a. develop in-home care system
b. parenting classes
c. classes for caregivers of elders
d. other
continuity of care:
a. coordination among providers
b. other
day care/respite:
a. child center
b. adult center
c. child respite services
d. adult respite services

e. volunteers
f. other

nursing care:
a. evaluation
b. schedule/provide services
c. coordination among providers
d. other

other community resources:
a. assisted living options
b. long term care options
c. advocate for community services
d. other

support group:
a. age/cultural/condition-specific groups for parents, adult caregivers, chronic/terminal illness, etc.
b. community-/facility-based services
c. reliable Internet sites
d. telephone information/reassurance
e. other

support system:
a. family/friends
b. spiritual/faith communities
c. schools
d. neighbors
e. work associates
f. other

transportation:
a. social service departments
b. public transportation
c. volunteers
d. drivers license testing
e. other

other:

Surveillance (suggested care planning/intervention guides)

bonding/attachment:
a. mutual responsiveness
b. eye contact
c. other

caretaking/parenting skills:
a. infant/child care
b. elder care
c. parent/infant interaction
d. caregiver/care recipient interaction
e. other

communication:
a. verbalization of feelings
b. other

continuity of care:
a. coordination among providers
b. other
coping skills:
a. adaptation/flexibility to demands
b. other
dietary management:
a. adequate/appropriate for age/physical status
b. other
discipline:
a. methods
b. appropriate
c. consistent
d. other
feeding procedures:
a. techniques
b. other
growth/development care:
a. realistic expectations
b. other
medical/dental care:
a. receives care when scheduled
b. adequate/appropriate
c. follows plan of care
d. other
nursing care:
a. receives care when scheduled
b. adequate/appropriate
c. follows plan of care
d. other
rest/sleep:
a. appropriate for age/condition
b. consistent patterns
c. other
safety:
a. environmental safety
b. presence of safety hazards
c. appropriate supervision
d. other
sickness/injury care:
a. recognize need for care and follow-up
b. other
support group:
a. participation
b. other
support system:
a. involvement
b. other
other:

Problem Rating Scale for Outcomes

Knowledge

1-No knowledge
  Example: unaware of safety hazards
2-Minimal knowledge
  Example: interested in information about safety hazards
3-Basic knowledge
  Example: understands safety hazards, but no solutions
4-Adequate knowledge
  Example: understands safety hazards and some solutions
5-Superior knowledge
  Example: understands safety hazards and reasonable solutions

Behavior

1-Not appropriate behavior
  Example: does not provide physical care; relates in hostile manner
2-Rarely appropriate behavior
  Example: provides minimal physical care; relates in indifferent manner
3-Inconsistently appropriate behavior
  Example: provides adequate physical care some of time; sometimes shows nurturing behavior
4-Usually appropriate behavior
  Example: provides adequate physical care most of time; often shows nurturing behavior
5-Consistently appropriate behavior
  Example: provides adequate physical care consistently and nurtures consistently

Status

1-Extreme signs/symptoms
  Example: consistently anxious, negative about caretaking/parenting
2-Severe signs/symptoms
  Example: frequently anxious, negative about caretaking/parenting
3-Moderate signs/symptoms
  Example: expresses some positive feelings about caretaking/parenting
4-Minimal signs/symptoms
  Example: usually positive about caretaking/parenting
5-No signs/symptoms
  Example: consistently positive about caretaking/parenting

NEGLECT

Problem Classification Scheme

Definition. Child or adult deprived of minimally accepted standards of food, shelter, clothing, or care.

Modifiers (select one):

Health Promotion
Example: church group asks social worker to conduct class about care for dependent adults.
Potential
Example: home with small children has open, unprotected stairway in living area.

Actual

Example: sign/symptom *lacks necessary supervision* suggested by the statement "2-year-old left with 6-year-old brother."

Signs/Symptoms of Actual (select those that apply):

- lacks adequate physical care
- lacks emotional nurturance/support
- lacks appropriate stimulation/cognitive experiences
- inappropriately left alone
- lacks necessary supervision
- inadequate/delayed medical care
- other

Related Medical Diagnoses. Mental Disorders (290-319). Injury and Poisoning (800-999). V Codes Supplementary Classification of Factors Influencing Health Status and Contact with Health Services (V01-V83). E Codes Supplementary Classification of External Causes of Injury and Poisoning (E800-E999).

Intervention Scheme

Teaching, Guidance, and Counseling (suggested care planning/intervention guides)

behavior modification:

a. new skills for new roles
b. make choices to promote health
c. recognize/change personal patterns
d. identify positive role models
e. guided imagery
f. other

bonding/attachment:

a. activities to promote
b. other

caretaking/parenting skills:

a. long-range planning/decision making
b. support in-home care system
c. infant/child care
d. elder care
e. telephone information/reassurance
f. other

discipline:

a. age-appropriate discipline
b. limit setting
c. clear expectations
d. reduce distractions/annoyances in environment
e. other

growth/development care:

a. realistic expectations
b. other

safety:

a. appropriate supervision
b. age/condition related safety concerns
c. drive car/operate hazardous outdoor equipment

d. electrical appliances
e. lock/security/alert systems
f. wander/fall alert systems
g. poison/medication control
h. appropriate furniture/placement
i. car seats/seat belts
j. other

sickness/injury care:
a. recognition/care of sick child/adult
b. temperature taking
c. routine/emergency care plans
d. other

stimulation/nurturance:
a. verbal
b. visual
c. tactile
d. day trips/outings
e. pet therapy
f. music/art/physical activity programs
g. educational programs
h. hobbies/crafts
i. games/play/toys
j. other

support group:
a. options
b. benefits
c. other

support system:
a. benefits
b. strategies
c. other

other:

Treatments and Procedures (suggested care planning/intervention guides)

other:

Case Management (suggested care planning/intervention guides)

day care/respite:
a. consider options
b. select most appropriate site
c. communication between family and provider
d. other

finances:
a. crisis intervention/short-range planning
b. long-range planning/decision making
c. budgeting
d. community resources
e. family resources
f. other

legal system:

a. governmental child-adult protective services
b. attorney referral service
c. public defender
d. legal assistance
e. guardian/conservator
f. other

nursing care:
a. evaluation
b. schedule/provide services
c. coordination among providers
d. other

social work/counseling care:
a. evaluation
b. schedule/provide services
c. coordination among providers
d. other

support group:
a. age/cultural/condition-specific group for those who were neglected, parents, caregivers, etc.
b. community-/facility-based services
c. reliable Internet sites
d. telephone information/reassurance
e. other

support system:
a. family/friends
b. spiritual/faith communities
c. schools
d. neighbors
e. work associates
f. other

other:

Surveillance (suggested care planning/intervention guides)

continuity of care:
a. coordination among providers
b. other

discipline:
a. methods
b. appropriate
c. consistent
d. other

safety:
a. appropriate supervision
b. home safety assessment
c. make changes
d. appropriate care
e. other

sickness/injury care:
a. recognize need for care and follow-up
b. other

signs/symptoms—mental/emotional:
a. behavior inappropriate for age
b. behavioral extremes
c. low self-esteem
d. depression
e. withdrawal
f. other
signs/symptoms—physical:
a. evidence of malnutrition
b. inappropriate clothing
c. poor personal hygiene
d. skin breakdown
e. developmental delay
f. untreated illness/disease/infection
g. other
other:

Problem Rating Scale for Outcomes

Knowledge
1-No knowledge
Example: does not understand need for visual, auditory, and tactile stimulation
2-Minimal knowledge
Example: interested in learning about stimulation needs
3-Basic knowledge
Example: understands need but no methods for providing stimulation
4-Adequate knowledge
Example: knows a few methods, materials, and timing for providing stimulation
5-Superior knowledge
Example: knows various methods, materials, and timing for providing stimulation

Behavior
1-Not appropriate behavior
Example: frail elder receiving very little physical care
2-Rarely appropriate behavior
Example: frail elder receiving minimal physical care
3-Inconsistently appropriate behavior
Example: frail elder receiving adequate physical care some of time
4-Usually appropriate behavior
Example: frail elder receiving adequate physical care most of time
5-Consistently appropriate behavior
Example: frail elder receiving adequate physical care consistently

Status
1-Extreme signs/symptoms
Example: toddler frequently left alone
2-Severe signs/symptoms
Example: toddler left alone for short/5- to 10-minute periods approximately once a week
3-Moderate signs/symptoms

Example: toddler left alone for short/5- to 10-minute periods approximately once a month
4-Minimal signs/symptoms
Example: no evidence for 1 month that toddler unsupervised
5-No signs/symptoms
Example: toddler consistently supervised

ABUSE

Problem Classification Scheme

Definition. Child or adult subjected to nonaccidental physical, emotional, or sexual violence or injury.

Modifiers (select one):

Health Promotion

Example: neighborhood association schedules session to increase recognition of abuse/domestic violence.

Potential

Example: partner fails to attend court-ordered conflict resolution/anger management class.

Actual

Example: child has "cigarette burn on chest" or adult has "unexplained black eye and bruises on face" indicating the signs/symptoms *welts/bruises/burns/other injuries* and *questionable explanation of injury*.

SIGNS/SYMPTOMS OF ACTUAL (select those that apply):

- harsh/excessive discipline
- welts/bruises/burns/other injuries
- questionable explanation of injury
- attacked verbally
- fearful/hypervigilant behavior
- violent environment
- consistent negative messages
- assaulted sexually
- other

PSY

Related Medical Diagnoses. Mental Disorders (290-319). Injury and Poisoning (800-999). V Codes Supplementary Classification of Factors Influencing Health Status and Contact with Health Services (V01-V83). E Codes Supplementary Classification of External Causes of Injury and Poisoning (E800-E999).

Intervention Scheme

Teaching, Guidance, and Counseling (suggested care planning/intervention guides)

anger management:
a. strategies
b. benefits
c. other

behavior modification:
a. new skills for new roles
b. make choices to promote health
c. recognize/change personal patterns

d. identify positive role models
e. guided imagery
f. other

discipline:

a. age-appropriate discipline
b. limit setting
c. clear expectations
d. reduce distractions/annoyances in environment
e. other

interaction:

a. appropriate with family/friends
b. appropriate at work/community
c. other

legal system:

a. options
b. procedures to obtain services
c. benefits
d. other

safety:

a. appropriate supervision
b. safety plan
c. concerns for each stage of development/condition
d. drive car/operate hazardous outdoor equipment
e. lock/security/alert systems
f. wander/fall alert systems
g. poison/medication control
h. appropriate furniture/placement
i. car seats/seat belts
j. other

sickness/injury care:

a. recognition/care of sick child/adult
b. temperature taking
c. routine/emergency care plans
d. other

signs/symptoms—mental/emotional:

a. effects of domestic violence on children/adults
b. depression
c. withdrawal
d. behavioral extremes
e. other

support system:

a. active listening
b. emotional support
c. realistic expectations
d. other

other:

Treatments and Procedures (suggested care planning/intervention guides)

other:

Case Management (suggested care planning/intervention guides)

day care/respite:

a. coordinate with provider
b. other

finances:

a. crisis intervention/short-range planning
b. long-range planning/decision making
c. budgeting
d. community resources
e. family resources
f. other

home:

a. options
b. other

legal system:

a. governmental child-adult protective services
b. attorney referral service
c. public defender
d. legal assistance
e. guardian/conservator
f. other

nursing care:

a. evaluation
b. schedule/provide services
c. coordination among providers
d. other

other community resources:

a. resource options
b. referral process
c. other

sickness/injury care:

a. recognize need for care and follow-up
b. other

social work/counseling:

a. evaluation
b. schedule/provide services
c. coordination among providers
d. other

support group:

a. age/cultural/condition-specific group for those who were abused, have special needs, etc.
b. community-/facility-based services
c. reliable Internet sites
d. telephone information/reassurance
e. other

support system:

a. family/friends
b. spiritual/faith communities
c. schools
d. neighbors

e. work associates
f. other
other:

Surveillance (suggested care planning/intervention guides)
continuity of care:
a. coordination among providers
b. other
discipline:
a. methods
b. appropriate
c. consistent
d. other
safety:
a. monitor safety plan
b. appropriate supervision
c. home safety assessment
d. make changes
e. appropriate care
f. other

signs/symptoms—mental/emotional:
a. wariness of physical contact
b. behavior inappropriate for age
c. behavioral extremes
d. fear of abuser
e. diminishing self-esteem
f. unable to participate in activities
g. other
signs/symptoms—physical:
a. welts
b. bruises
c. burns
d. lacerations
e. fractures
f. unexplained genital/urinary infections
g. unexplained injuries
h. evidence of disease/infection
i. other
other:

Problem Rating Scale for Outcomes

Knowledge

1-No knowledge

Example: does not know difference between usual interpersonal relationship and abusive behavior

2-Minimal knowledge

Example: expresses interest in learning about usual interpersonal relationship and abusive behavior

3-Basic knowledge

Example: describes what constitutes abusive behavior, but does not understand appropriate relationship interaction
4-Adequate knowledge
Example: understands appropriate relationship interaction, but not what to do if abused
5-Superior knowledge
Example: understands relationship concepts and knows safety resources to use if abused

Behavior
1-Not appropriate behavior
Example: too passive and fearful of caregiver; extremely disruptive or withdrawn
2-Rarely appropriate behavior
Example: too passive and fearful of caregiver; frequently disruptive or withdrawn
3-Inconsistently appropriate behavior
Example: not usually passive or fearful of caregiver; occasionally disruptive or withdrawn
4-Usually appropriate behavior
Example: occasionally positive relationship with caregiver; seldom disruptive or withdrawn
5-Consistently appropriate behavior
Example: positive relationship with caregiver consistently

Status
1-Extreme signs/symptoms
Example: many injuries
2-Severe signs/symptoms
Example: injuries in various stages of healing
3-Moderate signs/symptoms
Example: no new injuries but old injuries evident
4-Minimal signs/symptoms
Example: no evidence of injuries for 1 month
5-No signs/symptoms
Example: no evidence of injuries

GROWTH AND DEVELOPMENT

Problem Classification Scheme

Definition. Progressive physical, emotional, and social maturation along the age continuum from birth to death.

Modifiers (select one):

Health Promotion

Example: mixed age church group schedules series of six sessions about physical, emotional, and sexual aspects of aging.

Potential

Example: individual is at 75th percentile for weight.

Actual

Example: "2-year-old child does not walk without assistance," suggesting the sign/symptom *age-inappropriate behavior*.

Signs/Symptoms of Actual (select those that apply):

- abnormal results of developmental screening tests
- abnormal weight/height/head circumference in relation to growth/age standards
- age-inappropriate behavior
- inadequate achievement/maintenance of developmental tasks
- other

Related Medical Diagnoses. Mental Disorders (290-319). Complications of Pregnancy, Childbirth, and the Puerperium (630-677). Congenital Anomalies (740-759). Certain Conditions Originating in the Perinatal Period (760-779). Symptoms, Signs, and Ill-Defined Conditions (780-799). Injury and Poisoning (800-999). V Codes Supplementary Classification of Factors Influencing Health Status and Contact with Health Services (V01-V82). E Codes Supplementary Classification of External Causes of Injury and Poisoning (E800-E999).

Intervention Scheme

Teaching, Guidance, and Counseling (suggested care planning/intervention guides)

anatomy/physiology:
a. age/condition-appropriate
b. development/use of speech
c. other

anger management:
a. strategies
b. benefits
c. other

communication:
a. use non-verbal communication
b. other

discipline:
a. parent/caregiver's preferences/experiences
b. age/condition-appropriate measures
c. limit setting
d. clear expectations
e. reduce distractions/annoyances in environment
f. other

education:
a. school readiness
b. consistent interaction with school
c. assisting with homework
d. special needs programs/classes
e. work/study programs
f. community options
g. other

growth/development care:
a. growth spurts
b. developmental tasks

c. condition-specific options
d. realistic expectations
e. other

personal hygiene:
a. age/condition-appropriate independent behaviors
b. toileting
c. other

rest/sleep:
a. amount needed
b. planned rest
c. conducive environment
d. day/night schedule
e. other

safety:
a. appropriate supervision
b. age/condition-appropriate precautions
c. concerns for each stage of development/condition
d. drive car/operate hazardous outdoor equipment
e. electrical appliances
f. lock/security/alert systems
g. wander/fall alert systems
h. poison/medication control
i. appropriate furniture/placement
j. car seats/seat belts
k. environmental hazards
l. other

screening procedures:
a. self-screening
b. observe for age/condition symptoms
c. need for further developmental evaluation
d. other

signs/symptoms—physical:
a. height
b. weight
c. head circumference
d. physical problems
e. other

stimulation/nurturance:
a. light, textures, and color in environment
b. age/condition-appropriate games/toys/media
c. age/condition-appropriate exercises
d. speech/verbal stimulation
e. appropriate touching, holding, cuddling, and containing
f. other

support group:
a. emotional support
b. active listening
c. others' experiences
d. other

support system:
a. benefits
b. strategies
c. other

wellness:
a. lifestyle includes physical/emotional/spiritual activities
b. importance of routine preventive evaluations
c. well child/adult immunizations
d. influenza and pneumonia vaccinations
e. routine dental care
f. avoid areas that are high-risk for infection
g. other

other:

Treatments and Procedures (suggested care planning/intervention guides)

screening procedures:
a. standardized assessment guides/diagnostic tests for growth, depression, etc.
b. other

other:

Case Management (suggested care planning/intervention guides)

community outreach worker services:
a. evaluation
b. schedule/provide services
c. coordination among providers
d. other

medical/dental care:
a. evaluation
b. schedule/provide services
c. coordination among providers
d. other

nursing care:
a. evaluation
b. schedule/provide services
c. coordination among providers
d. other

occupational therapy care:
a. evaluation
b. schedule/provide services
c. coordination among providers
d. other

physical therapy care:
a. evaluation
b. schedule/provide services
c. coordination among providers
d. other

recreational therapy care:
a. evaluation
b. schedule/provide services

c. coordination among providers
d. other

social work/counseling care:
a. evaluation
b. schedule/provide services
c. coordination among providers
d. other

support group:
a. age/cultural/condition-specific group for parents, grandparents, chronic/terminal illness, etc.
b. community-/facility-based services
c. reliable Internet sites
d. telephone reassurance
e. other

support system:
a. family/friends
b. spiritual/faith communities
c. schools
d. neighbors
e. work associates
f. other

other:

Surveillance (suggested care planning/intervention guides)

bonding/attachment:
a. responses to parent/caregiver's stimulation/nurturance
b. other

communication:
a. expression of needs
b. expressive language
c. receptive language
d. other

continuity of care:
a. coordination among providers
b. other

discipline:
a. methods
b. appropriate
c. consistent
d. other

education:
a. appropriateness of grade level/program
b. client's attitude about progress
c. parent/caregiver's attitude toward client's progress
d. other

growth/development care:
a. appropriate growth pattern for family/group status
b. appropriate developmental tasks for age/condition
c. other

rest/sleep:
a. appropriate for age/condition
b. consistent patterns
c. other
safety:
a. appropriate precautions for age/condition
b. consistency
c. other
screening procedures:
a. developmental
b. behavioral
c. cognitive
d. gross/fine motor
e. speech/language
f. problem solving
g. personal/social
h. other
signs/symptoms—mental/emotional:
a. difficulty with interaction
b. difficulty with communication
c. difficulty adjusting to situations
d. difficulty participating in activities
e. behavior inappropriate for age
f. behavioral extremes
g. other
signs/symptoms—physical:
a. height
b. weight
c. head circumference
d. physical delays/issues
e. other
stimulation/nurturance:
a. environmental conditions
b. age/condition appropriate games/toys/media
c. physical/mental exercises
d. language development
e. social activities
f. other
support group:
a. participation
b. benefits
c. other
support system:
a. involvement
b. benefits
c. other
wellness:
a. appropriate contacts with providers
b. receives appropriate care

c. immunizations
d. influenza and pneumonia vaccinations
e. other
other:

Problem Rating Scale for Outcomes

Knowledge
1-No knowledge
Example: unwilling to learn about developmental needs of elderly parent
2-Minimal knowledge
Example: willing to learn about developmental needs of elderly parent
3-Basic knowledge
Example: describes minimal knowledge about developmental needs of elderly parent
4-Adequate knowledge
Example: understands developmental needs of elderly parent, but not how to meet those needs
5-Superior knowledge
Example: understands developmental needs of elderly parent and several ways to meet those needs

Behavior
1-Not appropriate behavior
Example: 10-year-old wets bed regularly
2-Rarely appropriate behavior
Example: 6-year-old wets bed regularly
3-Inconsistently appropriate behavior
Example: 5-year-old wets bed occasionally following high-stress days
4-Usually appropriate behavior
Example: 5-year-old wet bed twice since birth of sibling
5-Consistently appropriate behavior
Example: no bedwetting after child is toilet trained during the day

Status
1-Extreme signs/symptoms
Example: developmental screening results show severe delays in several areas
2-Severe signs/symptoms
Example: developmental screening results show delays ranging from minimal to moderate to severe
3-Moderate signs/symptoms
Example: developmental screening results show one or two minimal to moderate delays
4-Minimal signs/symptoms
Example: developmental screening results show one minimal delay
5-No signs/symptoms
Example: developmental screening results within normal limits

Physiological Domain

HEARING

Problem Classification Scheme

Definition. Perception of sound by the ears.
Modifiers (select one):

Health Promotion

Example: job counselor asks public health nurse to conduct a class about hearing protection for people seeking employment.

Potential

Example: frequent respiratory and ear infections.

Actual

Example: standardized or informal methods such as audiometric or whisper tests are used to diagnose partial deafness and suggest *abnormal results of hearing screening test*.

SIGNS/SYMPTOMS OF ACTUAL (select those that apply):

- difficulty hearing normal speech tones
- difficulty hearing speech in large group settings
- difficulty hearing high frequency sounds
- absent/abnormal response to sound
- abnormal results of hearing screening test
- other

Related Medical Diagnoses. Infectious and Parasitic Diseases (001-139). Diseases of the Nervous System and Sense Organs (320-326). Diseases of the Respiratory System (460-519). Congenital Anomalies (740-759). V Codes Supplementary Classification of Factors Influencing Health Status and Contact with Health Services (V01-V83).

Intervention Scheme

Teaching, Guidance, and Counseling (suggested care planning/intervention guides)

anatomy/physiology:

a. ear
b. other

communication:

a. compensatory techniques
b. assistive devices
c. interpretation of hearing tests
d. other

coping skills:

a. disease process
b. other

durable medical equipment:

a. care of hearing aid
b. test batteries
c. other

personal hygiene:
a. cleanse ears
b. irrigation
c. injury prevention
d. other

safety:
a. activity precautions
b. infection prevention
c. medical alert bracelet
d. security/weather alarms
e. other

signs/symptoms—physical:
a. evidence of disease/infection
b. pain
c. increased hearing loss/other changes
d. when to notify providers
e. other

other:

Treatments and Procedures (suggested care planning/intervention guides)

screening procedures:
a. audiometric threshold test
b. hearing assessment
c. other

other:

Case Management (suggested care planning/intervention guides)

medical/dental care:
a. evaluation
b. schedule/provide services
c. coordination among providers
d. other

other community resources:
a. audiologist
b. telephone company
c. school system
d. sources of specialized equipment
e. library
f. guides dogs trained for clients with hearing loss
g. volunteers
h. reliable Internet sites
i. day care
j. assisted living
k. other

speech and language pathology care:
a. evaluation
b. schedule/provide services
c. coordination among providers
d. other

other:

Surveillance (suggested care planning/intervention guides)

communication:

a. assistive devices
b. communication techniques
c. other

coping skills:

a. adequacy
b. physical/emotional/social difficulties
c. managing with environment
d. other

medical/dental care:

a. receives care when scheduled
b. adequate/appropriate
c. follows plan of care
d. other

medication administration:

a. correct technique
b. correct schedule
c. other

screening procedures:

a. hearing loss
b. other

signs/symptoms—physical:

a. evidence of disease/infection
b. hearing loss
c. pain
d. presence of wax
e. other

other:

Problem Rating Scale for Outcomes

Knowledge

1-No knowledge

Example: no knowledge about hearing problems, related anatomy/physiology, or corrections/treatments

2-Minimal knowledge

Example: interested in information about hearing problems, related anatomy/physiology, and corrections/treatments

3-Basic knowledge

Example: describes early signs/symptoms of hearing problems, but does not understand related anatomy/physiology or corrections/treatments

4-Adequate knowledge

Example: describes early signs/symptoms of hearing problems and related anatomy/physiology, but not corrections/treatments

5-Superior knowledge

Example: describes early signs/symptoms of hearing problems, related anatomy/physiology, and appropriate corrections/treatments

Behavior
1-Not appropriate behavior
Example: unwilling to obtain hearing aid
2-Rarely appropriate behavior
Example: has hearing aid, uses rarely
3-Inconsistently appropriate behavior
Example: uses hearing aid occasionally, batteries need to be replaced, and aid and hearing need to be re-tested
4-Usually appropriate behavior
Example: uses hearing aid with new batteries, had aid re-tested, unwilling to have hearing retested
5-Consistently appropriate behavior
Example: wears hearing aid with new batteries appropriately and consistently; has hearing retested regularly

Status
1-Extreme signs/symptoms
Example: severe loss bilaterally
2-Severe signs/symptoms
Example: minimal correction with hearing aid
3-Moderate signs/symptoms
Example: moderate correction with hearing aid
4-Minimal signs/symptoms
Example: good correction, malfunctions of hearing aid not repaired promptly
5-No signs/symptoms
Example: good correction with hearing aid

VISION

Problem Classification Scheme

Definition. Act or power of sensing with the eyes.
Modifiers (select one):

Health Promotion
Example: interested in lighting conducive to good working conditions.
Potential
Example: mother and grandfather had glaucoma.
Actual
Example: elementary school teacher reports that student "cannot read materials on the walls" suggesting the sign/symptom *difficulty seeing distant objects.*

Signs/Symptoms of Actual (select those that apply):

- difficulty seeing small print/calibrations
- difficulty seeing distant objects
- difficulty seeing close objects
- absent/abnormal response to visual stimuli
- abnormal results of vision screening test
- squinting/blinking/tearing/blurring
- floaters/flashes

- difficulty differentiating colors
- other

Related medical diagnoses. Infectious and Parasitic Diseases (001-139). Diseases of the Nervous System and Sense Organs (320-326). Congenital Anomalies (740-759). V Codes Supplementary Classification of Factors Influencing Health Status and Contact with Health Services (V01-V83).

Intervention Scheme

Teaching, Guidance, and Counseling (suggested care planning/intervention guides)

anatomy/physiology:
a. eye
b. diseases/conditions that diminish vision
c. other

communication:
a. compensatory techniques
b. assistive devices
c. interpretation of vision tests
d. other

coping skills:
a. managing disease process
b. managing signs/symptoms
c. other

dressing change/wound care:
a. eye dressings
b. eye patch/shield
c. other

durable medical equipment:
a. use/care of prosthesis
b. use/care of glasses/contact lenses
c. other

safety:
a. activity precautions
b. infection prevention
c. medical alert bracelet
d. security/weather alarms
e. other

screening procdures:
a. central vision test
b. visual assessment
c. other

signs/symptoms—physical:
a. evidence of disease/infection
b. swelling
c. pain
d. diminished vision/other changes
e. when to notify providers
f. other

other:

Treatments and Procedures (suggested care planning/intervention guides)

dressing change/wound care:
a. eye dressings
b. other

durable medical equipment:
a. insertion/care of prosthesis
b. insertion/care of contact lenses
c. other

other:

Case Management (suggested care planning/intervention guides)

dietary management:
a. home-delivered meals
b. community options such as group meal sites
c. other

durable medical equipment:
a. visual aids
b. security and alert systems
c. sources of specialized equipment
d. prosthesis
e. other

education:
a. Braille instruction
b. classroom accommodations
c. other

homemaking/housekeeping:
a. evaluation
b. schedule services
c. other

medical/dental care:
a. evaluation
b. schedule/provide services
c. coordination among providers
d. other

occupational therapy care:
a. evaluation
b. schedule/provide services
c. coordination among providers
d. other

other community resources:
a. governmental/private organizations such as Society for the Blind
b. guide dogs trained for clients with vision loss
c. media/materials such as Radio Talking Books
d. reliable Internet sites
e. volunteers
f. day care

g. assisted living
h. other

transportation:

a. identify resources
b. how to use
c. other

other:

Surveillance (suggested care planning/intervention guides)

communication:

a. assistive devices
b. communication techniques
c. other

coping skills:

a. adequacy
b. physical/emotional/social difficulties
c. managing the environment
d. other

durable medical equipment:

a. prosthesis care
b. other

medical/dental care:

a. receives care when scheduled
b. adequate/appropriate
c. follows plan of care
d. other

signs/symptoms—physical:

a. evidence of disease/infection
b. swelling
c. pain
d. diminished vision
e. other

other:

Problem Rating Scale for Outcomes

Knowledge

1-No knowledge

Example: not aware of relationship between diabetes and vision, or any symptoms of acute vision problems

2-Minimal knowledge

Example: not aware of relationship between diabetes and vision; recognizes symptoms of acute vision problems

3-Basic knowledge

Example: minimal awareness of relationship between diabetes and vision; recognizes symptoms of acute vision problems and appropriate action

4-Adequate knowledge

Example: moderate awareness of relationship between diabetes and vision; recognizes symptoms of acute and chronic vision problems but only appropriate action for acute signs/symptoms

5-Superior knowledge
Example: describes relationship between diabetes and vision, and ways to prevent, detect, and resolve acute and chronic signs/symptoms

Behavior
1-Not appropriate behavior
Example: unwilling to wear corrective lenses
2-Rarely appropriate behavior
Example: wears corrective lenses rarely
3-Inconsistently appropriate behavior
Example: wears corrective lenses some of the time
4-Usually appropriate behavior
Example: wears corrective lenses most of the time
5-Consistently appropriate behavior
Example: wears corrective lenses consistently and appropriately

Status
1-Extreme signs/symptoms
Example: has severe vision loss
2-Severe signs/symptoms
Example: limited vision, cannot read
3-Moderate signs/symptoms
Example: able to read large print only
4-Minimal signs/symptoms
Example: unable to see small calibrations
5-No signs/symptoms
Example: vision is nearly 20/20 with corrective lenses/surgery

SPEECH AND LANGUAGE

Problem Classification Scheme

Definition. Use of articulated vocal sounds, symbols, signs, or gestures for communication.
Modifiers (select one):
Health Promotion
Example: day care staff members distribute materials to parents each month about ways to encourage healthy children to speak.
Potential
Example: has hearing loss.
Actual
Example: elder who has "aphasia and a receptive speech impairment" demonstrates the sign/symptom *absent/abnormal ability to understand.*
Signs/Symptoms of Actual (select those that apply):
- absent/abnormal ability to speak/vocalize
- absent/abnormal ability to understand
- lacks alternative communication skills/gestures
- inappropriate sentence structure
- limited enunciation/clarity
- inappropriate word usage
- other

Related Medical Diagnoses. Infectious and Parasitic Diseases (001-139). Mental Disorders (290-319). Diseases of the Nervous System and Sense Organs (320-326). Congenital Anomalies (740-759). Symptoms, Signs, and Ill-Defined Conditions (780-799). V Codes Supplementary Classification of Factors Influencing Health Status and Contact with Health Services (V01-V83).

Intervention Scheme

Teaching, Guidance, and Counseling (suggested care planning/intervention guides)

anatomy/physiology:
a. oropharyngeal
b. speech
c. disease process
d. other

caretaking/parenting skills:
a. encourage practice
b. speak to child/adult and others frequently
c. avoid answering for child/adult
d. model correct language
e. communicate with media such as pictures and signing
f. other

communication:
a. compensatory strategies
b. eliciting verbal responses
c. eliciting nonverbal responses
d. visual/motor, writing, and numeric processes
e. other

coping skills:
a. disease process
b. signs/symptoms of disease/condition
c. evaluate behavior patterns
d. other

durable medical equipment:
a. communication devices such as switches, computer programs, and other electronic devices
b. communication boards such as flash cards, choice boards, and writing boards
c. adaptive eating devices
d. other

exercises:
a. swallowing/positioning
b. thermal or tactile stimulation
c. orofacial exercises
d. tongue strengthening and range of motion
e. base of tongue and pharyngeal region exercises
f. bolus control
g. techniques to elicit phonation
h. control of drooling
i. other

feeding procedures:
a. liquids
b. solids

c. feeding/nutrition products
d. other
positioning:
a. for specific activities
b. to improve quality/volume of voice production
c. other
other:

Treatments and Procedures (suggested care planning/intervention guides)
feeding procedures:
a. liquids
b. solids
c. feeding/nutrition products
d. other
speech and language pathology care:
a. thermal or tactile stimulation
b. orofacial exercises
c. tongue strengthening
d. base of tongue and pharyngeal region
e. bolus control
f. techniques to elicit phonation
g. control of drooling
h. other
other:

Case Management (suggested care planning/intervention guides)
durable medical equipment:
a. communication devices such as switches, computer programs, and other electronic devices
b. communication boards such as flash cards, choice boards, and writing boards
c. adaptive eating devices
d. other
medical/dental care:
a. evaluation
b. schedule/provide services
c. coordination among providers
d. other
nutritionist care:
a. evaluation
b. schedule/provide services
c. coordination among providers
d. other
other community resources:
a. governmental health/social service assistance
b. coordinate with early childhood/special education services
c. schools
d. private organizations
e. other

speech and language pathology care:
a. evaluation
b. schedule/provide services
c. coordination among providers
d. other

support group:
a. age/cultural/condition-specific group for stroke, stuttering, laryngectomy, etc.
b. community-/facility-based services
c. reliable Internet sites
d. telephone information/reassurance
e. other

support system:
a. family/friends
b. spiritual/faith communities
c. schools
d. neighbors
e. work associates
f. other

other:

Surveillance (suggested care planning/intervention guides)

caretaking/parenting skills:
a. modified practices
b. other

communication:
a. speech/language abilities
b. nonverbal
c. voice disorders
d. other

coping skills:
a. disease process
b. managing signs/symptoms
c. other

exercises:
a. follows plan of care
b. other

feeding procedures:
a. ability to chew
b. ability to swallow
c. bolus control
d. other

medical/dental care:
a. receives care when scheduled
b. adequate/appropriate
c. follows plan of care
d. other

positioning:
a. for specific activities

b. to improve quality/volume of voice production
c. other
other:

Problem Rating Scale for Outcomes

Knowledge
1-No knowledge
Example: has no knowledge of speech development or rehabilitation
2-Minimal knowledge
Example: interested in entering early intervention/rehabilitation program
3-Basic knowledge
Example: knows some speech exercises
4-Adequate knowledge
Example: remembers and understands most speech exercises
5-Superior knowledge
Example: understands all prescribed speech exercises consistently

Behavior
1-Not appropriate behavior
Example: unwilling to participate in speech program
2-Rarely appropriate behavior
Example: participates in speech program for only short periods
3-Inconsistently appropriate behavior
Example: participates with speech and language pathologist, no practice
4-Usually appropriate behavior
Example: participates with speech and language pathologist, occasionally practices
5-Consistently appropriate behavior
Example: participates in speech sessions, practices exercises consistently

Status
1-Extreme signs/symptoms
Example: unable to express words or sounds; severe receptive impairment
2-Severe signs/symptoms
Example: minimal expression of words and/or sounds; some receptive impairment
3-Moderate signs/symptoms
Example: moderate expression of words and/or sounds; no receptive impairment
4-Minimal signs/symptoms
Example: usually able to express words and sound; occasionally forgets words
5-No signs/symptoms
Example: speaks/articulates clearly; understands when spoken to

ORAL HEALTH

Problem Classification Scheme

Definition. Condition of the mouth and gums and the number, type, and arrangement of the teeth.

Modifiers (select one):
Health Promotion
Example: principal asks the school nurse to conduct class about care of teeth.

Potential

Example: smokes, uses alcohol, and/or has chronic health problems.

Actual

Example: the sign/symptom *ill-fitting/missing dentures* is evidenced by the elder who "only eats soft foods and liquids since getting dentures."

SIGNS/SYMPTOMS OF ACTUAL (select those that apply):

- missing/broken/malformed teeth
- caries
- excess tartar
- sore/swollen/bleeding gums
- malocclusion
- ill-fitting/missing dentures
- sensitivity to hot or cold
- other

Related Medical Diagnoses. Diseases of the Digestive System (520-579). Congenital Anomalies (740-759). Symptoms, Signs, and Ill-Defined Conditions (780-799).

Intervention Scheme

Teaching, Guidance, and Counseling (suggested care planning/intervention guides)

anatomy/physiology:

a. mouth, gums, and teeth
b. other

dietary management:

a. recommended diet
b. balanced intake of food and fluids
c. other

durable medical equipment:

a. dentures
b. electric toothbrushes
c. other

infection precautions:

a. identify sources of infection
b. hand washing
c. disposal of soiled/contaminated materials
d. clean environment
e. other

medical/dental care:

a. prevention/routine maintenance
b. gum disease
c. tooth decay
d. dentures
e. benefits of regular care
f. other

personal hygiene:

a. frequent brushing and flossing
b. denture care
c. other

signs/symptoms—physical:
a. when to notify providers
b. pain
c. bleeding
d. other
supplies
a. toothbrushes
b. toothpaste/denture cleansers
c. dental floss
d. other
other:

Treatments and Procedures (suggested care planning/intervention guides)
medical/dental care:
a. preventive care/cleaning
b. extractions
c. fill caries
d. replace/repair damaged teeth
e. braces/other orthodontia
f. dentures
g. other
personal hygiene:
a. oral care
b. other
other:

Case Management (suggested care planning/intervention guides)
medical/dental care:
a. evaluation
b. schedule/provide services
c. coordination among providers
d. other
nutritionist care:
a. evaluation
b. schedule/provide services
c. coordination among providers
d. other
other:

Surveillance (suggested care planning/intervention guides)
dietary management:
a. adequate/appropriate for age/physical status
b. other
medical/dental care:
a. receives care when scheduled
b. adequate/appropriate
c. follows plan of care
d. other

signs/symptoms—physical:
a. evidence of disease/infection
b. pain
c. lesions
d. rash
e. odor
f. other
other:

Problem Rating Scale for Outcomes

Knowledge
1-No knowledge
Example: unaware of proper oral hygiene and risk factors
2-Minimal knowledge
Example: willing to learn about oral hygiene and risk factors
3-Basic knowledge
Example: understands when and how to brush teeth
4-Adequate knowledge
Example: understands when and how to brush and floss teeth, and relationship of risk factors to oral health
5-Superior knowledge
Example: understands proper oral hygiene and preventive dental care

Behavior
1-Not appropriate behavior
Example: no teeth or dentures
2-Rarely appropriate behavior
Example: considering obtaining dentures
3-Inconsistently appropriate behavior
Example: wears dentures when eating; does not care for them consistently
4-Usually appropriate behavior
Example: wears dentures when eating and some other times; cares for them inconsistently
5-Consistently appropriate behavior
Example: wears dentures and cares for them consistently

Status
1-Extreme signs/symptoms
Example: extreme decay, gingivitis, and tartar, missing/broken teeth, lesions
2-Severe signs/symptoms
Example: moderate decay and gingivitis, extreme tartar, no missing/broken teeth or lesions
3-Moderate signs/symptoms
Example: mild decay and gingivitis, extreme tartar
4-Minimal signs/symptoms
Example: mild tartar, no caries, little/no gingivitis
5-No signs/symptoms
Example: teeth, gums, and mouth appear clean, healthy, and well cared for

COGNITION

Problem Classification Scheme

Definition. Ability to think and use information.
Modifiers (select one):

Health Promotion

Example: pattern of daily stimulating mental activities such as crossword/other puzzles, reading, and discussions.

Potential

Example: new diagnosis of stroke.

Actual

Example: the signs/symptoms *limited recall of recent events* and *limited concentration* are applicable for "cannot remember to turn stove/oven off or use it safely."

SIGNS/SYMPTOMS OF ACTUAL (select those that apply):

- diminished judgment
- disoriented to time/place/person
- limited recall of recent events
- limited recall of long past events
- limited calculating/sequencing skills
- limited concentration
- limited reasoning/abstract thinking ability
- impulsiveness
- repetitious language/behavior
- wanders
- other

Related Medical Diagnoses. Mental Disorders (290-319). Diseases of the Nervous System and Sense Organs (320-389). Symptoms, Signs, and Ill-Defined Conditions (780-799).

Intervention Scheme

Teaching, Guidance, and Counseling (suggested care planning/intervention guides)

anatomy/physiology:

a. neurological disease processes
b. other

anger management:

a. strategies
b. benefits
c. other

caretaking/parenting skills:

a. long-range planning/decision making
b. support in-home care system
c. telephone reassurance
d. other

continuity of care:

a. simplified routine
b. mild-mannered caregivers
c. consistency
d. other

coping skills:
a. disease process
b. adjustment to illness
c. crisis intervention
d. planned time away
e. other

dietary management:
a. safe preparation options
b. pre-prepared foods
c. other

durable medical equipment:
a. communication devices such as switches, computer programs, and other electronic devices
b. communication boards such as flash cards, choice boards, and writing boards
c. adaptive eating devices
d. memory book
e. labels for personal and household items
f. other

medication action/side effects:
a. important to take as prescribed
b. purpose/benefits
c. changes to note and report in timely manner
d. need for timely laboratory tests
e. other

personal hygiene:
a. evaluate/monitor abilities
b. daily routine care needs
c. other

safety:
a. appropriate supervision
b. drives car/operates hazardous outdoor equipment
c. electrical appliances
d. lock/security/alert systems
e. wander/fall alert systems
f. poison/medication control
g. appropriate furniture/placement
h. adaptive equipment
i. other

signs/symptoms—mental/emotional:
a. when to notify providers
b. orientation
c. confusion
d. memory/recall
e. behavioral changes
f. other

stimulation/nurturance:
a. orientation/re-orientation
b. written materials/media
c. music/art/physical activity programs

d. games/puzzles
e. hobbies/crafts
f. interaction/discussion
g. pet therapy
h. other

support group:
a. options
b. how to access
c. benefits
d. active listening
e. other

support system:
a. benefits
b. options
c. other

other:

Treatments and Procedures (suggested care planning/intervention guides)

other:

Case Management (suggested care planning/intervention guides)

continuity of care:
a. coordination among providers
b. other

day care/respite:
a. options
b. adult/specialized day care
c. governmental health/social service assistance
d. private day care
e. respite services
f. other

dietary management:
a. home-delivered meals
b. group meal sites
c. community options
d. other

durable medical equipment:
a. communication devices such as switches, computer programs, and other electronic devices
b. communication boards such as flash cards, choice boards, and writing boards
c. adaptive eating devices
d. other

legal system:
a. governmental mental health organizations
b. governmental adult protective services
c. legal assistance
d. guardian/conservator
e. law enforcement
f. other

medical/dental care:
a. evaluation
b. schedule/provide services
c. coordination among providers
d. other

medication coordination/ordering:
a. obtains refills in a timely manner
b. communicate with pharmacist/other providers
c. other

nursing care:
a. evaluation
b. schedule/provide services
c. coordination among providers
d. other

paraprofessional/aide care:
a. evaluation
b. schedule/provide services
c. coordination among providers
d. other

recreational therapy care:
a. evaluation
b. schedule/provide services
c. coordination among providers
d. other

support group:
a. age/cultural/condition-specific group for Alzheimer's disease, dementia, etc.
b. community-/facility-based services
c. reliable Internet sites
d. telephone information/reassurance
e. other

support system:
a. family/friends
b. spiritual/faith communities
c. schools
d. neighbors
e. work associates
f. other

transportation:
a. options
b. other

other:

Surveillance (suggested care planning/intervention guides)

anger management:
a. adequacy
b. other

medical/dental care:
a. receives care when scheduled
b. adequate/appropriate

c. follows plan of care
d. other

medication action/side effects:
a. takes as prescribed
b. notes and reports changes/side effects in timely manner
c. timely laboratory tests
d. other

nursing care:
a. receives care when scheduled
b. adequate/appropriate
c. follows plan of care
d. other

paraprofessional/aide care:
a. receives care when scheduled
b. adequate/appropriate
c. follows plan of care
d. other

recreational therapy care:
a. receives care when scheduled
b. adequate/appropriate
c. follows plan of care
d. other

signs/symptoms—mental/emotional:
a. orientation
b. memory/recall
c. behavioral changes
d. affect
e. other

other:

Problem Rating Scale for Outcomes

Knowledge

1-No knowledge

Example: unaware of cause, prognosis, treatment, or needed modifications for Alzheimer's disease or other forms of dementia

2-Minimal knowledge

Example: expresses interest in obtaining information about Alzheimer's disease or other forms of dementia

3-Basic knowledge

Example: has knowledge about cause and prognosis of Alzheimer's disease or other forms of dementia, but not treatment or modification options

4-Adequate knowledge

Example: aware of probable causes, prognosis, and treatment of Alzheimer's disease or other forms of dementia, but not modification options

5-Superior knowledge

Example: describes probable causes, prognosis, and treatment options of Alzheimer's disease or other forms of dementia, and ways to modify environment and social interaction

Behavior
1-Not appropriate behavior
Example: gets lost regularly when walking or driving the car
2-Rarely appropriate behavior
Example: alone for extended periods; finds keys and uses car occasionally
3-Inconsistently appropriate behavior
Example: alone for extended periods; does not have access to car or keys
4-Usually appropriate behavior
Example: occasionally unsupervised; does not have access to car or keys
5-Consistently appropriate behavior
Example: consistently supervised and wears a wander alert bracelet; does not have access to car or keys

Status
1-Extreme signs/symptoms
Example: disoriented to time and place; unable to recognize family
2-Severe signs/symptoms
Example: disoriented to time and place; occasionally recognizes family
3-Moderate signs/symptoms
Example: disoriented to time, but oriented to place; knows some or all of family
4-Minimal signs/symptoms
Example: occasionally disoriented to time, but oriented to place and recognizes family consistently
5-No signs/symptoms
Example: consistently oriented and recognizes family

PAIN

Problem Classification

Definition. Unpleasant sensory and emotional experience associated with actual or potential tissue damage.

Modifiers (select one):

Health Promotion

Example: healthy young woman knows older women who have experience due to osteoporosis and arthritis; she requests information about lifestyle choices to minimize her pain symptoms in future.

Potential

Example: recently diagnosed sarcoma.

Actual

Example: the sign/symptom *expresses discomfort/pain* is appropriate for "reports aching in knees when awakens each morning."

SIGNS/SYMPTOMS OF ACTUAL (select those that apply):

- expresses discomfort/pain
- elevated pulse/respirations/blood pressure
- compensated movement/guarding
- restless behavior

- facial grimaces
- pallor/perspiration
- other

Related Medical Diagnoses. Neoplasms (140-239). Diseases of the Nervous System and Sense Organs (320-389). Diseases of the Circulatory System (390-459). Diseases of the Respiratory System (460-519). Diseases of the Digestive System (520-579). Diseases of the Genitourinary System (580-629). Complications of Pregnancy, Childbirth, and the Puerperium (630-677). Diseases of the Musculoskeletal System and Connective Tissue (710-739). Symptoms, Signs, and Ill-Defined Conditions (780-799). Injury and Poisoning (800-999). E Codes Supplementary Classification of External Causes of Injury and Poisoning (E800-E999).

Intervention Scheme

Teaching, Guidance, and Counseling (suggested care planning/intervention guides)

anatomy/physiology:
a. pain
b. other

dietary management:
a. recommended diet
b. high protein
c. supplemental vitamins and minerals
d. herbs
e. macrobiotics
f. fluid balance
g. other

durable medical equipment:
a. oxygen use
b. braces/splints/wraps
c. specialty beds
d. electrical stimulation (TENS)
e. other

end-of-life care:
a. recognition/acceptance
b. plans
c. no code (no resuscitation)
d. other

exercises:
a. stretching
b. range of motion
c. weight lifting
d. other

medication action/side effects:
a. important to take as prescribed
b. purpose/benefits
c. changes to note and report in timely manner
d. need for timely laboratory tests
e. other

physical therapy care:
a. electrical stimulation (TENS)
b. massage
c. body mechanics
d. other

relaxation/breathing techniques:
a. guided imagery
b. music
c. breathing techniques
d. yoga
e. progressive muscle relaxation
f. other

signs/symptoms—physical:
a. location
b. severity
c. frequency/duration
d. when to notify providers
e. vital signs/blood pressure
f. other

other:

Treatments and Procedures (suggested care planning/intervention guides)

durable medical equipment:
a. administer oxygen
b. other

physical therapy care:
a. ultrasound
b. massage/relaxation techniques
c. traction/joint mobilization
d. electrical stimulation (TENS)
e. stretching
f. heat/cold applications
g. exercise program
h. positioning
i. weight lifting
j. other

other:

Case Management (suggested care planning/intervention guides)

medical/dental care:
a. evaluation
b. schedule/provide services
c. coordination among providers
d. other

medication coordination/ordering:
a. obtains refills in a timely manner
b. communicate with pharmacist/other providers
c. other

nursing care:
a. evaluation
b. schedule/provide services
c. coordination among providers
d. other
other community resources:
a. pain clinic
b. other
physical therapy care:
a. evaluation
b. schedule/provide services
c. coordination among providers
d. other
other:

Surveillance (suggested care planning/intervention guides)
medical/dental care:
a. receives care when scheduled
b. adequate/appropriate
c. follows plan of care
d. other
medication action/side effects:
a. takes as prescribed
b. notes and reports changes/side effects in timely manner
c. timely laboratory tests
d. other
nursing care:
a. receives care when scheduled
b. adequate/appropriate
c. follows plan of care
d. other
physical therapy care:
a. receives care when scheduled
b. adequate/appropriate
c. follows plan of care
d. other
signs/symptoms—physical:
a. location
b. pain scale to determine severity
c. frequency/duration
d. vital signs/blood pressure
e. effectiveness of all control measures
f. other
other:

Problem Rating Scale for Outcomes

Knowledge
1-No knowledge
Example: lacks knowledge about pain source or treatment

2-Minimal knowledge
Example: limited knowledge about pain source or treatment
3-Basic knowledge
Example: knows which medications relieve pain
4-Adequate knowledge
Example: knows which medications relieve pain as well as when and how to take them
5-Superior knowledge
Example: describes pain etiology, multiple effective treatment methods, and how to optimize effects of treatment

Behavior
1-Not appropriate behavior
Example: unwilling to participate in pain control program
2-Rarely appropriate behavior
Example: takes medication only in presence of severe pain
3-Inconsistently appropriate behavior
Example: refuses narcotic, accepts less effective non-narcotic; will not use non-pharmacological measures for pain control
4-Usually appropriate behavior
Example: uses appropriate medications and other therapeutic techniques for pain control most of the time
5-Consistently appropriate behavior
Example: consistently uses appropriate medications and other therapeutic techniques for pain control

Status
1-Extreme signs/symptoms
Example: regularly exhibits signs/symptoms of severe pain
2-Severe signs/symptoms
Example: regularly exhibits signs/symptoms of moderately severe pain
3-Moderate signs/symptoms
Example: regularly exhibits signs/symptoms of moderate pain
4-Minimal signs/symptoms
Example: regularly exhibits signs/symptoms of mild pain; rarely in severe pain
5-No signs/symptoms
Example: pain signs/symptoms controlled

CONSCIOUSNESS

Problem Classification Scheme

Definition. Awareness of and responsiveness to stimuli and the surroundings.
Modifiers (select one):

Health Promotion
Example: requests information regarding diabetic coma.
Potential
Example: in early stage of terminal illness.
Actual
Example: "rarely shows any response" or "does not acknowledge voices of family members," suggesting the sign/symptom *unresponsive* during coma/late stage of terminal illness.

SIGNS/SYMPTOMS OF ACTUAL (select those that apply):

- lethargic
- stuporous
- unresponsive
- comatose
- other

Related Medical Diagnoses. Infectious and Parasitic Diseases (001-139). Diseases of the Nervous System and Sense Organs (320-389). Symptoms, Signs, and Ill-Defined Conditions (780-799).

Intervention Scheme

Teaching, Guidance, and Counseling (suggested care planning/intervention guides)

anatomy/physiology:

a. disease process
b. other

end-of-life care:

a. recognition/acceptance
b. plans
c. control light, noise, and odors
d. no code (no resuscitation)
e. other

feeding procedures:

a. assess swallowing
b. sips/chips
c. other

medication action/side effects:

a. important to take as prescribed
b. purpose/benefits
c. changes to note and report in timely manner
d. need for timely laboratory tests
e. other

personal hygiene:

a. mouth care
b. skin care
c. toileting
d. other

positioning:

a. frequent position change
b. use of pillows/other support to maintain position
c. other

safety:

a. special bed/side rails
b. restraints
c. supervision
d. alert system
e. other

signs/symptoms—physical:

a. when to notify providers

b. level of consciousness
c. other

spiritual care:
a. allow expression of existential/faith preferences
b. offer active/passive prayer
c. other

stimulation/nurturance:
a. talking
b. touch/massage
c. other

other:

Treatments and Procedures (suggested care planning/intervention guides)

other:

Case Management (suggested care planning/intervention guides)

durable medical equipment:
a. special bed/side rails
b. toileting equipment
c. other

end-of-life care:
a. funeral home/morgue
b. memorial services
c. burial/cremation
d. other

medical/dental care:
a. evaluation
b. schedule/provide services
c. coordination among providers
d. other

medication coordination/ordering:
a. obtains refills in a timely manner
b. communicate with pharmacist/other providers
c. other

nursing care:
a. evaluation
b. schedule/provide services
c. coordination among providers
d. other

paraprofessional/aide care:
a. evaluation
b. schedule/provide services
c. coordination among providers
d. other

supplies:
a. mouth swabs and solution
b. other

other:

Surveillance (suggested care planning/intervention guides)

medication action/side effects:

a. takes as prescribed
b. notes and reports changes/side effects in timely manner
c. timely laboratory tests
d. other

signs/symptoms—physical:

a. scale to determine level of consciousness
b. skin integrity
c. measure pain even if cannot communicate
d. adequacy of comfort measures
e. other

other:

Problem Rating Scale for Outcomes

Knowledge

1-No knowledge
Example: family cannot recognize change in status

2-Minimal knowledge
Example: family cannot explain symptoms/status but recognizes a change in responsiveness

3-Basic knowledge
Example: family understands present symptoms/status but has unrealistic future expectations

4-Adequate knowledge
Example: family understands present symptoms/status; knows what to anticipate some of the time

5-Superior knowledge
Example: family understands present symptoms/status and anticipates future changes consistently

Behavior

1-Not appropriate behavior
Example: family unwilling to provide physical care or talk to client

2-Rarely appropriate behavior
Example: family provides inconsistent physical care but will not talk to client

3-Inconsistently appropriate behavior
Example: family provides more consistent care; talks to client rarely

4-Usually appropriate behavior
Example: family provides good physical care and talks to client occasionally

5-Consistently appropriate behavior
Example: family talks to client and provides adequate, consistent physical care

Status

1-Extreme signs/symptoms
Example: comatose; no response to deep pain stimuli

2-Severe signs/symptoms
Example: unresponsive most of the time; does not respond to stimulation

3-Moderate signs/symptoms
Example: lethargic; sleeps most of the time but can be aroused
4-Minimal signs/symptoms
Example: occasional periods of unresponsiveness
5-No signs/symptoms
Example: alert, oriented

SKIN

Problem Classification Scheme

Definition. Natural covering of the body.
Modifiers (select one):

Health Promotion
Example: young teen expresses concerns about skin care and use of make-up.
Potential
Example: uses wheelchair.
Actual
Example: individual is confined to bed and has "small open areas on both heels," indicating the presence of *lesion/pressure ulcer.*

SIGNS/SYMPTOMS OF ACTUAL (select those that apply):

- lesion/pressure ulcer
- rash
- excessively dry
- excessively oily
- inflammation
- pruritus
- drainage
- bruising
- hypertrophy of nails
- delayed incisional healing
- other

Related Medical Diagnoses. Neoplasms (140-239). Diseases of the Skin and Subcutaneous Tissue (680-709). Congenital Anomalies (740-759). Symptoms, Signs, and Ill-Defined Conditions (780-799). Injury and Poisoning (800-999). Persons Encountering Health Services for Specific Procedures and Aftercare (V50-V59).

Intervention Scheme

Teaching, Guidance, and Counseling (suggested care planning/intervention guides)

anatomy/physiology:
a. skin
b. maintaining tissue perfusion/oxygen supply
c. healing process
d. other

coping skills:
a. body image
b. other

dietary management:
a. recommended diet

b. high protein
c. supplemental vitamins and minerals
d. herbs
e. macrobiotics
f. fluid balance
g. other

dressing change/wound care:
a. recommended technique
b. maintain schedule
c. other

durable medical equipment:
a. pressure reducing devices/materials
b. special/pressure reduction bed
c. telehealth monitor
d. other

infection precautions:
a. hand washing
b. disposal of dressings
c. clean environment
d. protect lesion/incision
e. nonconstricting clothing
f. avoid others with infections
g. avoid moisture from body fluids
h. other

laboratory findings:
a. interpretation of culture results
b. other

mobility/transfers:
a. avoid shearing/friction
b. safe transfer techniques/body mechanics
c. splint wound/injured area
d. other

positioning:
a. frequent position change
b. use of pillows/other support
c. proper postural alignment
d. other

signs/symptoms—physical:
a. evidence of disease/infection
b. change in depth/diameter of lesion
c. control pain
d. intake and output
e. when to notify providers
f. other

skin care:
a. prevent breakdown/keep dry
b. check decreased circulation
c. check changed temperature/sensation
d. massage

e. lotion
f. hygiene
g. other
other:

Treatments and Procedures (suggested care planning/intervention guides)
dressing change/wound care:
a. recommended technique
b. remove sutures/staples
c. ultraviolet light therapy
d. protective dressing/Unna boot for stasis ulcers
e. soaks and wraps
f. wound irrigation using tanks/pulsed lavage
g. other
personal hygiene:
a. nail care
b. other
specimen collection:
a. culture
b. other
other:

Case Management (suggested care planning/intervention guides)
dietary management:
a. home-delivered meals
b. group meal sites
c. community options
d. other
durable medical equipment:
a. pressure reducing devices/materials
b. special/pressure reduction bed
c. telehealth monitor
d. other
medical/dental care:
a. evaluation
b. schedule/provide services
c. coordination among providers
d. other
nursing care:
a. evaluation
b. schedule/provide services
c. coordination among providers
d. other
paraprofessional/aide care:
a. evaluation
b. schedule/provide services
c. coordination among providers
d. other

physical therapy care:
a. evaluation
b. schedule/provide services
c. coordination among providers
d. other

supplies:
a. dressing supplies
b. moleskin
c. other

other:

Surveillance (suggested care planning/intervention guides)

continuity of care:
a. coordination among providers
b. photos of lesions/pressure ulcers/incisions
c. other

dietary management:
a. follows recommended diet
b. other

dressing change/wound care:
a. recommended technique
b. other

laboratory findings:
a. interpretation of culture results
b. other

medical/dental care:
a. receives care when scheduled
b. adequate/appropriate
c. follows plan of care
d. other

nursing care:
a. receives care when scheduled
b. adequate/appropriate
c. follows plan of care
d. other

paraprofessional/aide care
a. receives care when scheduled
b. adequate/appropriate
c. follows plan of care
d. other

physical therapy care:
a. receives care when scheduled
b. adequate/appropriate
c. follows plan of care
d. other

signs/symptoms—physical:
a. evidence of disease/infection or healing
b. drainage type, color, amount, and odor

c. wound diameter/depth
d. vital signs/blood pressure
e. discomfort/pain
f. telehealth monitor
g. intake and output
h. other

other:

Problem Rating Scale for Outcomes

Knowledge

1-No knowledge
Example: cannot describe cause, severity, or treatment of lesion
2-Minimal knowledge
Example: recognizes severity of lesion but neither cause nor treatment
3-Basic knowledge
Example: recognizes severity and treatment of lesion, but not cause or stages of healing
4-Adequate knowledge
Example: describes cause, severity, treatment, and healing stages of lesion with partial accuracy
5-Superior knowledge
Example: accurately describes cause, severity, treatment, and healing stages of lesion

Behavior

1-Not appropriate behavior
Example: unwilling to care for surgical incision
2-Rarely appropriate behavior
Example: willing to learn to care for surgical incision
3-Inconsistently appropriate behavior
Example: attempts to care for surgical incision, but technique is frequently inappropriate
4-Usually appropriate behavior
Example: usually cleanses and dresses surgical incision using appropriate technique
5-Consistently appropriate behavior
Example: consistently cleanses and dresses surgical incision using appropriate technique

Status

1-Extreme signs/symptoms
Example: serious pressure sore/decubitus ulcer that involves underlying muscle, tendons, and bone (stage IV lesion)
2-Severe signs/symptoms
Example: serious pressure sore/decubitus ulcer that extends through all layers of skin (stage III lesion)
3-Moderate signs/symptoms
Example: pressure sore/decubitus ulcer stage characterized by a broken or unbroken blister; more extensive than superficial (stage II lesion)
4-Minimal signs/symptoms
Example: lesion characterized by reddening of unbroken skin (stage I lesion)
5-No signs/symptoms
Example: skin intact

NEURO-MUSCULO-SKELETAL FUNCTION

Problem Classification Scheme

Definition. Ability of nerves, muscles, and bones to perform or coordinate specific movement, sensation, or regulation.

Modifiers (select one):

Health Promotion

Example: public health nurses, city officials, and other providers collaborate to create and promote "walk-for-wellness" routes in the community.

Potential

Example: history of falls although no/minor injury occurred.

Actual

Example: "unable to walk without assistance" or "falls and is injured," suggests the signs/symptoms *decreased muscle strength, decreased balance*, and *gait/ambulation disturbance*.

Signs/Symptoms of Actual (select those that apply):

- limited range of motion
- decreased muscle strength
- decreased coordination
- decreased muscle tone
- increased muscle tone
- decreased sensation
- increased sensation
- decreased balance
- gait/ambulation disturbance
- difficulty transferring
- fractures
- tremors/seizures
- difficulty with thermoregulation
- other

PHY

Related Medical Diagnoses. Diseases of the Nervous System and Sense Organs (320-326). Diseases of the Musculoskeletal System and Connective Tissue (710-739). Congenital Anomalies (740-759). Symptoms, Signs, and Ill-Defined Conditions (780-799). V Codes Supplementary Classification of Factors Influencing Health Status and Contact with Health Services (V01-V83). E Codes Supplementary Classification of External Causes of Injury and Poisoning (E800-999).

Intervention Scheme

Teaching, Guidance, and Counseling (suggested care planning/intervention guides):

anatomy/physiology:

a. body structure and function
b. other

caretaking/parenting skills:

a. safe transfer techniques
b. bicycle helmets/safety measures
c. other

cast care:
a. injury precautions
b. condition of cast/tissue
c. condition of splint/tissue
d. elevate extremity
e. other

coping skills:
a. body image
b. dealing with disease process
c. permanent loss of function
d. other

dietary management:
a. recommended diet
b. high protein
c. supplemental vitamins and minerals
d. herbs
e. macrobiotics
f. fluid balance
g. other

durable medical equipment:
a. shower/bath chair
b. special/pressure reduction bed
c. toileting equipment
d. ambulation equipment
e. assistive devices such as reachers and long-handled shoe horns
f. pressure reducing devices/materials
g. safety devices such as grab bars
h. lift
i. telehealth monitor
j. other

end-of-life care:
a. recognition/acceptance
b. plans
c. no code (no resuscitation)
d. other

exercises:
a. passive
b. assistive
c. active
d. resistive
e. balance activities
f. range of motion
g. water/aquatics therapy
h. axial mobility program
i. other

gait training:
a. gait techniques
b. stair management
c. ambulate with assistive device

d. orthosis/prosthesis training
e. other

home:
a. modify for functional limitations
b. other

laboratory findings:
a. interpretation of blood tests
b. other

medication action/side effects:
a. important to take as prescribed
b. purpose/benefits
c. changes to note and report in timely manner
d. need for timely laboratory tests
e. other

mobility/transfers:
a. bed mobility
b. transportation options/skills
c. safe transfer techniques/body mechanics
d. avoid shearing/friction
e. splint wound/injured area
f. energy conservation
g. other

personal hygiene:
a. assistive devices
b. assistance with bathing/toileting
c. other

positioning:
a. frequent position change
b. proper postural alignment
c. elevation of extremity
d. use of pillows/other support
e. other

relaxation/breathing techniques:
a. massage
b. guided imagery
c. yoga
d. progressive muscle relaxation
e. other

safety:
a. falls prevention/environmental hazards
b. seizure precautions
c. other

signs/symptoms—physical:
a. when to notify providers
b. tolerance to activity
c. recognize abnormal body temperature
d. other

skin care:
a. prevent skin breakdown/keep dry

b. check decreased circulation
c. check changed temperature/sensation
d. massage
e. lotion
f. hygiene
g. other

support group:

a. options
b. how to participate
c. benefits
d. active listening
e. other

support system:

a. benefits
b. options
c. other

other:

Treatments and Procedures (suggested care planning/intervention guides)

exercises:

a. passive
b. assistive
c. active
d. resistive
e. range of motion
f. balance activities
g. water/aquatics therapy
h. axial mobility program
i. other

feeding procedures:

a. liquids
b. solids
c. feeding/nutrition products
d. other

gait training:

a. gait techniques
b. manage stairs
c. ambulate with assistive device
d. orthosis/prosthesis training
e. other

mobility/transfers:

a. transfer training
b. other

specimen collection:

a. blood
b. other

other:

Case Management (suggested care planning/intervention guides)

dietary management:
a. home-delivered meals
b. group meal sites
c. schools
d. community options
e. other

durable medical equipment:
a. shower/bath chair
b. special/pressure reduction bed
c. toileting equipment
d. ambulation equipment
e. assistive devices such as reachers and long-handled shoe horns
f. pressure reducing devices/materials
g. safety devices such as grab bars
h. cooling or warming blanket
i. telehealth monitor
j. other

medical/dental care:
a. evaluation
b. schedule/provide services
c. coordination among providers
d. other

medication coordination/ordering:
a. obtains refills in a timely manner
b. communicate with pharmacist/other providers
c. other

nursing care:
a. evaluation
b. schedule/provide services
c. coordination among providers
d. other

occupational therapy care:
a. evaluation
b. schedule/provide services
c. coordination among providers
d. other

paraprofessional/aide care:
a. evaluation
b. schedule/provide services
c. coordination among providers
d. other

physical therapy care:
a. evaluation
b. schedule/provide services
c. coordination among providers
d. other

speech and language pathology care:
a. evaluation

b. schedule/provide services
c. coordination among providers
d. other

support group:
a. age/cultural/condition-specific groups for cerebral palsy, stroke, arthritis, etc.
b. community-/facility-based services
c. reliable Internet sites
d. telephone information/reassurance
e. other

support system:
a. family/friends
b. spiritual/faith communities
c. schools
d. neighbors
e. work associates
f. other

transportation:
a. options
b. other

other:

Surveillance (suggested care planning/intervention guides)

exercises:
a. follows recommended regimen
b. other

gait training:
a. follows recommended regimen
b. other

laboratory findings:
a. interpretation of blood tests
b. other

medical/dental care:
a. receives care when scheduled
b. adequate/appropriate
c. follows plan of care
d. other

medication action/side effects:
a. takes as prescribed
b. notes and reports changes/side effects in timely manner
c. timely laboratory tests
d. other

mobility/transfers:
a. follows recommended regimen
b. gait/ambulation
c. transfers/body mechanics
d. bed mobility
e. other

nursing care:
a. receives care when scheduled

b. adequate/appropriate
c. follows plan of care
d. other

occupational therapy care:
a. receives care when scheduled
b. adequate/appropriate
c. follows plan of care
d. other

paraprofessional/aide care:
a. receives care when scheduled
b. adequate/appropriate
c. follows plan of care
d. other

physical therapy care:
a. receives care when scheduled
b. adequate/appropriate
c. follows plan of care
d. other

positioning:
a. proper alignment
b. follows recommended regimen
c. other

safety:
a. falls prevention/environmental hazards
b. mobility
c. other

sign/symptoms–mental/emotional:
a. coping mechanisms
b. other

signs/symptoms—physical:
a. balance
b. tremors
c. range of motion
d. muscle strength and endurance
e. coordination
f. seizures
g. skin
h. prevent injuries from falls
i. abnormal body temperature
j. telehealth monitor findings
k. other

other:

Problem Rating Scale for Outcomes

Knowledge

1-No knowledge
Example: unaware of appropriate/recommended exercises

2-Minimal knowledge
Example: able to describe a few exercises

3-Basic knowledge
Example: knows most exercises, but not benefits
4-Adequate knowledge
Example: knows all exercises and some benefits
5-Superior knowledge
Example: can describe full exercise program and its benefits

Behavior
1-Not appropriate behavior
Example: unwilling to use gait assistive devices/walker
2-Rarely appropriate behavior
Example: willing to try using gait assistive devices/walker
3-Inconsistently appropriate behavior
Example: uses gait assistive devices/walker on occasion; technique rarely correct
4-Usually appropriate behavior
Example: uses gait assistive devices/walker most of the time; technique occasionally correct
5-Consistently appropriate behavior
Example: uses gait assistive devices/walker consistently and correctly

Status
1-Extreme signs/symptoms
Example: no active range of motion
2-Severe signs/symptoms
Example: minimal functional level of activity
3-Moderate signs/symptoms
Example: activity restricted due to loss of range of motion/strength
4-Minimal signs/symptoms
Example: functional in most activities with minimal loss of range of motion/strength
5-No signs/symptoms
Example: full functional active range of motion/strength

RESPIRATION

Problem Classification Scheme

Definition. Inhaling and exhaling air into the body and exchanging oxygen.
Modifiers (select one):

Health Promotion
Example: community campaign conducted about the value and techniques of radon detection.

Potential
Example: 5 year history of smoking.

Actual
Example: "rhonchi (gurgles)" indicate the presence of *abnormal breath sounds.*

SIGNS/SYMPTOMS OF ACTUAL (select those that apply):

- abnormal breath patterns
- unable to breathe independently

- cough
- unable to cough/expectorate independently
- cyanosis
- abnormal sputum
- noisy respirations
- rhinorrhea/nasal congestion
- abnormal breath sounds
- abnormal respiratory laboratory results
- other

Related Medical Diagnoses. Infectious and Parasitic Diseases (001-139). Neoplasms (140-239). Diseases of the Respiratory System (460-519). Congenital Anomalies (740-759). Symptoms, Signs, and Ill-Defined Conditions (780-799). V Codes Supplementary Classification of Factors Influencing Health Status and Contact with Health Services: Persons Encountering Health Services for Specific Procedures and Aftercare (V50-V59).

Intervention Scheme

Teaching, Guidance, and Counseling (suggested care planning/intervention guides)

anatomy/physiology:

a. respiratory system
b. other

coping skills:

a. dealing with disease process
b. body image
c. other

dietary management:

a. recommended diet
b. high protein/carbohydrate
c. fluid balance
d. supplemental vitamins and minerals
e. small, frequent feedings
f. avoid extreme temperatures
g. decrease gas-forming foods
h. herbs
i. macrobiotics
j. other

dressing change/wound care:

a. tracheostomy dressing
b. chest tube dressing
c. other

durable medical equipment:

a. oxygen
b. ventilator
c. apnea monitor
d. artificial larynx
e. telehealth monitor
f. pulse oximeter
g. spirometer

h. vaporizer/humidifier
i. nebulizer
j. other

end-of-life care:
a. recognition/acceptance
b. plans
c. no code (no resuscitation)
d. other

exercises:
a. recommended activity program
b. balanced rest/activity
c. pacing activities
d. aquatics/pool therapy
e. percussion and vibration
f. other

infection precautions:
a. hand washing
b. cover nose and mouth
c. dispose of dressings
d. clean environment
e. protect incision
f. avoid others with infections
g. influenza and pneumonia vaccinations
h. other

laboratory findings:
a. interpretation of sputum and blood tests
b. other

medication action/side effects:
a. important to take as prescribed
b. purpose/benefits
c. changes to note and report in timely manner
d. need for timely laboratory tests
e. other

mobility/transfers:
a. balanced rest/activity
b. pacing activities
c. energy conservation
d. safe transfer techniques/body mechanics
e. other

positioning:
a. to improve air exchange
b. other

relaxation/breathing techniques:
a. guided imagery
b. music
c. breathing techniques
d. yoga
e. progressive muscle relaxation
f. other

respiratory care:
a. mouth/nose care
b. turn, cough, and deep breathe
c. medical alert bracelet/chain
d. avoid allergens, smoking/other substance use, second-hand smoke, and temperature extremes
e. sexual activity
f. tracheostomy care
g. suction
h. percussion/postural drainage
i. nebulizer
j. other

safety:
a. medical alert bracelet/chain
b. oxygen precautions
c. other

signs/symptoms—physical:
a. evidence of disease/infection
b. shortness of breath
c. change in sputum color, amount, and characteristics
d. telehealth monitor findings
e. oxygen saturation less than 96% on room air
f. intake and output
g. when to notify providers
h. other

supplies:
a. tracheostomy supplies
b. other

other:

Treatments and Procedures (suggested care planning/intervention guides)

dressing change/wound care:
a. tracheostomy dressing change
b. other

durable medical equipment:
a. for administering oxygen
b. pulse oximeter
c. nebulizer
d. peak flow meter
e. spirometer
f. other

medication administration:
a. nebulizer
b. bronchodilators
c. oxygen
d. other

screening procedures:
a. pulmonary function tests
b. pulse oximetry

c. other

specimen collection:

a. sputum
b. blood
c. other

respiratory care:

a. tracheostomy/stoma care
b. suction
c. percussion/postural drainage
d. nebulizer
e. mouth/nose care
f. weaning procedures
g. other

other:

Case Management (suggested care planning/intervention guides)

continuity of care:

a. coordination among providers
b. follows plan of care
c. other

dietary management:

a. home-delivered meals
b. group meal sites
c. community options
d. other

durable medical equipment:

a. oxygen
b. ventilator
c. apnea monitor
d. artificial larynx
e. telehealth monitor
f. pulse oximeter
g. nebulizer
h. peak flow meter
i. other

medical/dental care:

a. evaluation
b. schedule/provide services
c. coordination among providers
d. other

medication coordination/ordering:

a. obtains refills in a timely manner
b. communicate with pharmacist/other providers
c. other

nursing care:

a. evaluation
b. schedule/provide services
c. coordination among providers
d. other

occupational therapy care:
a. evaluation
b. schedule/provide services
c. coordination among providers
d. other

respiratory therapy care:
a. evaluation
b. schedule/provide services
c. coordination among providers
d. other

supplies:
a. tracheostomy supplies
b. other

support group:
a. age/cultural/condition-specific group for lung disease, cystic fibrosis, etc.
b. community-/facility-based services
c. reliable Internet sites
d. telephone information/reassurance
e. other

support system:
a. family/friends
b. spiritual/faith communities
c. schools
d. neighbors
e. work associates
f. other

transportation:
a. options
b. other

other:

Surveillance (suggested care planning/intervention guides)

dietary management:
a. follows recommended diet
b. other

laboratory findings:
a. interpretation of sputum and blood tests
b. other

medical/dental care:
a. receives care when scheduled
b. adequate/appropriate
c. follows plan of care
d. other

medication action/side effects:
a. takes as prescribed
b. notes and reports changes/side effects in timely manner
c. timely laboratory tests
d. other

mobility/transfers:

a. balance rest/activity
b. pacing activities
c. energy conservation
d. transfers/body mechanics
e. other

nursing care:
a. receives care when scheduled
b. adequate/appropriate
c. follows plan of care
d. other

occupational therapy care:
a. receives care when scheduled
b. adequate/appropriate
c. follows plan of care
d. other

respiratory care:
a. tracheostomy/stoma status
b. follows recommended treatments
c. weaning procedures
d. other

respiratory therapy care:
a. receives care when scheduled
b. adequate/appropriate
c. follows plan of care
d. other

sign/symptoms—mental/emotional:
a. coping mechanisms
b. other

signs/symptoms—physical:
a. evidence of disease/infection
b. lung sounds
c. sputum color, amount, and characteristics
d. skin color
e. telehealth monitor findings
f. results of peak flow meter, spirometer, and pulse oximeter recordings
g. intake and output
h. other

other:

Problem Rating Scale for Outcomes

Knowledge

1-No knowledge
Example: does not know about oxygen or breathing exercises

2-Minimal knowledge
Example: willing to learn about using oxygen and breathing exercises

3-Basic knowledge
Example: describes some steps for using oxygen and breathing exercises, but requires prompting

4-Adequate knowledge

Example: describes steps for using oxygen and breathing exercises accurately most of the time
5-Superior knowledge
Example: describes steps for using oxygen and breathing exercises consistently and accurately; knows use will increase comfort and endurance

Behavior
1-Not appropriate behavior
Example: unwilling to use inhalers
2-Rarely appropriate behavior
Example: not using inhalers but willing to learn
3-Inconsistently appropriate behavior
Example: uses inhalers for severe symptoms only; inconsistent technique
4-Usually appropriate behavior
Example: usually uses inhalers for symptoms and sometimes for prophylaxis; reasonable technique
5-Consistently appropriate behavior
Example: uses inhalers consistently as recommended

Status
1-Extreme signs/symptoms
Example: respiration rate above 40 per minute; short of breath at rest, rales halfway up lungs bilaterally; coarse rhonchi
2-Severe signs/symptoms
Example: minimal activity causes shortness of breath; cannot climb stairs; rales in lung bases
3-Moderate signs/symptoms
Example: becomes short of breath with usual activities; has a few crackles or scattered rhonchi throughout lungs
4-Minimal signs/symptoms
Example: becomes short of breath with moderate exercise; lungs clear
5-No signs/symptoms
Example: respirations and breath sounds within normal limits; no shortness of breath

CIRCULATION

Problem Classification Scheme

Definition. Pumping blood in adequate amounts and pressure throughout the body.
Modifiers (select one):

Health Promotion
Example: healthy child/adult seeks information about low cholesterol diet.
Potential
Example: family history of hypertension.
Actual
Example: "complains of crushing feeling in left chest," suggesting the sign/symptom *anginal pain.*

Signs/Symptoms of Actual (select those that apply):

- edema
- cramping/pain of extremities

- decreased pulses
- discoloration of skin/cyanosis
- temperature change in affected area
- varicosities
- syncopal episodes (fainting)/dizziness
- abnormal blood pressure reading
- pulse deficit
- irregular heart rate
- excessively rapid heart rate
- excessively slow heart rate
- anginal pain
- abnormal heart sounds/murmurs
- abnormal clotting
- abnormal cardiac laboratory results
- other

Related Medical Diagnoses. Infectious and Parasitic Diseases (001-139). Neoplasms (140-239). Diseases of the Blood and Blood-Forming Organs (280-289). Diseases of the Circulatory System (390-459). Congenital Anomalies (740-759). Symptoms, Signs, and Ill-Defined Conditions (780-799). V Codes Supplementary Classification of Factors Influencing Health Status and Contact with Health Services: Persons Encountering Health Services for Specific Procedures and Aftercare (V50-V59).

Intervention Scheme

Teaching, Guidance, and Counseling (suggested care planning/intervention guides)

anatomy/physiology:
a. circulatory system
b. other

cardiac care:
a. relief of edema
b. medical alert bracelet/chain
c. identify/change factors that increase symptoms
d. sexual activity
e. avoid valsalva maneuver
f. cardiac rehabilitation program
g. pacemaker check
h. support hose
i. other

coping skills:
a. dealing with disease process
b. dealing with fear/anxiety/helplessness
c. body image
d. other

dietary management:
a. recommended diet
b. foods to avoid
c. fluid restriction
d. supplemental vitamins and minerals
e. small, frequent feedings

f. avoid extreme temperatures
g. decrease gas-forming foods
h. herbs
i. macrobiotics
j. other

durable medical equipment:
a. oxygen
b. support hose
c. cardiac monitor
d. telehealth monitor
e. pulse oximeter
f. other

end-of-life care:
a. recognition/acceptance
b. plans
c. no code (no resuscitation)
d. other

exercises:
a. recommended activity/rehabilitation program
b. balanced rest/activity
c. pacing activities
d. aquatics/pool therapy
e. other

infection precautions:
a. hand washing
b. disposal of dressings
c. clean environment
d. protect incision
e. avoid others with infections
f. influenza and pneumonia vaccinations
g. other

laboratory findings:
a. interpretation of blood and urine tests
b. other

medication action/side effects:
a. important to take as prescribed
b. purpose/benefits
c. changes to note and report in timely manner
d. need for timely laboratory tests
e. other

mobility/transfers:
a. energy conservation
b. safe transfer techniques/body mechanics
c. other

personal hygiene:
a. foot care
b. nail care
c. bathing
d. other

relaxation/breathing techniques:
a. guided imagery
b. music
c. breathing techniques
d. yoga
e. progressive muscle relaxation
f. massage
g. other

safety:
a. oxygen precautions
b. other

signs/symptoms—physical:
a. edema
b. vital signs/blood pressure
c. height
d. weight
e. pain
f. telehealth monitor findings
g. intake and output
h. when to notify providers
i. other

other:

Treatments and Procedures (suggested care planning/intervention guides)

cardiac care:
a. apply support hose
b. set-up/change pulmonary artery catheter/arterial line
c. calibration of pulmonary artery catheter/arterial line
d. electrocardiogram
e. other

dressing change:
a. arterial line site
b. pulmonary artery catheter site
c. other

specimen collection:
a. blood
b. urine
c. other

other:

Case Management (suggested care planning/intervention guides)

continuity of care:
a. coordination among providers
b. follow plan of care
c. other

dietary management:
a. home-delivered meals
b. group meal sites

c. community options
d. other

durable medical equipment:
a. cardiac monitor
b. electrocardiogram
c. telehealth monitor
d. other

finances:
a. coordination among resources
b. other options/resources
c. other

medical/dental care:
a. evaluation
b. schedule/provide services
c. coordination among providers
d. other

medication coordination/ordering:
a. obtains refills in timely manner
b. communicate with pharmacist/other providers
c. other

nursing care:
a. evaluation
b. schedule/provide services
c. coordination among providers
d. other

occupational therapy care:
a. evaluation
b. schedule/provide services
c. coordination among providers
d. other

physical therapy care:
a. evaluation
b. schedule/provide services
c. coordination among providers
d. other

support group:
a. age/cultural/condition-specific group for heart disease, etc.
b. community-/facility-based services
c. reliable Internet sites
d. telephone information/reassurance
e. other

support system:
a. family/friends
b. spiritual/faith communities
c. schools
d. neighbors
e. work associates
f. other

transportation:
a. options
b. other
other:

Surveillance (suggested care planning/intervention guides)
cardiac care:
a. adequate/appropriate
b. pacemaker check
c. support hose
d. cardiac output/ejection fraction
e. cardiac rhythm
f. circulatory pressures (blood pressure, pulmonary artery, central venous)
g. chest pain
h. other
dietary management:
a. follows recommended diet
b. fluid balance
c. other
laboratory findings:
a. interpretation of blood and urine tests
b. other
medical/dental care:
a. receives care when scheduled
b. adequate/appropriate
c. follows plan of care
d. other
medication action/side effects:
a. takes as prescribed
b. notes and reports changes/side effects in timely manner
c. timely laboratory tests
d. other
medication administration:
a. correct technique
b. correct schedule
c. other
mobility/transfers:
a. recommended activity
b. balance rest/exercise
c. pacing activities
d. energy conservation
e. transfers/body mechanics
f. other
nursing care:
a. receives care when scheduled
b. adequate/appropriate
c. follows plan of care
d. other

occupational therapy care:
a. receives care when scheduled
b. adequate/appropriate
c. follows plan of care
d. other

sign/symptoms—mental/emotional:
a. adjustment/coping mechanisms
b. status of fear/anxiety/helplessness
c. other

signs/symptoms—physical:
a. weight
b. edema
c. skin color
d. shortness of breath
e. vital signs/blood pressure
f. telehealth monitor findings
g. results of pulse oximeter recordings
h. intake and output
i. evidence of disease/infection
j. other

other:

Problem Rating Scale for Outcomes

Knowledge

1-No knowledge
Example: does not know symptoms, etiology, or treatment for heart condition

2-Minimal knowledge
Example: describes symptoms, but does not understand etiology or treatment for heart condition

3-Basic knowledge
Example: describes symptoms and etiology; understands the basics about the treatment of cardiac disease

4-Adequate knowledge
Example: describes symptoms, etiology, and minimal treatment options; knows when to call a health care provider

5-Superior knowledge
Example: describes symptoms, etiology, and the relationship among diet, medication, exercise, and lifestyle changes to improve condition; knows when to call a health care provider

Behavior

1-Not appropriate behavior
Example: unwilling to weigh self or take pulse each morning as recommended

2-Rarely appropriate behavior
Example: weighs self and takes pulse 1 time per week; does not record either and usually cannot remember

3-Inconsistently appropriate behavior
Example: weighs self and takes pulse sporadically; sometimes records one or both

4-Usually appropriate behavior

Example: weighs self and takes pulse in the morning about 5 times per week; usually records one or both

5-Consistently appropriate behavior

Example: weighs self, takes pulse, and records both each morning

Status

1-Extreme signs/symptoms

Example: unable to complete physical activity without discomfort; symptoms may be present even at rest (New York Heart Association class IV disability); pitting edema of feet, ankles, and lower extremities

2-Severe signs/symptoms

Example: marked limitation of physical activity; comfortable at rest but minimal physical activity causes fatigue, palpitation, dyspnea, or anginal pain (class III disability); pitting edema of feet and ankles

3-Moderate signs/symptoms

Example: slight limitation of physical activity; comfortable at rest, but usual physical activity results in fatigue, palpitation, dyspnea, or anginal pain (class II disability); moderate edema of feet and ankles

4-Minimal signs/symptoms

Example: no limitation on physical activity; usual physical activity does not cause undue fatigue, palpitation, dyspnea, or anginal pain (class I disability); slight edema of feet

5-No signs/symptoms

Example: usual physical activity and some exertion does not cause symptoms; feet, ankles, and lower extremities-no edema, all warm to touch

DIGESTION-HYDRATION

Problem Classification Scheme

Definition. Process of converting food into forms that can be absorbed and assimilated, and maintaining fluid balance.

Modifiers (select one):

Health Promotion

Example: nurse presents class to 20- and 30-year-olds about relationship between stress, ulcers, and ulcerative colitis.

Potential

Example: elderly man takes aspirin four times daily for rheumatoid arthritis.

Actual

Example: individual who has a medical diagnosis of hiatal hernia complains of "excessive belching and epigastric pain after large meals" indicating the sign/symptom *indigestion.*

SIGNS/SYMPTOMS OF ACTUAL (select those that apply):

- nausea/vomiting
- difficulty/inability to chew/swallow/digest
- indigestion
- reflux
- anorexia
- anemia
- ascites

- jaundice/liver enlargement
- decreased skin turgor
- cracked lips/dry mouth
- electrolyte imbalance
- other

Related Medical Diagnoses. Infectious and Parasitic Diseases (001-139). Neoplasms (140-239). Endocrine, Nutritional, and Metabolic Diseases, and Immunity Disorders (240-279). Diseases of the Digestive System (520-579). Congenital Anomalies (740-759). Symptoms, Signs, and Ill-Defined Conditions (780-799). Injury and Poisoning (800-999). V Codes Supplementary Classification of Factors Influencing Health Status and Contact with Health Services: Persons Encountering Health Services for Specific Procedures and Aftercare (V50-V59).

Intervention Scheme

Teaching, Guidance, and Counseling (suggested care planning/intervention guides)

anatomy/physiology:
a. digestive system function
b. other

coping skills:
a. body image
b. disease process
c. other

dietary management:
a. recommended diet
b. fluid balance
c. other

durable medical equipment:
a. suction
b. pump
c. other

end-of-life care:
a. recognition/acceptance
b. plans
c. no code (no resuscitation)
d. other

feeding procedures:
a. tube feeding/care
b. nasogastric tube insertion
c. parenteral feeding (TPN)
d. formula preparation/storage
e. other

infection precautions:
a. hand washing
b. disposal of dressings
c. clean environment
d. protect incision
e. avoid others with infections
f. other

laboratory findings:
a. interpretation of stool, blood, urine, and gastric contents tests
b. other
medication action/side effects:
a. takes as prescribed
b. notes and reports changes/side effects in timely manner
c. timely laboratory tests
d. other
positioning:
a. to facilitate feeding/digestion
b. for comfort
c. other
signs/symptoms—physical:
a. dehydration
b. aspiration
c. height
d. weight
e. skin color
f. ascites/edema
g. nausea/vomiting
h. intake and output
i. when to notify providers
j. other
skin care:
a. nose
b. stoma
c. mouth
d. other
other:

Treatments and Procedures (suggested care planning/intervention guides)
dressing change/wound care:
a. tube insertion sites
b. other
feeding procedures:
a. tube placement/patency
b. tube insertion/change
c. tube removal
d. enteral nutrition
e. parenteral nutrition
f. liquids
g. solids
h. feeding/nutrition products
i. other
specimen collection:
a. stool
b. blood
c. urine

d. gastric contents
e. other
other:

Case Management (suggested care planning/intervention guides)
continuity of care:
a. coordination among providers
b. follow plan of care
c. other
dietary management:
a. home-delivered meals
b. group meal sites
c. community options
d. other
durable medical equipment:
a. pumps
b. other
medical/dental care:
a. evaluation
b. schedule/provide services
c. coordination among providers
d. other
medication coordination/ordering:
a. obtains refills in timely manner
b. communicate with pharmacist/other providers
c. other
nursing care:
a. evaluation
b. schedule/provide services
c. coordination among providers
d. other
nutritionist care:
a. evaluation
b. schedule/provide services
c. coordination among providers
d. other
speech and language therapy care:
a. evaluation
b. schedule/provide services
c. coordination among providers
d. other
supplies:
a. formula
b. feeding tube
c. other
support group:
a. age/cultural/condition-specific groups for Crohn's disease, cancer, etc.
b. community-/facility-based services
c. reliable Internet sites

d. telephone information/reassurance
e. other
support system:
a. family/friends
b. spiritual/faith communities
c. schools
d. neighbors
e. work associates
f. other
transportation:
a. options
b. other
other:

Surveillance (suggested care planning/intervention guides)
dietary management:
a. fluid balance
b. weight
c. malnutrition
d. follows recommended diet
e. other
feeding procedures:
a. administration technique
b. other
laboratory findings:
a. interpretation of stool, blood, urine, and gastric contents tests
b. other
medical/dental care:
a. receives care when scheduled
b. adequate/appropriate
c. follows plan of care
d. other
medication action/side effects:
a. takes as prescribed
b. notes and reports changes/side effects in timely manner
c. timely laboratory tests
d. other
nursing care:
a. receives care when scheduled
b. adequate/appropriate
c. follows plan of care
d. other
signs/symptoms—mental/emotional:
a. coping mechanisms
b. other
signs/symptoms—physical:
a. upper gastrointestinal bleeding
b. tube insertion site
c. edema/ascites

d. nausea/vomiting
e. skin turgor
f. indigestion
g. dysphagia
h. appetite
i. skin color
j. vital signs/blood pressure
k. intake and output
l. evidence of disease/infection
m. other

skin care:

a. nose
b. mouth
c. stoma
d. other

other:

Problem Rating Scale for Outcomes

Knowledge

1-No knowledge

Example: parent does not recognize severity of child's acute diarrhea or how to manage

2-Minimal knowledge

Example: parent recognizes severity, but not how to manage symptoms

3-Basic knowledge

Example: parent knows some details about selecting fluids and foods to manage symptoms, but not how to schedule

4-Adequate knowledge

Example: parent knows details about selecting and scheduling fluids and foods to manage symptoms

5-Superior knowledge

Example: parent knows details about selecting and scheduling fluids and foods to manage symptoms, and methods of prevention

Behavior

1-Not appropriate behavior

Example: no fluid intake

2-Rarely appropriate behavior

Example: takes only sips of water

3-Inconsistently appropriate behavior

Example: occasionally follows prescribed regimen for prevention of dehydration

4-Usually appropriate behavior

Example: usually follows prescribed regimen for prevention of dehydration

5-Consistently appropriate behavior

Example: consistently follows prescribed regimen for prevention of dehydration

Status

1-Extreme signs/symptoms

Example: severe nausea and vomiting; needs intravenous or tube feedings

2-Severe signs/symptoms
Example: frequent nausea and vomiting; needs occasional intravenous or tube feedings
3-Moderate signs/symptoms
Example: occasional nausea and vomiting; able to eat small amounts of selected foods
4-Minimal signs/symptoms
Example: infrequent nausea and vomiting precipitated by certain foods or large meal
5-No signs/symptoms
Example: no nausea and vomiting; selects type, size, and timing of food and fluids freely

BOWEL FUNCTION

Problem Classification Scheme

Definition. Transporting food through the gastrointestinal tract to eliminate wastes.
Modifiers (select one):

Health Promotion
Example: group of healthy, active adults requests information about high fiber diet.
Potential
Example: history of occasional constipation.
Actual
Example: young child has "four liquid stools daily." This indicates the sign/symptom *abnormal frequency/consistency of stool.*

SIGNS/SYMPTOMS OF ACTUAL (select those that apply):
- abnormal frequency/consistency of stool
- painful defecation
- decreased bowel sounds
- blood in stools
- abnormal color
- cramping/abdominal discomfort
- incontinent of stool
- other

Related Medical Diagnoses: Infectious and Parasitic Diseases (001-139). Neoplasms (140-239). Diseases of the Digestive System (520-579). Congenital Anomalies (740-759). Symptoms, Signs, and Ill-Defined Conditions (780-799). Injury and Poisoning (800-999). V Codes Supplementary Classification of Factors Influencing Health Status and Contact with Health Services: Persons Encountering Health Services for Specific Procedures and Aftercare (V50-V59).

Intervention Scheme

Teaching, Guidance, and Counseling (suggested care planning/intervention guides)

anatomy/physiology:
a. bowel function
b. other

bowel care:
a. bowel training program
b. medical alert bracelet/chain
c. sexual activity

d. identify/change factors that increase symptoms
e. other

coping skills:
a. dealing with disease process
b. body image
c. other

dietary management:
a. recommended diet
b. high fiber
c. fluid balance
d. low residue
e. supplemental vitamins and minerals
f. decrease gas-forming foods
g. herbs
h. macrobiotics
i. other

end-of-life care:
a. recognition/acceptance
b. plans
c. no code (no resuscitation)
d. other

exercises:
a. stimulation of bowel function
b. regular activity program
c. other

laboratory findings:
a. interpretation of stool and blood tests
b. other

medication action/side effects:
a. takes as prescribed
b. notes and reports changes/side effects in timely manner
c. timely laboratory tests
d. other

ostomy care:
a. appliance care and change
b. irrigation
c. odor control
d. medication management
e. identify/change factors that increase symptoms
f. sexual activity
g. other

signs/symptoms—physical:
a. when to notify providers
b. evidence of disease/infection
c. abdominal distention
d. dehydration
e. change in color, consistency, and frequency of stools
f. incontinence

g. intake and output
h. other

skin care:
a. stoma care
b. perineal care
c. keep area clean and dry
d. other

other:

Treatments and Procedures (suggested care planning/intervention guides)

bowel care:
a. remove impaction
b. enema
c. digital stimulation
d. change pads/diapers
e. other

ostomy care:
a. change appliance/bag
b. irrigate
c. other

specimen collection:
a. stool
b. blood
c. other

other:

Case Management (suggested care planning/intervention guides)

dietary management:
a. home-delivered meals
b. group meal sites
c. community options
d. other

durable medical equipment:
a. toileting equipment including commodes
b. other

medical/dental care:
a. evaluation
b. schedule/provide services
c. coordination among providers
d. other

medication coordination/ordering:
a. obtains refills in timely manner
b. communicate with pharmacist/other providers
c. other

nursing care:
a. evaluation
b. schedule/provide services
c. coordination among providers
d. other

nutritionist care:
a. evaluation
b. schedule/provide services
c. coordination among providers
d. other

supplies:
a. ostomy supplies
b. enema supplies
c. pads/diapers
d. other

support group:
a. age/cultural/condition-specific groups for ostomies, etc.
b. community-/facility-based services
c. reliable Internet sites
d. telephone information/reassurance
e. other

support system:
a. family/friends
b. spiritual/faith communities
c. schools
d. neighbors
e. work associates
f. other

other:

Surveillance (suggested care planning/intervention guides)

bowel care:
a. fluid balance-intake/output
b. follows recommended diet
c. other

laboratory findings:
a. interpretation of stool and blood tests
b. other

medical/dental care:
a. receives care when scheduled
b. adequate/appropriate
c. follows plan of care
d. other

medication action/side effects:
a. takes as prescribed
b. notes and reports changes/side effects in timely manner
c. timely laboratory tests
d. other

nursing care:
a. receives care when scheduled
b. adequate/appropriate
c. follows plan of care
d. other

ostomy care:
a. appliance care/change
b. irrigation
c. other

signs/symptoms—mental/emotional:
a. coping mechanisms
b. other

signs/symptoms—physical:
a. bleeding
b. constipation
c. diarrhea or encopresis
d. impaction
e. bowel sounds
f. color, consistency, and frequency of stools
g. pain/tenderness
h. distention
i. continence
j. vital signs/blood pressure
k. intake and output
l. redness and irritation near stoma site
m. evidence of disease/infection
n. other

other:

Problem Rating Scale for Outcomes

Knowledge

1-No knowledge
Example: cannot describe cause of abnormal bowel function or ways to improve

2-Minimal knowledge
Example: knows that medications affect bowel function but does not know ways to improve

3-Basic knowledge
Example: aware that food and medications affect bowel function

4-Adequate knowledge
Example: knows that medications, high fiber foods, and fluids promote normal bowel function

5-Superior knowledge
Example: describes type, amount, and timing of food and fluids and behavior patterns that promote normal bowel function

Behavior

1-Not appropriate behavior
Example: overdoses on multiple laxatives; not willing to modify diet

2-Rarely appropriate behavior
Example: consistently uses laxatives; diet low in fiber and fluids

3-Inconsistently appropriate behavior
Example: relies on laxatives; occasionally eats high fiber foods

4-Usually appropriate behavior
Example: attempts to follow diet; usually does not need laxatives

5-Consistently appropriate behavior
Example: selects fluids and high-fiber food consistently; does not need laxatives

Status
1-Extreme signs/symptoms
Example: infant has green stools with occasional traces of blood, distended abdomen, cries much of day
2-Severe signs/symptoms
Example: infant's green stools continue but without traces of blood, moderately distended abdomen and frequent crying
3-Moderate signs/symptoms
Example: infant alternates between green and normal color stools, abdomen slightly distended and cries occasionally
4-Minimal signs/symptoms
Example: most of infant's stools are normal in color/frequency/consistency with occasional green stools; abdomen not distended; rare periods of excessive fussiness and crying
5-No signs/symptoms
Example: infant's stools are normal color/frequency/consistency

URINARY FUNCTION

Problem Classification Scheme

Definition. Production and excretion of urine.
Modifiers (select one):
Health Promotion
Example: young women learn importance of practicing pelvic floor exercises (Kegel) regularly.
Potential
Example: history of bladder infections.
Actual
Example: has the sign/symptom *incontinent of urine*, suggested by "bed wet at time of dressing change" or "Foley catheter continues to leak."
SIGNS/SYMPTOMS OF ACTUAL (select those that apply):

- burning/painful urination
- incontinent of urine
- urgency/frequency
- difficulty initiating urination
- difficulty emptying bladder
- abnormal amount
- hematuria/abnormal color
- nocturia
- abnormal urinary laboratory results
- other

Related Medical Diagnoses. Neoplasms (140-239). Diseases of the Genitourinary System (580-629). Congenital Anomalies (740-759). Symptoms, Signs, and Ill-Defined Conditions (780-799). V Codes Supplementary Classification of Factors Influencing Health Status and Contact with Health Services (V01-V83).

Intervention Scheme

Teaching, Guidance, and Counseling (suggested care planning/intervention guides)

anatomy/physiology:
a. urinary system function
b. other

bladder care:
a. bladder training
b. catheter irrigation
c. catheter care
d. self-catheterization
e. medication management
f. medical alert bracelet/chain
g. identify/decrease factors that increase symptoms
h. sexual activity
i. other

coping skills:
a. dealing with disease process
b. body image
c. other

dietary management:
a. recommended diet
b. fluid balance
c. cranberry juice
d. supplemental vitamins and minerals
e. herbs
f. macrobiotics
g. other

end-of-life care:
a. recognition/acceptance
b. plans
c. no code (no resuscitation)
d. other

exercises:
a. pelvic floor muscle strengthening/Kegel exercises
b. electrical stimulation
c. other

infection precautions:
a. follow catheter care plan of care
b. hand washing
c. disposal of soiled materials
d. clean environment
e. correct perineal wiping technique
f. nonconstricting clothing
g. avoid others with infections
h. keep area clean and dry
i. other

laboratory findings:
a. interpretation of urine tests
b. other

medication action/side effects:
a. takes as prescribed
b. notes and reports changes/side effects in timely manner
c. timely laboratory tests
d. other

ostomy care:
a. appliance care and change
b. other

signs/symptoms—physical:
a. urine color, frequency, and amount
b. intake and output
c. when to notify providers
d. other

skin care:
a. peristomal care
b. perineal care
c. other

specimen collection:
a. urine
b. other

other:

Treatments and Procedures (suggested care planning/intervention guides)

bladder care:
a. catheter insertion/change
b. catheter removal
c. catheter irrigation
d. change pads/diapers
e. other

ostomy care:
a. change and care of appliance
b. other

specimen collection:
a. urine
b. other

other:

Case Management (suggested care planning/intervention guides)

continuity of care:
a. coordination among providers
b. follows plan of care
c. other

dietary management:
a. home-delivered meals
b. group meal sites
c. other

medical/dental care:
a. evaluation
b. schedule/provide services

c. coordination among providers
d. other

medication coordination/ordering:
a. obtains refills in timely manner
b. communicate with pharmacist/other providers
c. other

nutritionist care:
a. evaluation
b. schedule/provide services
c. coordination among providers
d. other

nursing care:
a. evaluation
b. schedule/provide services
c. coordination among providers
d. other

physical therapy care:
a. evaluation
b. schedule/provide services
c. coordination among providers
d. other

supplies:
a. ostomy supplies
b. catheter supplies
c. pads/diapers
d. other

support group:
a. age/cultural/condition-specific group for ostomies, interstitial cystitis, etc.
b. community-/facility-based services
c. reliable Internet sites
d. telephone information/reassurance
e. other

support system:
a. family/friends
b. spiritual/faith communities
c. schools
d. neighbors
e. work associates
f. other

other:

Surveillance (suggested care planning/intervention guides)

bladder care:
a. catheter function
b. catheter care
c. other

laboratory findings:
a. interpretation of urine tests
b. other

medical/dental care:
a. receives care when scheduled
b. adequate/appropriate
c. follows plan of care
d. other
medication action/side effects:
a. takes as prescribed
b. notes and reports changes/side effects in timely manner
c. timely laboratory tests
d. other
medication administration:
a. correct technique
b. correct schedule
c. other
nursing care:
a. receives care when scheduled
b. adequate/appropriate
c. follows plan of care
d. other
ostomy care:
a. ostomy care/function
b. other
physical therapy care:
a. receives care when scheduled
b. adequate/appropriate
c. follows plan of care
d. other
signs/symptoms—mental/emotional:
a. coping mechanisms
b. other
signs/symptoms—physical:
a. evidence of urinary tract infection
b. urine color, frequency, and amount
c. intake and output
d. retention
e. incontinence/enuresis
f. pain/tenderness
g. distention
h. vital signs/blood pressure
i. evidence of disease
j. other
skin care:
a. stoma
b. other
other:

Problem Rating Scale for Outcomes

Knowledge
1-No knowledge

Example: unwilling to learn how to empty drainage bag or irrigate catheter
2-Minimal knowledge
Example: willing to learn how to empty drainage bag or irrigate catheter
3-Basic knowledge
Example: understands need to know how to empty drainage bag and irrigate catheter, but does not know steps
4-Adequate knowledge
Example: describes how and when to empty drainage bag and some of steps to irrigate catheter
5-Superior knowledge
Example: consistently describes how and when to empty drainage bag and irrigate catheter

Behavior
1-Not appropriate behavior
Example: not using any methods to manage incontinence
2-Rarely appropriate behavior
Example: uses pads/diapers
3-Inconsistently appropriate behavior
Example: uses pads/diapers, starting to regulate 24 hour fluid intake
4-Usually appropriate behavior
Example: uses pads/diapers, regulates 24 hour fluid intake and urination and does Kegel exercises some of the time
5-Consistently appropriate behavior
Example: follows bladder training/control regimen consistently and successfully

Status
1-Extreme signs/symptoms
Example: no bladder control, strong urine smell, bed/clothing soaked
2-Severe signs/symptoms
Example: usually catheter in place; needs assistance to manage catheter care
3-Moderate signs/symptoms
Example: manages catheter independently; clamps catheter as part of bladder training program
4-Minimal signs/symptoms
Example: usually does not use catheter; may have some residual urine when catheterized
5-No signs/symptoms
Example: incontinence controlled with no incontinence

REPRODUCTIVE FUNCTION

Problem Classification Scheme

Definition. Condition of the genital organs and breasts and the ability to reproduce.
Modifiers (select one):
Health Promotion
Example: health department staff members work with local teens to develop an effective infection prevention media campaign.

Potential

Example: not able to become pregnant.

Actual

Example: woman or man has the sign/symptom *abnormal lumps/swelling/tenderness of genital organs or breasts*, suggested by "cancerous lump in breast."

SIGNS/SYMPTOMS OF ACTUAL (select those that apply):

- abnormal discharge
- abnormal menstrual pattern
- difficulty managing menopause/andropause
- abnormal lumps/swelling/tenderness of genital organs or breasts
- pain during or after sexual intercourse
- infertility
- impotency
- other

Related Medical Diagnoses. Neoplasms (140-239). Diseases of the Genitourinary System (580-629). Congenital Anomalies (740-759). Symptoms, Signs, and Ill-Defined Conditions (780-799). V Codes Supplementary Classification of Factors Influencing Health Status and Contact with Health Services (V01-V83).

Intervention Scheme

Teaching, Guidance, and Counseling (suggested care planning/intervention guides)

anatomy/physiology:

a. reproductive system
b. breasts
c. other

behavior modification:

a. safe sex behaviors
b. other

coping skills:

a. dealing with disease process
b. body image
c. other

end-of-life care:

a. recognition/acceptance
b. plans
c. no code (no resuscitation)
d. other

genetics:

a. family history
b. resources for testing/screening
c. other

infection precautions:

a. correct perineal wiping technique
b. safe sex behaviors
c. other

laboratory findings:

a. interpretation of fluids and blood tests
b. other

screening procedures:
a. breast self-examination
b. testicular self-examination
c. Papanicolaou test
d. mammogram
e. gynecological examination
f. prostate-specific antigen test (PSA)
g. other

signs/symptoms—physical:
a. evidence of disease/infection
b. menstrual pattern
c. sexual intercourse pattern
d. when to notify providers
e. other

other:

Treatments and Procedures (suggested care planning/intervention guides)

specimen collection:
a. Papanicolaou smear
b. blood
c. drainage
d. other

other:

Case Management (suggested care planning/intervention guides)

medical/dental care:
a. evaluation
b. schedule/provide services
c. coordination among providers
d. other

nursing care:
a. evaluation
b. schedule/provide services
c. coordination among providers
d. other

support group:
a. age/cultural/condition-specific group for cancer, etc.
b. community-/facility-based services
c. reliable Internet sites
d. telephone information/reassurance
e. other

support system:
a. family/friends
b. spiritual/faith communities
c. schools
d. neighbors
e. work associates
f. other

other:

Surveillance (suggested care planning/intervention guides)

genetics:
a. receives care when scheduled
b. results
c. other

laboratory findings:
a. interpretation of fluids and blood tests
b. other

medical/dental care:
a. receives care when scheduled
b. adequate/appropriate
c. follows plan of care
d. other

nursing care:
a. receives care when scheduled
b. adequate/appropriate
c. follows plan of care
d. other

signs/symptoms—mental/emotional:
a. coping mechanisms
b. body image
c. dealing with diagnosis
d. other

signs/symptoms—physical:
a. evidence of disease/infection
b. lump/swelling/pain/tenderness
c. vaginal drainage, color, consistency, and odor
d. menstruation changes
e. vital signs/blood pressure
f. other

other:

Problem Rating Scale for Outcomes

Knowledge

1-No knowledge
Example: not aware of breast self-examination purpose or technique

2-Minimal knowledge
Example: interested in learning about breast self-examination purpose and technique

3-Basic knowledge
Example: knows basic information about breast self-examination purpose and technique

4-Adequate knowledge
Example: knows basic information and describes some correct steps/technique for breast self-examination

5-Superior knowledge
Example: knows purpose and need for monthly breast self-examination; describes correct steps/technique consistently

Behavior
1-Not appropriate behavior
Example: noticed lump in right testicle but does not want to see provider
2-Rarely appropriate behavior
Example: will consider seeing provider for lump
3-Inconsistently appropriate behavior
Example: saw provider for lump, but is not willing to receive needed treatment
4-Usually appropriate behavior
Example: saw provider for lump, received needed treatment, but has not returned for follow up visits
5-Consistently appropriate behavior
Example: sees provider regularly for comprehensive care involving lump

Status
1-Extreme signs/symptoms
Example: woman has foul-smelling vaginal discharge, itching, and painful intercourse
2-Severe signs/symptoms
Example: foul-smelling vaginal discharge and itching; intercourse occasionally painful
3-Moderate signs/symptoms
Example: occasional foul-smelling vaginal discharge and itching
4-Minimal signs/symptoms
Example: minimal vaginal discharge and itching; inflamed vagina
5-No signs/symptoms
Example: no vaginal discharge, itching, or painful intercourse

PREGNANCY

Problem Classification Scheme

Definition. Period from conception to childbirth.
Modifiers (select one):
Health Promotion
Example: couple who are planning pregnancy request information about labor and delivery.
Potential
Example: had preterm labor with previous pregnancy.
Actual
Example: "eats only one meal a day" to limit weight gain indicates the sign/symptom *difficulty with prenatal exercise/rest/diet/behaviors.*

SIGNS/SYMPTOMS OF ACTUAL (select those that apply):
- difficulty bonding with unborn baby
- difficulty coping with body changes
- difficulty with prenatal exercise/rest/diet/behaviors
- fears delivery procedure
- prenatal complications/preterm labor
- inadequate social support
- other

Related Medical Diagnoses. Endocrine, Nutritional, and Metabolic Diseases, and Immunity Disorders (240-279). Complications of Pregnancy, Childbirth, and the Puerperium (630-677).

Certain Conditions Originating in the Perinatal Period (760-779). V Codes Supplementary Classification of Factors Influencing Health Status and Contact with Health Services (V01-V83).

Intervention Scheme

Teaching, Guidance, and Counseling (suggested care planning/intervention guides)

anatomy/physiology:
a. normal pregnancy changes
b. fetal growth and development
c. pregnancy variations
d. common discomforts
e. reproductive system
f. lactation preparation
g. other

bladder care:
a. risk for urinary tract infection
b. preventive measures
c. manage incontinence
d. other

bonding/attachment:
a. attitudes about pregnancy/emotional readiness
b. preparation for baby's physical needs
c. other

bowel care:
a. risk for constipation/hemorrhoids
b. prevention of constipation/hemorrhoids
c. other

coping skills:
a. expected emotional changes
b. plan for life changes
c. community resources including financial
d. personal assistance during labor and delivery
e. other

dietary management:
a. appropriate weight gain
b. recommended food and fluid intake
c. measures to prevent heartburn/indigestion
d. measures to prevent morning sickness
e. prenatal vitamins and minerals
f. other

durable medical equipment:
a. fetal telemetry
b. blood glucose monitor
c. other

environment:
a. exposure to rubella/communicable diseases
b. exposure to cat feces
c. occupational hazards
d. appropriate cautions
e. other

exercises:
a. appropriate mode, frequency, and duration for stage of pregnancy
b. pelvic floor muscle strengthening/Kegel exercises
c. activities to avoid/body mechanics
d. other

genetics:
a. family history
b. resources for testing/screening
c. other

laboratory findings:
a. interpretation of blood tests
b. other

medical/dental care:
a. prenatal care
b. other

nursing care:
a. prenatal care
b. other

relaxation/breathing techniques:
a. breathing exercises
b. guided imagery
c. music
d. yoga
e. progressive muscle relaxation
f. other

rest/sleep:
a. elevation of legs
b. need for increased rest
c. positioning for comfort
d. other

safety:
a. use of seatbelts
b. recommendations for travel
c. x-ray exposure
d. accident/injury prevention
e. other

screening procedures:
a. pregnancy test
b. blood/Rh type
c. rubella titer
d. amniocentesis
e. ultrasound
f. gestational diabetes test
g. other

signs/symptoms—physical:
a. height
b. weight
c. vital signs/blood pressure
d. danger signs of pregnancy

e. onset of labor
f. when to notify providers
g. other

substance use cessation:
a. effects of smoking on fetus
b. effects of alcohol use on fetus
c. effects of drug use on fetus
d. prescribed medication use
e. other

other:

Treatments and Procedures (suggested care planning/intervention guides)

medical/dental care:
a. labor and delivery
b. other

nursing care:
a. labor and delivery
b. other

specimen collection:
a. blood
b. other

other:

Case Management (suggested care planning/intervention guides)

continuity of care:
a. coordination among providers
b. follow plan of care
c. other

durable medical equipment:
a. fetal telemetry
b. other

finances:
a. governmental health/social service assistance
b. private insurance
c. charitable organizations
d. budgeting
e. other

medical/dental care:
a. evaluation
b. schedule/provide services
c. coordination among providers
d. other

nursing care:
a. evaluation
b. schedule/provide services
c. coordination among providers
d. other

social work/counseling care:
a. evaluation
b. schedule/provide services

c. coordination among providers
d. other

supplies:
a. clothing
b. bottles/formula
c. furniture
d. car seat
e. infant care supplies
f. other

support group:
a. age/cultural/condition-specific groups for pregnancy, labor, etc.
b. community-/facility-based services
c. reliable Internet sites
d. telephone information/reassurance
e. other

support system:
a. family/friends
b. spiritual/faith communities
c. schools
d. neighbors
e. work associates
f. other

other:

Surveillance (suggested care planning/intervention guides)

coping skills:
a. emotional responses
b. body image
c. anticipate responsibilities of infant care
d. relationships with partner/family
e. other

exercises:
a. appropriate mode, frequency, and duration
b. other

dietary management:
a. follows recommended diet
b. weight
c. other

laboratory findings:
a. interpretation of blood tests
b. other

medical/dental care:
a. receives care when scheduled
b. adequate/appropriate
c. follows plan of care
d. other

nursing care:
a. receives care when scheduled
b. adequate/appropriate

c. follows plan of care
d. other

signs/symptoms—physical:
a. vital signs/blood pressure
b. fetal heart tones/movements
c. danger signs
d. onset of labor
e. evidence of infection
f. injuries/accidents
g. other

social work/counseling care:
a. receives care when scheduled
b. adequate/appropriate
c. follows plan of care
d. other

substance use cessation:
a. actions
b. other

other:

Problem Rating Scale For Outcomes

Knowledge

1-No knowledge
Example: does not know about appropriate rest, exercise, and diet patterns

2-Minimal knowledge
Example: interested in information about appropriate rest, exercise, and diet patterns

3-Basic knowledge
Example: knows some recommendations for appropriate rest, exercise, and diet patterns, but does not understand rationale or potential consequences

4-Adequate knowledge
Example: knows recommendations and rationale for appropriate rest, exercise, and diet patterns, but not potential consequences or application to herself

5-Superior knowledge
Example: understands appropriate rest, exercise, and diet patterns, and their relationship to positive outcome of pregnancy

Behavior

1-Not appropriate behavior
Example: no prenatal care; high-risk behaviors including smoking

2-Rarely appropriate behavior
Example: no prenatal care; listens to information but not willing to change high-risk behaviors

3-Inconsistently appropriate behavior
Example: irregular prenatal care; listens to information, does not smoke, and wants to change other high-risk behaviors

4-Usually appropriate behavior
Example: prenatal care most of the time; few risk behaviors and does not allow smoking in residence

5-Consistently appropriate behavior
Example: regular prenatal care; follows recommendations for healthy pregnancy

Status
1-Extreme signs/symptoms
Example: hospitalized for pregnancy complications including excessive weight gain, pitting edema, and elevated blood pressure
2-Severe signs/symptoms
Example: bed rest at home with complications; condition warrants close monitoring
3-Moderate signs/symptoms
Example: restricted activity; complications interfere with daily activity
4-Minimal signs/symptoms
Example: works limited hours; minimal complications
5-No signs/symptoms
Example: healthy pregnancy with mild discomforts that do not interfere with daily activities

POSTPARTUM

Problem Classification Scheme

Definition. Six-week period following childbirth.

Modifiers (select one):

Health Promotion
Example: woman who is pregnant for the first time requests information about a breastfeeding support group.

PHY

Potential
Example: pregnant woman reports having postpartum depression following birth of her first child.

Actual
Example: "nursing mother has breast infection," indicating the signs/symptoms *difficulty breast-feeding* and *postpartum complications.*

SIGNS/SYMPTOMS OF ACTUAL (select those that apply):

- difficulty breast-feeding
- difficulty coping with postpartum changes
- difficulty with postpartum exercise/rest/diet/behaviors
- abnormal bleeding/vaginal discharge
- postpartum complications
- abnormal depressed feelings
- other

Related Medical Diagnoses. Endocrine, Nutritional, and Metabolic Diseases, and Immunity Disorders (240-279). Complications of Pregnancy, Childbirth, and the Puerperium (630-677). Certain Conditions Originating in the Perinatal Period (760-779). V Codes Supplementary Classification of Factors Influencing Health Status and Contact with Health Services (V01-V83).

Intervention Scheme

Teaching, Guidance, and Counseling (suggested care planning/intervention guides)

anatomy/physiology:

a. normal physiological changes
b. physiological variations
c. common discomforts

d. lactation
e. reproductive system
f. other

bonding/attachment:
a. parent-child interaction
b. recognize cues
c. involve others including siblings
d. process of becoming a parent
e. special needs child
f. other

dietary management:
a. expected weight changes
b. lactation needs
c. recommended food and fluid intake
d. flexible eating schedule
e. postnatal vitamins and minerals
f. other

dressing change/wound care:
a. episiotomy care
b. Cesarean section care
c. hemorrhoid care
d. other

exercises:
a. appropriate mode, frequency, and duration for stage of postpartum
b. pelvic floor muscle strengthening/Kegel exercises
c. other

family planning care:
a. resume sexual activity
b. appropriate methods
c. other

laboratory findings:
a. interpretation of blood and other tests
b. other

personal hygiene:
a. breast/nipple care
b. skin care
c. bathing precautions
d. appropriate clothing
e. pads
f. other

relaxation/breathing techniques:
a. guided imagery
b. music
c. yoga
d. progressive muscle relaxation
e. other

rest/sleep:
a. naps
b. need for increased rest

c. need for assistance from family/others
d. other

screening procedures:
a. blood/Rh type
b. hearing
c. routine infant testing (e.g., PKU, T_4, bilirubin)
d. Papanicolaou test
e. breast self-examination
f. other

signs/symptoms—mental/emotional
a. expected emotional changes
b. current and predicted life changes
c. baby blues
d. postpartum depression
e. other

signs/symptoms—physical:
a. height
b. weight
c. expected physiological changes
d. evidence of breast/vaginal/urinary/other infection
e. constipation/hemorrhoids
f. when to notify providers
g. other

substance use cessation:
a. dangers to self, baby, and others
b. other

other:

Treatments and Procedures (suggested care planning/intervention guides)

specimen collection:
a. blood
b. other

other

Case Management (suggested care planning/intervention guides)

continuity of care:
a. coordination among providers
b. follow plan of care
c. special needs child
d. other

finances:
a. governmental health/social service assistance
b. private insurance
c. charitable organizations
d. budgeting
e. other

medical/dental care:
a. evaluation
b. schedule/provide services

c. coordination among providers
d. other

nursing care:
a. evaluation
b. schedule/provide services
c. coordination among providers
d. other

social work/counseling care:
a. evaluation
b. schedule/provide services
c. coordination among providers
d. other

supplies:
a. clothing
b. bottles/formula
c. furniture
d. car seat
e. infant care supplies
f. dressings
g. nursing bra/pads
h. pads
i. other

support group:
a. age/cultural/condition-specific groups for new parents, etc.
b. community-/facility-based services
c. reliable Internet sites
d. telephone information/reassurance
e. other

support system:
a. family/friends
b. spiritual/faith communities
c. schools
d. neighbors
e. work associates
f. other

other:

Surveillance (suggested care planning/intervention guides)

bonding/attachment:
a. parent-child interaction
b. other

coping skills:
a. emotional responses
b. body image
c. other

dietary management:
a. follows recommended diet
b. weight
c. other

exercises:
a. appropriate mode, frequency, and duration for status
b. other
laboratory findings:
a. interpretation of blood and other tests
b. other
medical/dental care:
a. receives care when scheduled
b. adequate/appropriate
c. follows plan of care
d. other
nursing care:
a. receives care when scheduled
b. adequate/appropriate
c. follows plan of care
d. other
rest/sleep:
a. adequate/appropriate
b. other
signs/symptoms—mental/emotional:
a. baby blues
b. postpartum depression
c. other
signs/symptoms—physical:
a. engorged/infected breasts
b. heavy/excessive/foul smelling lochia
c. vital signs/blood pressure
d. other
social work/counseling care:
a. receives care when scheduled
b. adequate/appropriate
c. follows plan of care
d. other
substance use cessation:
a. actions
b. other
other:

Problem Rating Scale for Outcomes

Knowledge

1-No knowledge

Example: no knowledge about physical/emotional postpartum changes; believes inaccurate information/myths

2-Minimal knowledge

Example: knows some basic postpartum changes, but not specifically what to expect or why

3-Basic knowledge

Example: aware of common physical/emotional postpartum changes, but unsure if her experience is typical

4-Adequate knowledge
Example: understands physical/emotional postpartum changes; knows when to seek help
5-Superior knowledge
Example: understands physical/emotional postpartum changes, self care, and rationale; knows when, where, and how to seek help

Behavior
1-Not appropriate behavior
Example: has not read about postpartum and does not want information; sleeps little/irregularly, not exercising, eats mainly snack foods with little nutritional value
2-Rarely appropriate behavior
Example: listens to information about breastfeeding and accepts pamphlets about sleep, exercise, and diet
3-Inconsistently appropriate behavior
Example: has read some information about breastfeeding, attempts adequate sleep, exercise, and diet; considering using suggestions
4-Usually appropriate behavior
Example: has read some information; considering new parent support group meetings; adequate sleep and diet patterns most of the time; exercises occasionally
5-Consistently appropriate behavior
Example: reading, attending new parent support group meetings; consistently healthy sleep, exercise, and diet patterns

Status
1-Extreme signs/symptoms
Example: has untreated left-side breast infection and is trying to breast feed using right side
2-Severe signs/symptoms
Example: has severe breast engorgement, breastfeeding with extreme discomfort
3-Moderate signs/symptoms
Example: has occasional problems with infant latching on to breast
4-Minimal signs/symptoms
Example: has occasional nipple tenderness with infant latching on to breast successfully most of the time
5-No signs/symptoms
Example: breastfeeding well

COMMUNICABLE/INFECTIOUS CONDITION

Problem Classification Scheme

Definition. State in which organisms invade/infest and produce superficial or systemic illness with the potential for spreading or transmission.

Modifiers (select one):

Health Promotion
Example: public health nurses conduct campaign to encourage community residents to receive influenza vaccinations.

Potential
Example: others reside with an individual who has tuberculosis.

Actual

Example: infection or *infestation* is appropriate when "tuberculosis, head lice, AIDS, or methicillin-resistant Staphylococcus aureus (MRSA) diagnosis is confirmed."

SIGNS/SYMPTOMS OF ACTUAL (select those that apply):

- infection
- infestation
- fever
- biological hazards
- positive screening/culture/laboratory results
- inadequate supplies/equipment/policies to prevent transmission
- does not follow infection control regimen
- inadequate immunity
- other

Related Medical Diagnoses: Infectious and Parasitic Diseases (001-139). Diseases of the Nervous System and Sense Organs (320-389). Diseases of the Circulatory System (390-459). Diseases of the Respiratory System (460-579). Diseases of the Digestive System (520-579). V Codes Supplementary Classification of Persons with Potential Health Hazards related to Communicable Diseases (V01-V06).

Intervention Scheme

Teaching, Guidance, and Counseling (suggested care planning/intervention guides)

anatomy/physiology:
a. disease process
b. transmission
c. source of infection/infestation
d. other

anger management:
a. strategies
b. benefits
c. other

behavior modification:
a. make choices to promote health
b. recognize/change personal patterns
c. safe sex behaviors
d. use good technique to prevent spread/promote healing
e. other

coping skills:
a. dealing with disease process
b. body image
c. other

day care/respite:
a. restrictions for children/adults
b. restrictions for staff
c. staff education
d. reduce risk of transmission
e. other

dietary management:
a. food cleaning equipment
b. food preparation
c. food storage
d. follows recommended diet
e. fluid balance
f. other

dressing change/wound care:
a. site
b. other

education:
a. restrictions for students
b. restrictions for staff
c. staff education
d. reduce risk of transmission
e. other

employment:
a. restrictions
b. reduce risk of transmission
c. other

infection precautions:
a. hand washing
b. contact follow-up
c. correct perineal wiping technique
d. safe sex behaviors
e. clean environment
f. clean kitchen/food equipment
g. wear protective apparel as gown, mask, gloves, goggles, etc.
h. reporting procedures
i. other

laboratory findings:
a. interpretation of sputum, blood, stool, and drainage tests
b. other

medication action/side effects:
a. important to take as prescribed
b. purposes/benefits
c. changes to note and report in timely manner
d. need for timely laboratory tests
e. other

medication administration:
a. correct technique
b. correct schedule
c. directly observed therapy
d. obtain refills appropriately
e. other

personal hygiene:
a. hand washing
b. bathing

c. hair/scalp
d. other
screening procedures:
a. interpretation of tuberculin skin tests
b. x-rays
c. other
signs/symptoms—physical:
a. vital signs/blood pressure
b. height
c. weight
d. skin color
e. nausea and vomiting
f. evidence of disease/infection
g. when to notify providers
h. other
skin care:
a. nail care
b. other
other:

Treatments and Procedures (suggested care planning/intervention guides)
dressing change/wound care:
a. site
b. other
screening procedures:
a. tuberculin skin test
b. other
specimen collection:
a. sputum
b. blood
c. stool
d. drainage
e. other
other:

Case Management (suggested care planning/intervention guides)
community outreach worker services:
a. evaluation
b. schedule/provide services
c. coordination among providers
d. other
continuity of care:
a. coordination among providers
b. follows plan of care
c. reporting procedures
d. contact follow-up
e. other
finances:
a. crisis intervention/short-range planning

b. long-range planning/decision making
c. obtain medication samples
d. sources of lower cost medications/supplies
e. budgeting
f. community resources
g. family resources
h. other

medical/dental care:
a. evaluation
b. schedule/provide services
c. coordination among providers
d. other

medication coordination/ordering:
a. multiple medications
b. monitor supply
c. obtain refills in timely manner
d. communicate with pharmacist/other providers
e. other

nursing care:
a. evaluation
b. schedule/provide services
c. coordination among providers
d. other

social work/counseling care:
a. evaluation
b. schedule/provide services
c. coordination among providers
d. other

supplies:
a. gowns
b. masks
c. gloves
d. goggles
e. tuberculin skin tests and supplies
f. other

support group:
a. age/cultural/condition-specific group for hepatitis B, tuberculosis, etc.
b. community-/facility-based services
c. reliable Internet sites
d. telephone information/reassurance
e. other

support system:
a. family/friends
b. spiritual/faith communities
c. school
d. neighbors
e. work associates
f. other

other:

Surveillance (suggested care planning/intervention guides)

community outreach worker services:

a. receives care when scheduled
b. adequate/appropriate
c. follows plan of care
d. other

infection precautions:

a. hand washing
b. dispose dressings/waste
c. clean equipment
d. clean environment
e. wear protective apparel such as gown, mask, gloves, goggles, etc.
f. avoid others with infection
g. reporting procedures
h. contact follow-up
i. other

laboratory findings:

a. interpretation of sputum, blood, stool, and drainage tests
b. other

medical/dental care:

a. receives care when scheduled
b. adequate/appropriate
c. follows plan of care
d. other

medication action/side effects:

a. prescribed/recommended/over-the-counter medications
b. takes as prescribed
c. notes and reports changes/side effects in timely manner
d. timely laboratory tests
e. other

medication administration:

a. directly observed therapy
b. other

nursing care:

a. receives care when scheduled
b. adequate/appropriate
c. follows plan of care
d. other

screening procedures:

a. read/interpret tuberculin skin tests
b. other

signs/symptoms—mental/emotional:

a. coping mechanisms
b. body image
c. dealing with diagnosis
d. other

signs/symptoms—physical:

a. evidence of disease/infection
b. pain/tenderness

c. vital signs/blood pressure
d. other

social work/counseling care:
a. receives care when scheduled
b. adequate/appropriate
c. follows plan of care
d. other

substance use cessation:
a. actions
b. other

other:

Problem Rating Scale For Outcomes

Knowledge

1-No knowledge

Example: pregnant woman learns she is a hepatitis B carrier; does not know prevention measures for newborn and other contacts or consequences for self

2-Minimal knowledge

Example: pregnant woman knows she is a carrier; wants to learn about prevention and treatment measures

3-Basic knowledge

Example: pregnant woman knows she is a carrier and that newborn will need prevention measures at birth; does not know consequences for self or spread to others

4-Adequate knowledge

Example: pregnant woman knows she is a carrier, prevention measures for newborn, and some information about preventing spread to others; does not know consequences for self

5-Superior knowledge

Example: pregnant woman who is hepatitis B carrier understands prevention measures for newborn and others and importance of good health care for self

Behavior

1-Not appropriate behavior

Example: refuses to seek care, follow tuberculosis treatment plan, or infection control guidelines

2-Rarely appropriate behavior

Example: received a tuberculosis treatment plan and infection control guidelines from provider; has not taken medications and seldom disposes of sputum or nasal drainage appropriately

3-Inconsistently appropriate behavior

Example: agreed to participate in directly observed therapy medication program but is not home consistently; occasionally follows guidelines including appropriate disposal of sputum or nasal drainage

4-Usually appropriate behavior

Example: usually follows infection control guidelines and is home for directly observed therapy medication program

5-Consistently appropriate behavior

Example: follows treatment plan and infection control program accurately and consistently

Status

1-Extreme signs/symptoms

Example: individual with acquired immune deficiency syndrome (AIDS) experiences sudden/dramatic weight loss, fever, difficulty breathing and swallowing, diarrhea, rashes, and visual disturbances; CD4 cell count less than 200

2-Severe signs/symptoms

Example: individual with human immunodeficiency virus (HIV) experiences significant weight loss and rashes, but no other symptoms

3-Moderate signs/symptoms

Example: individual with HIV noticed moderate weight loss and occasional rashes during the last month, but no other symptoms

4-Minimal signs/symptoms

Example: individual with HIV feels well most of the time; rarely has rashes and no weight loss or other symptoms

5-No signs/symptoms

Example: individual has no communicable/infectious condition; CD4 cell count is between 500 and 1800

Health-Related Behaviors Domain

NUTRITION

Problem Classification Scheme

Definition. Select, consume, and use food and fluids for energy, maintenance, growth, and health.

Modifiers (select one):

Health Promotion

Example: reads nutrition labels to learn about the benefits and liabilities of food products.

Potential

Example: child's parents are overweight.

Actual

Example: "diet high in starches (e.g., potato chips, pastries, candy bars) with minimal inclusion of fruit" suggests the sign/symptom *unbalanced diet*.

SIGNS/SYMPTOMS OF ACTUAL (select those that apply):

- overweight: adult BMI 25.0 or more; child BMI 95th percentile or more
- underweight: adult BMI 18.5 or less; child BMI 5th percentile or less
- lacks established standards for daily caloric/fluid intake
- exceeds established standards for daily caloric/fluid intake
- unbalanced diet
- improper feeding schedule for age
- does not follow recommended nutrition plan
- unexplained/progressive weight loss
- unable to obtain/prepare food
- hypoglycemia
- hyperglycemia
- other

HRB

Related Medical Diagnoses. Endocrine, Nutritional, and Metabolic Diseases, and Immunity Disorders (240-279). Diseases of the Digestive System (520-579). Symptoms, Signs, and Ill-Defined Conditions (780-799). V Codes Supplementary Classification of Factors Influencing Health Status and Contact with Health Services (V01-V83).

Intervention Scheme

Teaching, Guidance, and Counseling (suggested care planning/intervention guides)

behavior modification:

a. alter eating habits
b. increase activity
c. environment conducive to eating
d. presentation of food
e. identify positive role models
f. guided imagery
g. other

dietary management:

a. recommended diet
b. dietary supplements/formulas

c. basic nutrition
d. fluid balance
e. meal planning
f. consumer buying
g. feeding schedule for age
h. food diary
i. ideal weight for height
j. supplemental vitamins and minerals
k. herbs
l. macrobiotics
m. other

durable medical equipment:

a. feeding aids such as special spoons and cups
b. telehealth monitor
c. other

exercises:

a. suggested activity program
b. balanced rest/activity
c. pacing activities
d. other

feeding procedures:

a. assess swallowing
b. solids
c. liquids
d. feeding/nutritional products
e. other

laboratory findings:

a. interpretation of blood and urine tests
b. other

medication action/side effects:

a. important to take as prescribed
b. purpose/benefits
c. changes to note and report in timely manner
d. need for timely laboratory tests
e. other

signs/symptoms—physical:

a. hypo-/hyperglycemia
b. height
c. weight
d. body mass index (BMI)
e. intake and output
f. when to notify providers
g. other

substance use cessation:

a. dangers to self/others
b. other

other:

Treatments and Procedures (suggested care planning/intervention guides)

specimen collection:
a. glucose monitoring
b. blood
c. urine
d. other

other:

Case Management (suggested care planning/intervention guides)

continuity of care:
a. coordination among providers
b. follows plan of care
c. other

dietary management:
a. home-delivered meals
b. group meal sites
c. community options
d. other

durable medical equipment:
a. glucose monitoring equipment
b. feeding aids such as special spoons and cups
c. telehealth monitor
d. other

medical/dental care:
a. evaluation
b. schedule/provide services
c. coordination among providers
d. other

medication coordination/ordering:
a. obtain refills in timely manner
b. communicate with pharmacist/other providers
c. other

nursing care:
a. evaluation
b. schedule/provide services
c. coordination among providers
d. other

nutritionist care:
a. evaluation
b. schedule/provide services
c. coordination among providers
d. other

support group:
a. age/cultural/condition-specific groups for weight control, diabetes, etc.
b. community-/facility-based services
c. reliable Internet sites
d. telephone information/reassurance
e. other

support system:
a. family/friends
b. spiritual/faith communities
c. schools
d. neighbors
e. work associates
f. other
other:

Surveillance (suggested care planning/intervention guides)

dietary management:
a. follows suggested diet
b. follows basic nutritional plan
c. diet history
d. other
laboratory findings:
a. interpretation of glucose monitoring
b. interpretation of blood and urine tests
c. other
medical/dental care:
a. receives care when scheduled
b. adequate/appropriate
c. follows plan of care
d. other
medication action/side effects:
a. takes as prescribed
b. notes and reports changes/side effects in timely manner
c. timely laboratory tests
d. other
nursing care:
a. receives care when scheduled
b. adequate/appropriate
c. follows plan of care
d. other
nutritionist care:
a. receives care when scheduled
b. adequate/appropriate
c. follows plan of care
d. other
signs/symptoms—physical:
a. height
b. weight
c. body mass index (BMI)
d. vital signs/blood pressure
e. fluid balance
f. intake and output
g. hyper-/hypoglycemia
h. evidence of disease/infection
i. other

specimen collection:
a. glucose monitoring technique
b. urine testing technique
c. other
other:

Problem Rating Scale for Outcomes

Knowledge
1-No knowledge
Example: no knowledge of suggested diet for newly diagnosed diabetes or current blood sugar level
2-Minimal knowledge
Example: minimum dietary knowledge, but willing to learn; does not know blood sugar level
3-Basic knowledge
Example: beginning to understand relationship of diet to blood sugar; remembers blood sugar level from 2 weeks ago
4-Adequate knowledge
Example: understands relationship of diet to blood sugar; usually recalls blood sugar levels
5-Superior knowledge
Example: understands dietary rationale, describes purpose and benefits of guidelines and restrictions, and reports daily blood sugar levels accurately

Behavior
1-Not appropriate behavior
Example: will not follow suggested nutritional plan; refuses to change food patterns
2-Rarely appropriate behavior
Example: follows suggested nutritional plan diet only if food planned or prepared by another person
3-Inconsistently appropriate behavior
Example: occasionally participates in planning meals and selecting foods that are part of nutritional plan
4-Usually appropriate behavior
Example: follows suggested nutritional plan when at home, but not when eating out
5-Consistently appropriate behavior
Example: plans meals and eats to meet nutritional goals consistently

Status
1-Extreme signs/symptoms
Example: gaining weight because nutritional intake exceeds standards for age and height; adult BMI 25.0 or more; child BMI 95th percentile or more
2-Severe signs/symptoms
Example: continues to gain some weight; nutritional intake is occasionally within recommend amounts for age and height
3-Moderate signs/symptoms
Example: little weight gain; nutritional intake within recommended amounts at least three days per week
4-Minimal signs/symptoms

Example: remains overweight, but lost considerable weight recently; nutritional intake within recommended amounts

5-No signs/symptoms

Example: maintains optimal weight for height and eats balanced nutritional intake; adult BMI between 18.6 and 24.9; child BMI between 6th and 94th percentiles

SLEEP AND REST PATTERNS

Problem Classification Scheme

Definition. Periods of suspended motor and sensory activity and periods of inactivity, repose, or mental calm.

Modifiers (select one):

Health Promotion

Example: interested in the relationship of rest to health.

Potential

Example: sleep patterns interrupted when job requires changing shifts/work hours.

Actual

Example: new parent "cannot return to sleep after getting up with baby," suggesting the sign/symptom *insufficient sleep/rest for age/physical condition.*

SIGNS/SYMPTOMS OF ACTUAL (select those that apply):

- sleep/rest pattern disrupts family
- frequently wakes during night
- sleepwalking
- insomnia
- nightmares
- insufficient sleep/rest for age/physical condition
- sleep apnea
- snoring
- other

Related Medical Diagnoses. Mental Disorders (290-319). Diseases of the Nervous System and Sense Organs (320-389). Symptoms, Signs, and Ill-Defined Conditions (780-799).

Intervention Scheme

Teaching, Guidance, and Counseling (suggested care planning/intervention guides)

coping skills:

a. disease process
b. adjustment to illness
c. managing responsibilities safely
d. other

durable medical equipment:

a. continuous positive airway pressure machine
b. other

medication action/side effects:

a. important to take as prescribed
b. purpose/benefits
c. changes to note and report in timely manner
d. need for timely laboratory tests
e. other

positioning:
a. comfort
b. bedding
c. other
relaxation/breathing techniques:
a. massage
b. guided imagery
c. yoga
d. progressive muscle relaxation
e. other
rest/sleep:
a. establish routine
b. sleep aids
c. for age
d. for physical condition
e. planned rest and naps
f. other
signs/symptoms—physical:
a. when to notify providers
b. sleep deprivation
c. narcolepsy
d. sleep apnea
e. use of substances
f. intake and output
g. other
other:

Treatments and Procedures (suggested care planning/intervention guides)
other:

Case Management (suggested care planning/intervention guides)
durable medical equipment:
a. special mattress/bedding
b. continuous positive airway pressure machine
c. other
medical/dental care:
a. evaluation
b. schedule/provide services
c. coordination among providers
d. other
medication coordination/ordering:
a. obtain refills in timely manner
b. communicate with pharmacist/other providers
c. other
other community resources:
a. sleep clinics
b. other
other:

Surveillance (suggested care planning/intervention guides)

medication action/side effects:
a. takes as prescribed
b. notes and reports changes/side effects in timely manner
c. timely laboratory tests
d. other

rest/sleep:
a. amount/intervals
b. other

signs/symptoms—mental/emotional:
a. coping mechanisms
b. other

signs/symptoms—physical:
a. exhaustion
b. restlessness
c. height
d. weight
e. vital signs/blood pressure
f. snoring
g. sleep walking
h. evidence of disease/infection
i. intake and output
j. other

other:

Problem Rating Scale for Outcomes

Knowledge

1-No knowledge
Example: no understanding about symptoms and sleep apnea

2-Minimal knowledge
Example: interested in learning about symptoms and sleep apnea

3-Basic knowledge
Example: understands symptoms and cause, but not treatment of sleep apnea

4-Adequate knowledge
Example: understands symptoms and cause, but only one sleep apnea treatment option

5-Superior knowledge
Example: understands the benefits of optimal weight and various treatment options to improve sleep pattern and daytime wakefulness

Behavior

1-Not appropriate behavior
Example: no routine for child's sleep

2-Rarely appropriate behavior
Example: sends child to bedroom at approximately the same time each night

3-Inconsistently appropriate behavior
Example: takes child to bed but follows no routine

4-Usually appropriate behavior
Example: follows bedtime routine, no nap routine

5-Consistently appropriate behavior
Example: follows nap and bedtime routines

Status
1-Extreme signs/symptoms
Example: no regular sleep pattern
2-Severe signs/symptoms
Example: rarely has adequate day/night sleep
3-Moderate signs/symptoms
Example: occasionally has adequate day/night sleep
4-Minimal signs/symptoms
Example: usually has adequate day/night sleep
5-No signs/symptoms
Example: adequate day/night sleep

PHYSICAL ACTIVITY

Problem Classification Scheme

Definition. State or quality of body movements during daily living.
Modifiers (select one):
Health Promotion
Example: healthy adult wants help developing exercise program.
Potential
Example: job requires using a computer all day long.
Actual
Example: individual with cardiac disease "spends most of day watching TV" while another individual with a similar diagnosis "uses steps even when having anginal pain" and "exceeds recommended activity according to wife." Both clients exhibit the sign/symptom *inappropriate type/amount of exercise for age/physical condition.*

SIGNS/SYMPTOMS OF ACTUAL (select those that apply):
- sedentary life style
- inadequate/inconsistent exercise routine
- inappropriate type/amount of exercise for age/physical condition
- other

Related Medical Diagnoses. Diseases of the Musculoskeletal System and Connective Tissue (710-739). Symptoms, Signs, and Ill-Defined Conditions (780-799). V Codes Supplementary Classification of Factors Influencing Health Status and Contact with Health Services: Persons Encountering Health Services for Specific Procedures and Aftercare (V50-V59). E Codes Supplementary Classification of External Causes of Injury and Poisoning (E800-E999).

Intervention Scheme

Teaching, Guidance, and Counseling (suggested care planning/intervention guides):
behavior modification:
a. make choices to promote health
b. review patterns
c. increase appropriate physical activity
d. decrease inappropriate physical activity

e. explore motivation
f. identify positive role models
g. other

exercises:
a. benefits
b. develop consistent routines
c. establish appropriate type/schedule
d. balance rest/activity
e. pacing activities
f. other

relaxation/breathing techniques:
a. massage
b. guided imagery
c. yoga
d. progressive muscle relaxation
e. other

other:

Treatments and Procedures (suggested care planning/intervention guides)

other:

Case Management (suggested care planning/intervention guides)

durable medical equipment:
a. exercise equipment
b. other

nutritionist care:
a. evaluation
b. schedule/provide services
c. coordination among providers
d. other

occupational therapy care:
a. evaluation
b. schedule/provide services
c. coordination among providers
d. other

other community resources:
a. health club/physical fitness center
b. other

physical therapy care:
a. evaluation
b. schedule/provide services
c. coordination among providers
d. other

support group:
a. age/cultural/condition-specific groups for exercise, wellness, etc.
b. community-/facility-based services
c. reliable Internet sites
d. telephone information/reassurance
e. other

support system:
a. family/friends
b. spiritual/faith communities
c. schools
d. neighbors
e. work associates
f. other
other:

Surveillance (suggested care planning/intervention guides)
exercises:
a. type/amount
b. consistency
c. other
other:

Problem Rating Scale for Outcomes

Knowledge
1-No knowledge
Example: believes there is no need to participate in cardiac activity program
2-Minimal knowledge
Example: aware that activity is important for health but does not relate it to cardiac status
3-Basic knowledge
Example: knows that a relationship exists between regular activity and cardiac status
4-Adequate knowledge
Example: knows some specific activities to promote health and reduce cardiac condition
5-Superior knowledge
Example: describes goals and potential benefits of regularly participating in cardiac activity program

Behavior
1-Not appropriate behavior
Example: does not engage in regular physical activity
2-Rarely appropriate behavior
Example: does some daily activities with encouragement
3-Inconsistently appropriate behavior
Example: does daily activities independently; insufficient exercise on a daily or weekly basis
4-Usually appropriate behavior
Example: does daily activities independently; usually follows exercise program
5-Consistently appropriate behavior
Example: does daily activities independently and engages in regular, appropriate exercise

Status
1-Extreme signs/symptoms
Example: student is completely sedentary when at home; spends leisure time watching television, using computer, and playing video games

2-Severe signs/symptoms

Example: usually sedentary when at home; spends most leisure time at home watching television, using computer, and playing video games

3-Moderate signs/symptoms

Example: participates in independent physical activity once per week; spends moderate leisure time watching television, using computer, and playing video games

4-Minimal signs/symptoms

Example: participates in independent physical activity three days per week; spends limited leisure time watching television, using computer, and playing video games

5-No signs/symptoms

Example: participates in independent and/or other physical activity on a daily basis

PERSONAL CARE

Problem Classification Scheme

Definition. Management of personal cleanliness and dressing.

Modifiers (select one):

Health Promotion

Example: school nurse talks to fourth graders about using soap, shampoo, and deodorant.

Potential

Example: regular caregiver is moving to a distant community next month.

Actual

Example: the sign/symptom *unwilling/unable/forgets to complete personal care activities* applies to the individual with recently diagnosed Alzheimer's disease who is "wearing same clothes as last week."

SIGNS/SYMPTOMS OF ACTUAL (select those that apply):

- difficulty laundering clothing
- difficulty with bathing
- difficulty with toileting activities
- difficulty dressing lower body
- difficulty dressing upper body
- foul body odor
- difficulty shampooing/combing hair
- difficulty brushing/flossing/mouth care
- unwilling/unable/forgets to complete personal care activities
- other

Related Medical Diagnoses. Mental Disorders (290-319). V Codes Supplementary Classification of Persons with a Condition Influencing their Health Status (V40-V49).

Intervention Scheme

Teaching, Guidance, and Counseling (suggested care planning/intervention guides):

caretaking/parenting skills:

a. cues for self care
b. pacing activities
c. recognize agitation
d. other

home:
a. modify for accessibility
b. modify for safety
c. other
homemaking/housekeeping:
a. care of clothing
b. care of residence
c. other
personal hygiene:
a. bathing
b. hair/scalp care
c. oral care
d. change clothing
e. other
skin care:
a. nail care
b. lotion/oil
c. massage
d. other
supplies:
a. soap
b. shampoo
c. lotion
d. oral care supplies
e. other
other:

Treatments and Procedures (suggested care planning/intervention guides)
paraprofessional/aide care:
a. provide appropriate personal care services
b. other
other:

Case Management (suggested care planning/intervention guides)
continuity of care:
a. coordination among providers
b. follows plan of care
c. other
durable medical equipment:
a. shower/bath chair
b. toileting equipment
c. assistive devices such as reachers and long-handled shoe horns
d. safety devices such as grab bars
e. lift
f. adaptive equipment
g. other
nursing care:
a. evaluation
b. schedule/provide services

c. coordination among providers
d. supervise paraprofessional/aide
e. other

occupational therapy care:
a. evaluation
b. schedule/provide services
c. coordination among providers
d. supervise paraprofessional/aide
e. other

paraprofessional/aide care:
a. evaluation
b. schedule services
c. coordination among providers
d. report to nurse and occupational therapist
e. other

supplies:
a. adaptive/modified clothing and shoes
b. soap
c. shampoo
d. lotion
e. oral care supplies
f. other

other:

Surveillance (suggested care planning/intervention guides)

nursing care:
a. receives care when scheduled
b. adequate/appropriate
c. follows plan of care
d. other

paraprofessional/aide care:
a. receives care when scheduled
b. adequate/appropriate
c. follows plan of care
d. other

personal hygiene:
a. body odor
b. body cleanliness
c. condition of clothing
d. other

other:

Problem Rating Scale for Outcomes

Knowledge

1-No knowledge

Example: does not understand the importance of good, consistent hygiene or need for supplies

2-Minimal knowledge
Example: willing to receive information about the importance of good hygiene and need for supplies
3-Basic knowledge
Example: limited understanding about the importance of good, consistent hygiene and need for supplies
4-Adequate knowledge
Example: knows importance of good hygiene and supplies, but does not understand need for consistency
5-Superior knowledge
Example: knows importance of good, consistent hygiene and need for supplies

Behavior
1-Not appropriate behavior
Example: rarely bathes, wears clean clothes, shampoos/combs hair, or completes mouth care
2-Rarely appropriate behavior
Example: occasionally bathes and wears clean clothes; shampoos/combs hair and completes mouth care infrequently
3-Inconsistently appropriate behavior
Example: occasionally bathes, wears clean clothes, and shampoos/combs hair; forgets mouth care frequently
4-Usually appropriate behavior
Example: usually bathes, wears clean clothes, and shampoos/combs hair; forgets mouth care infrequently
5-Consistently appropriate behavior
Example: regularly bathes, wears clean clothes, shampoos/combs hair, and completes mouth care

Status
1-Extreme signs/symptoms
Example: cannot dress self; does not use assistive devices or modified clothing
2-Severe signs/symptoms
Example: rarely dresses self using minimal assistive devices or modified clothing
3-Moderate signs/symptoms
Example: occasionally dresses self using assistive devices and modified clothing
4-Minimal signs/symptoms
Example: frequently dresses upper body using assistive devices and modified clothing; needs assistance for lower body
5-No signs/symptoms
Example: dresses self independently or with minimal assistance

SUBSTANCE USE

Problem Classification Scheme

Definition. Consumption of medicines, recreational drugs, or other materials likely to cause mood changes and/or psychological/physical dependence, illness, and disease.

Modifiers (select one):

Health Promotion

Example: community organizes campaign about the dangers of tobacco, alcohol, and "street" drug use.

Potential

Example: has parent who uses marijuana.

Actual

Example: "involved in automobile accident while driving under the influence of alcohol" suggests the signs/symptoms *abuses alcohol* and *difficulty performing normal routines.*

SIGNS/SYMPTOMS OF ACTUAL (select those that apply):

- abuses over-the-counter/prescription medications
- uses "street"-recreational drugs
- abuses alcohol
- smokes/uses tobacco products
- difficulty performing normal routines
- reflex disturbances
- behavior change
- exposure to cigarette/cigar smoke
- buys/sells illegal substances
- other

Related Medical Diagnoses: Mental Disorders (290-319). V Codes Supplementary Classification of Factors Influencing Health Status and Contact with Health Services (V01-V83). E Codes Supplementary Classification of External Causes of Injury and Poisoning (E800-E999).

Intervention Scheme

Teaching, Guidance, and Counseling (suggested care planning/intervention guides)

behavior modification:

a. motivate change
b. decrease/stop smoking/tobacco use
c. decrease/stop alcohol use
d. decrease/stop "street" drug use
e. decrease/stop prescription medication use
f. other

coping skills:

a. strategies to deal with behavior triggers
b. strategies to support behavior/lifestyle change
c. managing responsibilities safely
d. crisis intervention
e. other

dietary management:

a. effects from substance use
b. concerns related to treatment
c. dietary supplements/formulas
d. basic nutrition
e. fluid balance
f. meal planning
g. ideal weight for height

h. supplemental vitamins and minerals
i. herbs
j. macrobiotics
k. other

genetics:
a. family history
b. substance use history
c. resources for testing/screening
d. other

laboratory findings:
a. interpretation of blood, urine, and gastric contents tests
b. other

legal system:
a. legal consequences
b. law enforcement
c. other

medication action/side effects:
a. important to take as prescribed
b. purpose/benefits
c. changes to note and report in timely manner
d. need for timely laboratory tests
e. other

relaxation/breathing techniques:
a. massage
b. guided imagery
c. yoga
d. progressive muscle relaxation
e. other

signs/symptoms—physical:
a. height
b. weight
c. vital signs/blood pressure
d. when to notify providers
e. involve withdrawal
f. involve intoxication
g. involve "street" drug use
h. other

substance use cessation:
a. appropriate use of alcohol
b. effects of use on self
c. effects of use on others
d. treatment options
e. other

other:

Treatments and Procedures (suggested care planning/intervention guides)

specimen collection:
a. blood
b. urine

c. gastric contents
d. other
other:

Case Management (suggested care planning/intervention guides)

finances:
a. crisis intervention/short-range planning
b. long-range planning/decision making
c. budgeting
d. community resources
e. family resources
f. other

legal system:
a. attorney referral system
b. legal assistance organizations
c. governmental social service/adult-child protective services
d. guardian/conservator
e. courts
f. law enforcement
g. other

medical/dental care:
a. evaluation
b. schedule/provide services
c. coordination among providers
d. other

medication coordination/ordering:
a. obtain refills in timely manner
b. communicate with pharmacist/other providers
c. other

nursing care:
a. evaluation
b. schedule/provide services
c. coordination among providers
d. other

other community resources:
a. detoxification centers
b. treatment centers
c. other

social work/counseling care:
a. evaluation
b. schedule/provide services
c. coordination among providers
d. other

support group:
a. age/cultural/condition-specific groups for alcohol, drug, tobacco use, etc.
b. community/facility based services
c. reliable Internet sites
d. telephone information/reassurance
e. other

support system:
a. family/friends
b. spiritual/faith communities
c. schools
d. neighbors
e. work associates
f. other
other:

Surveillance (suggested care planning/intervention guides)
laboratory findings:
a. interpretation of blood, urine, and gastric contents tests
b. other
medical/dental care:
a. receives care when scheduled
b. adequate/appropriate
c. follows plan of care
d. other
medication action/side effects:
a. takes as prescribed
b. notes and reports changes/side effects in timely manner
c. timely laboratory tests
d. other
nursing care:
a. receives care when scheduled
b. adequate/appropriate
c. follows plan of care
d. other
screening procedures:
a. level of addiction
b. other
signs/symptoms—mental/emotional:
a. depression
b. anxiety
c. other
signs/symptoms—physical:
a. withdrawal/cravings
b. long-term effects/risk for illness/disease
c. other
social work/counseling care:
a. receives care when scheduled
b. adequate/appropriate
c. follows plan of care
d. other
substance use cessation:
a. use pattern
b. uses others to obtain substances
c. obtains medication prescriptions from multiple providers

d. ability to perform normal routines
e. ability to meet obligations (family, social, work)
f. other

other:

Problem Rating Scale for Outcomes

Knowledge

1-No knowledge

Example: unaware of negative effects of substance use on health status

2-Minimal knowledge

Example: knows some dangers of substance use to self and some treatment options

3-Basic knowledge

Example: knows treatment options, beginning to relate physiological status to substance use

4-Adequate knowledge

Example: understands danger of substance use to self, not others

5-Superior knowledge

Example: aware of dangers of substance use to self and others and treatment options

Behavior

1-Not appropriate behavior

Example: cannot control use of alcohol/tobacco/other drugs; increases use to obtain desired effects

2-Rarely appropriate behavior

Example: regular use of alcohol/tobacco/other drugs

3-Inconsistently appropriate behavior

Example: moderate/variable use of alcohol/tobacco/other drugs

4-Usually appropriate behavior

Example: occasional use of alcohol/tobacco/other drugs

5-Consistently appropriate behavior

Example: no use of substances

Status

1-Extreme signs/symptoms

Example: not interested in changing behavior or receiving treatment; not able to meet family, social, work obligations

2-Severe signs/symptoms

Example: considers changing behavior, investigates treatment options; meets a few family, social, work obligations

3-Moderate signs/symptoms

Example: prepares to change behavior, receives treatment sporadically; meets some family, social, work obligations

4-Minimal signs/symptoms

Example: taking appropriate action to change behavior, attending treatment program most of the time; meets most family, social, work obligations

5-No signs/symptoms

Example: not using substances; meets family, social, work obligations consistently

FAMILY PLANNING

Problem Classification Scheme

Definition. Practices designed to plan and space pregnancy within the context of values, attitudes, and beliefs.

Modifiers (select one):

Health Promotion

Example: woman is considering pregnancy in the future and requests information about folic acid to prevent child from having neural tube defects.

Potential

Example: pregnant adolescent has never used family planning method consistently.

Actual

Example: "wants to stop taking birth control pills" or "concerned about the effectiveness of condoms," indicating the sign/symptom *dissatisfied with present family planning method.*

Signs/Symptoms of Actual (select those that apply):

- inappropriate/insufficient knowledge about family planning methods
- inappropriate/insufficient knowledge about preconception health practices
- inaccurate/inconsistent use of family planning methods
- dissatisfied with present family planning method
- fears others' reactions regarding family planning choices
- difficulty obtaining family planning methods
- other

Related Medical Diagnoses. V Codes Supplementary Classification of Factors Influencing Health Status and Contact with Health Services (V01-V83).

HRB

Intervention Scheme

Teaching, Guidance, and Counseling (suggested care planning/intervention guides)

anatomy/physiology:

a. reproductive system
b. other

family planning care:

a. methods
b. preferences
c. barriers to using birth control
d. resources
e. safe sex methods
f. sexually transmitted disease prevention
g. other

finances:

a. sources of lower/no cost medications/supplies
b. other

genetics:

a. family history
b. resources for testing/screening
c. other

medication action/side effects:
a. important to take as prescribed
b. purpose/benefits
c. changes to note and report in timely manner
d. need for timely laboratory tests
e. other

screening procedures:
a. pregnancy testing
b. Papanicolaou test
c. provider and self breast examination
d. mammogram
e. other

other:

Treatments and Procedures (suggested care planning/intervention guides)

other:

Case Management (suggested care planning/intervention guides)

family planning care:
a. community clinics
b. private physician-nurse providers/clinics
c. other

medical/dental care:
a. evaluation
b. schedule/provide services
c. coordination among providers
d. other

medication coordination/ordering:
a. obtain refills in timely manner
b. communicate with pharmacist/other providers
c. other

nursing care:
a. evaluation
b. schedule/provide services
c. coordination among providers
d. other

social work/counseling care:
a. evaluation
b. schedule/provide services
c. coordination among providers
d. other

support group:
a. age/cultural/condition-specific groups for pregnancy prevention, infertility, etc.
b. community-/facility-based services
c. telephone information/reassurance
d. other

support system:
a. family/friends
b. spiritual/faith communities

c. schools
d. neighbors
e. work associates
f. other
other:

Surveillance (suggested care planning/intervention guides)
family planning care:
a. follow guidelines of method
b. adverse effects of method
c. other
medical/dental care:
a. receives care when scheduled
b. adequate/appropriate
c. follows plan of care
d. other
medication action/side effects:
a. takes as prescribed
b. notes and reports changes/side effects in timely manner
c. timely laboratory tests
d. other
nursing care:
a. receives care when scheduled
b. adequate/appropriate
c. follows plan of care
d. other
signs/symptoms—physical:
a. evidence of disease/infection
b. vital signs/blood pressure
c. height
d. weight
e. body changes
f. other
social work/counseling care:
a. receives care when scheduled
b. adequate/appropriate
c. follows plan of care
d. other
other:

Problem Rating Scale for Outcomes

Knowledge
1-No knowledge
Example: unaware of family planning methods
2-Minimal knowledge
Example: minimal knowledge about family planning methods, believes some myths
3-Basic knowledge
Example: knows family planning methods, but no side effects, contraindications, or efficacy

4-Adequate knowledge
Example: knows family planning methods and efficacy, not side effects or contraindications
5-Superior knowledge
Example: knows family planning methods, side effects, contraindications, and efficacy of each

Behavior
1-Not appropriate behavior
Example: no family planning method; sexually active but does not want to conceive
2-Rarely appropriate behavior
Example: seldom uses family planning method but does not want to conceive
3-Inconsistently appropriate behavior
Example: occasionally uses family planning method but does not want to conceive
4-Usually appropriate behavior
Example: usually uses family planning method but does not want to conceive
5-Consistently appropriate behavior
Example: uses birth control method consistently and appropriately with no side effects

Status
1-Extreme signs/symptoms
Example: has severe migraine headaches and increased systolic blood pressure since starting on oral contraceptives
2-Severe signs/symptoms
Example: increase in systolic blood pressure since starting on oral contraceptives
3-Moderate signs/symptoms
Example: moderate spotting continues after three months on oral contraceptives
4-Minimal signs/symptoms
Example: small weight gain since starting on oral contraceptives
5-No signs/symptoms
Example: no side effects since starting on oral contraceptives

HEALTH CARE SUPERVISION

Problem Classification Scheme

Definition. Management of the health care treatment plan by health care providers.
Modifiers (select one):

Health Promotion
Example: young adult requests information about appropriate medical/health care provider services for well individual.

Potential
Example: diagnosed with a new chronic condition.

Actual
Example: "parent repeatedly fails to take sick child to scheduled appointments," suggesting the sign/symptom *fails to return as requested to health care provider.*

SIGNS/SYMPTOMS OF ACTUAL (select those that apply):

- fails to obtain routine/preventive health care
- fails to seek care for symptoms requiring evaluation/treatment
- fails to return as requested to health care provider
- inability to coordinate multiple appointments/treatment plans

- inconsistent source of health care
- inadequate source of health care
- inadequate treatment plan
- other

Related Medical Diagnoses. V Codes Supplementary Classification of Factors Influencing Health Status and Contact with Health Services (V01-V83).

Intervention Scheme

Teaching, Guidance, and Counseling (suggested care planning/intervention guides)

continuity of care:
a. need for multiple providers
b. coordination among providers
c. follows plan of care
d. other

end-of-life care:
a. recognition/acceptance
b. plans
c. no code (no resuscitation)
d. other

medical/dental care:
a. preventive care
b. emergency care
c. chronic care
d. acute illness care
e. multiple problems
f. multiple health care providers
g. multiple medications
h. frequent episodes of instability
i. other

nursing care:
a. preventive
b. emergency care
c. chronic illness care
d. acute illness care
e. multiple problems
f. multiple health care providers
g. multiple medications
h. frequent episodes of instability
i. other

screening procedures:
a. self screening
b. standardized assessment guides/diagnostic tests
c. alert for age/condition symptoms
d. other

wellness:
a. lifestyle includes physical/emotional/spiritual activities
b. importance of routine preventive evaluations
c. immunizations

d. influenza and pneumonia vaccinations
e. routine dental care
f. avoid areas that are high-risk for infection
g. other
other:

Treatments and Procedures (suggested care planning/intervention guides)
other:

Case Management (suggested care planning/intervention guides)
continuity of care:
a. need for multiple providers
b. coordination among providers
c. follows plan of care
d. other
finances:
a. crisis intervention/short-range planning
b. long-range planning/decision making
c. budgeting
d. community resources
e. family resources
f. other
genetics:
a. family history
b. resources for testing/screening
c. other
medical/dental care:
a. evaluation
b. schedule/provide services
c. coordination among providers
d. other
medication coordination/ordering:
a. monitor multiple medications
b. monitor supply
c. communicate with pharmacist/other providers
d. other
nursing care:
a. evaluation
b. schedule/provide services
c. coordination among providers
d. other
transportation:
a. options
b. other
other:

Surveillance (suggested care planning/intervention guides)
medical/dental care:
a. receives care when scheduled
b. adequate/appropriate

c. follows plan of care
d. other

nursing care:

a. receives care when scheduled
b. adequate/appropriate
c. follows plan of care
d. other

signs/symptoms—mental/emotional:

a. coping mechanisms
b. behavioral changes
c. affect
d. other

signs/symptoms—physical:

a. when to notify providers
b. vital signs/blood pressure
c. evidence of disease/infection
d. height
e. weight
f. pain
g. mobility
h. other

other:

Problem Rating Scale for Outcomes

Knowledge

1-No knowledge

Example: does not know how and when to seek care

2-Minimal knowledge

Example: knows how and when to seek care for obvious medical emergencies, but not for chronic or acute illness or preventive care

3-Basic knowledge

Example: knows how and when to seek care for obvious medical emergencies; knows how and sometimes when to seek care for chronic and acute illness; does not know how or when to seek preventive care

4-Adequate knowledge

Example: knows how and when to seek care for obvious medical emergencies; knows how and usually when to seek care for chronic and acute illness; knows how but not when to seek preventive care

5-Superior knowledge

Example: knows when and how to seek emergency, chronic and acute illness, and preventive care

Behavior

1-Not appropriate behavior

Example: does not follow prescribed/recommended treatment plan

2-Rarely appropriate behavior

Example: follows a limited portion of prescribed/recommended treatment plan

3-Inconsistently appropriate behavior

Example: follows some of prescribed/recommended treatment plan after verifying information on authenticated Internet sites

4-Usually appropriate behavior

Example: follows most of prescribed/recommended treatment plan after discussing options with provider and verifying information on authenticated Internet sites

5-Consistently appropriate behavior

Example: follows prescribed/recommended treatment plan after discussing options with provider and verifying information on authenticated Internet sites

Status

1-Extreme signs/symptoms

Example: receives no health care

2-Severe signs/symptoms

Example: rarely receives appropriate, timely health care

3-Moderate signs/symptoms

Example: sometimes receives appropriate, timely health care

4-Minimal signs/symptoms

Example: usually receives appropriate, timely health care

5-No signs/symptoms

Example: receives appropriate, timely health care

MEDICATION REGIMEN

Problem Classification Scheme

Definition. Use or application of over-the-counter and prescribed/recommended medications and infusions to meet guidelines for therapeutic action, safety, and schedule.

Modifiers (select one):

HRB

Health Promotion

Example: healthy adult asks for information about immunizations, over-the-counter vitamins, and herbal supplements.

Potential

Example: indicates that medications are too expensive; has two month supply but not certain about obtaining refills after that.

Actual

Example: individual with cardiac disease "admits forgetting to take medications occasionally," indicating the sign/symptom *does not recommended dosage/schedule.*

SIGNS/SYMPTOMS OF ACTUAL (select those that apply):

- does not follow recommended dosage/schedule
- evidence of side effects/adverse reactions
- inadequate system for taking medication
- improper storage of medication
- fails to obtain refills appropriately
- fails to obtain immunizations
- inadequate medication regimen
- unable to take medications without help
- other

Related Medical Diagnoses. Injury and Poisoning (800-999). V Codes Supplementary Classification of Factors Influencing Health Status and Contact with Health Services (V01-V83). E Codes Supplementary Classification of External Causes of Injury and Poisoning (E800-E999).

Intervention Scheme

Teaching, Guidance, and Counseling (suggested care planning/intervention guides)

anatomy/physiology:
a. body structure and function
b. disease process
c. how medications effect symptoms/function
d. other

dressing change/wound care:
a. intravenous
b. other

durable medical equipment:
a. intravenous supplies/equipment
b. subcutaneous supplies/equipment
c. gastrostomy supplies/equipment
d. pump function
e. reminder/organizer/Mediset
f. telehealth monitor
g. other

finances:
a. sources of lower/no cost medications/supplies
b. other

laboratory findings:
a. interpretation of blood, urine, drainage, and gastric contents tests
b. other

medication action/side effects:
a. for oral medications
b. for injections
c. for infusions
d. for topical medications
e. for suppositories
f. for instillations
g. for inhalations
h. important to take as prescribed
i. purpose/benefits
j. changes to note and report in a timely manner
k. need for timely laboratory tests
l. other

medication administration:
a. follows correct technique
b. intravenous medications
c. intramuscular medications
d. subcutaneous medications
e. suppository
f. topical
g. instillation
h. inhalation
i. oral prescribed/recommended/over-the-counter
j. correct schedule
k. other

medication set-up:
a. reminder/organizer/Mediset
b. other
signs/symptoms—physical:
a. evidence of infection at administration site
b. evidence of other disease/infection
c. intake and output
d. when to notify providers
e. other
other:

Treatments and Procedures (suggested care planning/intervention guides)
dressing change/wound care:
a. intravenous site (Heplock, PICC, central line)
b. other
medication administration:
a. intravenous medications
b. intramuscular medications
c. subcutaneous medications
d. suppository
e. topical
f. instillation
g. inhalation
h. other
medication prescription:
a. for diagnosed condition
b. other
medication set-up:
a. reminder/organizer/Mediset
b. subcutaneous/intramuscular medications/syringe prefills
c. insert intravenous access device/tubing
d. insert gastric access device
e. other medication system
f. reconstitute medications
g. other
specimen collection:
a. blood
b. urine
c. drainage
d. gastric contents
e. other
other:

Case Management (suggested care planning/intervention guides)
continuity of care:
a. coordination among providers
b. follows plan of care
c. other

durable medical equipment:
a. automated medication dispensing devices/alarms
b. reminder/organizer/Mediset
c. telehealth monitor
d. other

finances:
a. crisis intervention/short-range planning
b. long-range planning/decision making
c. obtain medication samples
d. sources of lower cost medications/supplies
e. budgeting
f. community resources
g. family resources
h. other

medical/dental care:
a. evaluation
b. schedule/provide services
c. coordination among providers
d. other

medication coordination/ordering:
a. monitor multiple medications
b. monitor supply
c. obtain refills in a timely manner
d. communicate with pharmacist/other providers
e. other

medication prescription:
a. for diagnosed condition
b. renew prescription for refills
c. other

nursing care:
a. evaluation
b. schedule/provide services
c. coordination among providers
d. other

supplies:
a. dressing supplies
b. needles and syringes
c. other

support group:
a. age/cultural/condition-specific groups for specific diagnosis/treatment, etc.
b. community-/facility-based services
c. reliable Internet sites
d. telephone information/reassurance
e. other

support system:
a. family/friends
b. spiritual/faith communities
c. schools
d. neighbors

e. work associates
f. other
other:

Surveillance (suggested care planning/intervention guides)
durable medical equipment:
a. intravenous supplies/equipment
b. subcutaneous supplies/equipment
c. gastrostomy supplies/equipment
d. pump function
e. reminder/organizer/Mediset
f. telehealth monitor
g. other
finances:
a. ability to pay for medications/supplies
b. other
laboratory findings:
a. therapeutic drug levels
b. hematology
c. blood chemistry
d. renal function
e. liver function
f. other
medical/dental care:
a. receives care when scheduled
b. adequate/appropriate
c. follows plan of care
d. other
medication action/side effects:
a. takes as prescribed
b. notes and reports changes/side effects in timely manner
c. timely laboratory tests
d. other
medication administration:
a. takes medications as prescribed/recommended
b. correct technique
c. correct dose
d. correct frequency
e. correct storage precautions
f. other
medication coordination/ordering:
a. monitor multiple medications
b. monitor supply
c. obtains refills as recommended
d. communicate with pharmacist/other providers
e. other
medication set-up:
a. follows plan of care
b. other

nursing care:
a. receives care when scheduled
b. adequate/appropriate
c. follows plan of care
d. other

signs/symptoms—mental/emotional:
a. side effects
b. coping mechanisms
c. behavioral changes
d. affect
e. other

signs/symptoms—physical:
a. patent access device
b. site infection
c. side effects
d. intake and output
e. evidence of other disease/infection
f. other

other:

Problem Rating Scale for Outcomes

Knowledge
1-No knowledge
Example: does not know names, purpose, dose, side effects, or schedule of medications
2-Minimal knowledge
Example: does not know names, purpose, dose, or side effects of medications; describes only medication schedule
3-Basic knowledge
Example: describes schedule, name, purpose, dose, and side effects of some medications
4-Adequate knowledge
Example: describes schedule, name, purpose, dose, and side effects of most medications
5-Superior knowledge
Example: describes schedule, name, purpose, dose, and side effects of all medications

Behavior
1-Not appropriate behavior
Example: does not take medications as ordered
2-Rarely appropriate behavior
Example: rarely takes medications as ordered
3-Inconsistently appropriate behavior
Example: occasionally takes medications as ordered
4-Usually appropriate behavior
Example: usually takes medications as ordered
5-Consistently appropriate behavior
Example: consistently takes medications as ordered

Status

1-Extreme signs/symptoms
Example: no therapeutic effects from medication; severe side effects evident

2-Severe signs/symptoms
Example: some therapeutic effects from medication; many side effects evident

3-Moderate signs/symptoms
Example: moderate therapeutic effects from medication; occasional side effects evident

4-Minimal signs/symptoms
Example: good therapeutic effects from medication; some side effects evident

5-No signs/symptoms
Example: maximum therapeutic effects from medication; no side effects evident

SECTION

III

Appendixes

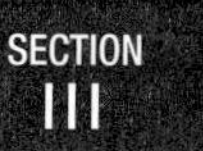

APPENDIX

A

The Omaha System

Revised 2005

The newly revised terms and definitions of the Omaha System (Problem Classification Scheme, Intervention Scheme, and Problem Rating Scale for Outcomes) are presented in this appendix. Important suggestions, examples, and guidelines for users are included in Chapters 1 to 6 and the User's Guide; application of the System is illustrated in the case studies in Appendix B; associations with conditions, medical diagnoses, and treatments are presented in Appendix C; details about the revision process and coding are in Appendixes D and E; and all definitions are provided in the Glossary. The Omaha System's structure, terms, and definitions are not copyrighted so that they would be equally accessible to all potential users. They do not represent new knowledge, but a systematic organization of what compassionate health care professionals need to know, do, and communicate.

For each of the 42 problems in the Problem Classification Scheme, the practitioner selects two modifiers: one that is *Individual, Family,* or *Community* and one that is *Health Promotion, Potential,* or *Actual.* For simplicity, the definitions of these modifiers are presented below and only the terms appear throughout this appendix.

Modifiers (select one):
Individual: A person who lives alone or a single-family member who experiences a health-related problem.
Family: A social unit or related group of individuals who live together and experience a health-related problem.
Community: The individuals and/or families who comprise a group, neighborhood, or other geographic district that experience a health-related problem.

Modifiers (select one):
Health Promotion: Client interest in increasing knowledge, behavior, and health expectations and developing more assets and resources that maintain or enhance well-being in the absence of risk factors, signs, or symptoms.
Potential: Client status characterized by the presence of certain health patterns, practices, behaviors, or risk factors that may preclude optimal health and the absence of signs and symptoms.
Actual: Client status characterized by one or more existing signs and symptoms that may preclude optimal health.

Problem Classification Scheme

ENVIRONMENTAL DOMAIN: Material resources and physical surroundings both inside and outside the living area, neighborhood, and broader community.

Income: Money from wages, pensions, subsidies, interest, dividends, or other sources available for living and health care expenses.

Modifiers: Individual/Family/Community *and* Health Promotion/Potential/Actual

SIGNS/SYMPTOMS OF ACTUAL

- low/no income
- uninsured medical expenses
- difficulty with money management
- able to buy only necessities
- difficulty buying necessities
- other

Sanitation: Environmental cleanliness and precautions against infection and disease.

Modifiers: Individual/Family/Community *and* Health Promotion/Potential/Actual

SIGNS/SYMPTOMS OF ACTUAL

- soiled living area
- inadequate food storage/disposal
- insects/rodents
- foul odor
- inadequate water supply
- inadequate sewage disposal
- inadequate laundry facilities
- allergens
- infectious/contaminating agents
- presence of mold
- excessive pets
- other

Residence: Living area.

Modifiers: Individual/Family/Community *and* Health Promotion/Potential/Actual

SIGNS/SYMPTOMS OF ACTUAL

- structurally unsound
- inadequate heating/cooling
- steep/unsafe stairs
- inadequate/obstructed exits/entries
- cluttered living space
- unsafe storage of dangerous objects/substances
- unsafe mats/throw rugs
- inadequate safety devices
- presence of lead-based paint
- unsafe appliances/equipment
- inadequate/crowded living space
- exposed wiring

- structural barriers
- homeless
- other

Neighborhood/workplace safety: Freedom from illness, injury, or loss in the community or place of employment.

Modifiers: Individual/Family/Community *and* Health Promotion/Potential/Actual

SIGNS/SYMPTOMS OF ACTUAL

- high crime rate
- high pollution level
- uncontrolled/dangerous/infected animals
- inadequate/unsafe play/exercise areas
- inadequate space/resources to foster health
- threats/reports of violence
- physical hazards
- vehicle/traffic hazards
- chemical hazards
- radiological hazards
- other

PSYCHOSOCIAL DOMAIN: Patterns of behavior, emotion, communication, relationships, and development.

Communication with community resources: Interaction between the individual/family/community and social service organizations, schools, and businesses in regard to services, information, and goods/supplies.

Modifiers: Individual/Family/Community *and* Health Promotion/Potential/Actual

SIGNS/SYMPTOMS OF ACTUAL

- unfamiliar with options/procedures for obtaining services
- difficulty understanding roles/regulations of service providers
- unable to communicate concerns to provider
- dissatisfaction with services
- inadequate/unavailable resources
- language barrier
- cultural barrier
- educational barrier
- transportation barrier
- limited access to care/services/goods
- unable to use/has inadequate communication devices/equipment
- other

Social contact: Interaction between the individual/family/community and others outside the immediate living area.

Modifiers: Individual/Family/Community *and* Health Promotion/Potential/Actual

SIGNS/SYMPTOMS OF ACTUAL

- limited social contact
- uses health care provider for social contact

- minimal outside stimulation/leisure time activities
- other

Role change: Additions to or removal of a set of expected behavioral characteristics.

Modifiers: Individual/Family/Community *and* Health Promotion/Potential/Actual

SIGNS/SYMPTOMS OF ACTUAL

- involuntary role reversal
- assumes new role
- loses previous role
- other

Interpersonal relationship: Associations or bonds between the individual/family/community and others.

Modifiers: Individual/Family/Community *and* Health Promotion/Potential/Actual

SIGNS/SYMPTOMS OF ACTUAL

- difficulty establishing/maintaining relationships
- minimal shared activities
- incongruent values/goals/expectations/schedules
- inadequate interpersonal communication skills
- prolonged, unrelieved tension
- inappropriate suspicion/manipulation/control
- physically/emotionally abusive to partner
- difficulty problem solving without conflict
- other

Spirituality: Beliefs and practices that involve faith, religion, values, the spirit, and/or the soul.

Modifiers: Individual/Family/Community *and* Health Promotion/Potential/Actual

SIGNS/SYMPTOMS OF ACTUAL

- expresses spiritual concerns
- disrupted spiritual rituals
- disrupted spiritual trust
- conflicting spiritual beliefs and medical/health care regimen
- other

Grief: Suffering and distress associated with loss.

Modifiers: Individual/Family/Community *and* Health Promotion/Potential/Actual

SIGNS/SYMPTOMS OF ACTUAL

- fails to recognize stages of grief/process of healing
- difficulty coping with grief responses
- difficulty expressing grief responses
- conflicting stages of grief among individuals/families
- other

Mental health: Development and use of mental/emotional abilities to adjust to life situations, interact with others, and engage in activities.

Modifiers: Individual/Family/Community *and* Health Promotion/Potential/Actual

SIGNS/SYMPTOMS OF ACTUAL

- sadness/hopelessness/decreased self-esteem
- apprehension/undefined fear
- loss of interest/involvement in activities/self-care
- narrowed to scattered attention/focus
- flat affect
- irritable/agitated/aggressive
- purposeless/compulsive activity
- difficulty managing stress
- difficulty managing anger
- somatic complaints/fatigue
- delusions
- hallucinations/illusions
- expresses suicidal/homicidal thoughts
- attempts suicide/homicide
- self-mutilation
- mood swings
- flash-backs
- other

Sexuality: Attitudes, feelings, and behaviors related to intimacy and sexual activity.

Modifiers: Individual/Family/Community *and* Health Promotion/Potential/Actual

SIGNS/SYMPTOMS OF ACTUAL

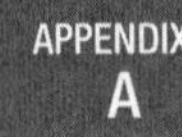

- difficulty recognizing consequences of sexual behavior
- difficulty expressing intimacy
- sexual identity confusion
- sexual value confusion
- dissatisfied with sexual relationships
- unsafe sexual practices
- sexual acting out/provocative behaviors/harassment
- sexual perpetration/assault
- other

Caretaking/parenting: Providing support, nurturance, stimulation, and physical care for dependent child or adult.

Modifiers: Individual/Family/Community *and* Health Promotion/Potential/Actual

SIGNS/SYMPTOMS OF ACTUAL

- difficulty providing physical care/safety
- difficulty providing emotional nurturance
- difficulty providing cognitive learning experiences and activities
- difficulty providing preventive and therapeutic health care
- expectations incongruent with stage of growth and development
- dissatisfaction/difficulty with responsibilities
- difficulty interpreting or responding to verbal/nonverbal communication
- neglectful

- abusive
- other

Neglect: Child or adult deprived of minimally accepted standards of food, shelter, clothing, or care.

Modifiers: Individual/Family/Community *and* Health Promotion/Potential/Actual

SIGNS/SYMPTOMS OF ACTUAL

- lacks adequate physical care
- lacks emotional nurturance/support
- lacks appropriate stimulation/cognitive experiences
- inappropriately left alone
- lacks necessary supervision
- inadequate/delayed medical care
- other

Abuse: Child or adult subjected to nonaccidental physical, emotional, or sexual violence or injury.

Modifiers: Individual/Family/Community *and* Health Promotion/Potential/Actual

SIGNS/SYMPTOMS OF ACTUAL

- harsh/excessive discipline
- welts/burns/other injuries
- questionable explanation of injury
- attacked verbally
- fearful/hypervigilant behavior
- violent environment
- consistent negative messages
- assaulted sexually
- other

APPENDIX A

Growth and development: Progressive physical, emotional, and social maturation along the age continuum from birth to death.

Modifiers: Individual/Family/Community *and* Health Promotion/Potential/Actual

SIGNS/SYMPTOMS OF ACTUAL

- abnormal results of developmental screening tests
- abnormal weight/height/head circumference in relation to growth/age standards
- age-inappropriate behavior
- inadequate achievement/maintenance of developmental tasks
- other

PHYSIOLOGICAL DOMAIN: Functions and processes that maintain life.

Hearing: Perception of sound by the ears.

Modifiers: Individual/Family/Community *and* Health Promotion/Potential/Actual

Signs/Symptoms of Actual

- difficulty hearing normal speech tones
- difficulty hearing speech in large group settings
- difficulty hearing high frequency sounds
- absent/abnormal response to sound
- abnormal results of hearing screening test
- other

Vision: Act or power of sensing with the eyes.

Modifiers: Individual/Family/Community *and* Health Promotion/Potential/Actual

Signs/Symptoms of Actual

- difficulty seeing small print/calibrations
- difficulty seeing distant objects
- difficulty seeing close objects
- absent/abnormal response to visual stimuli
- abnormal results of vision screening test
- squinting/blinking/tearing/blurring
- floaters/flashes
- difficulty differentiating colors
- other

Speech and language: Use of articulated vocal sounds, symbols, signs, or gestures for communication.

Modifiers: Individual/Family/Community *and* Health Promotion/Potential/Actual

Signs/Symptoms of Actual

- absent/abnormal ability to speak/vocalize
- absent/abnormal ability to understand
- lacks alternative communication skills/gestures
- inappropriate sentence structure
- limited enunciation/clarity
- inappropriate word usage
- other

Oral health: Condition of the mouth and gums and the number, type, and arrangement of the teeth.

Modifiers: Individual/Family/Community *and* Health Promotion/Potential/Actual

Signs/Symptoms of Actual

- missing/broken/malformed teeth
- caries
- excess tartar
- sore/swollen/bleeding gums
- malocclusion
- ill-fitting/missing dentures
- sensitivity to hot or cold
- other

Cognition: Ability to think and use information.

Modifiers: Individual/Family/Community *and* Health Promotion/Potential/Actual

Signs/Symptoms of Actual

- diminished judgment
- disoriented to time/place/person
- limited recall of recent events
- limited recall of long past events
- limited calculating/sequencing skills
- limited concentration
- limited reasoning/abstract thinking ability
- impulsiveness
- repetitious language/behavior
- wanders
- other

Pain: Unpleasant sensory and emotional experience associated with actual or potential tissue damage.

Modifiers: Individual/Family/Community *and* Health Promotion/Potential/Actual

Signs/Symptoms of Actual

- expresses discomfort/pain
- elevated pulse/respirations/blood pressure
- compensated movement/guarding
- restless behavior
- facial grimaces
- pallor/perspiration
- other

Consciousness: Awareness of and responsiveness to stimuli and the surroundings.

Modifiers: Individual/Family/Community *and* Health Promotion/Potential/Actual

Signs/Symptoms of Actual

- lethargic
- stuporous
- unresponsive
- comatose
- other

Skin: Natural covering of the body.

Modifiers: Individual/Family/Community *and* Health Promotion/Potential/Actual

Signs/Symptoms of Actual

- lesion/pressure ulcer
- rash
- excessively dry
- excessively oily
- inflammation
- pruritus
- drainage
- bruising
- hypertrophy of nails
- delayed incisional healing
- other

Neuro-musculo-skeletal function: Ability of nerves, muscles, and bones to perform or coordinate specific movement, sensation, or regulation.

Modifiers: Individual/Family/Community *and* Health Promotion/Potential/Actual

SIGNS/SYMPTOMS OF ACTUAL

- limited range of motion
- decreased muscle strength
- decreased coordination
- decreased muscle tone
- increased muscle tone
- decreased sensation
- increased sensation
- decreased balance
- gait/ambulation disturbance
- difficulty transferring
- fractures
- tremors/seizures
- difficulty with thermoregulation
- other

Respiration: Inhaling and exhaling air into the body and exchanging oxygen.

Modifiers: Individual/Family/Community *and* Health Promotion/Potential/Actual

SIGNS/SYMPTOMS OF ACTUAL

- abnormal breath patterns
- unable to breathe independently
- cough
- unable to cough/expectorate independently
- cyanosis
- abnormal sputum
- noisy respirations
- rhinorrhea/nasal congestion
- abnormal breath sounds
- abnormal respiratory laboratory results
- other

Circulation: Pumping blood in adequate amounts and pressure throughout the body.

Modifiers: Individual/Family/Community *and* Health Promotion/Potential/Actual

SIGNS/SYMPTOMS OF ACTUAL

- edema
- cramping/pain of extremities
- decreased pulses
- discoloration of skin
- temperature change in affected area
- varicosities
- syncopal episodes (fainting)/dizziness
- abnormal blood pressure reading
- pulse deficit

- irregular heart rate
- excessively rapid heart rate
- excessively slow heart rate
- anginal pain
- abnormal heart sounds/murmurs
- abnormal clotting
- abnormal cardiac laboratory results
- other

Digestion-hydration: Process of converting food into forms that can be absorbed and assimilated, and maintaining fluid balance.

Modifiers: Individual/Family/Community *and* Health Promotion/Potential/Actual

SIGNS/SYMPTOMS OF ACTUAL

- nausea/vomiting
- difficulty/inability to chew/swallow/digest
- indigestion
- reflux
- anorexia
- anemia
- ascites
- jaundice/liver enlargement
- decreased skin turgor
- cracked lips/dry mouth
- electrolyte imbalance
- other

Bowel function: Transporting food through the gastrointestinal tract to eliminate wastes.

Modifiers: Individual/Family/Community *and* Health Promotion/Potential/Actual

SIGNS/SYMPTOMS OF ACTUAL

- abnormal frequency/consistency of stool
- painful defecation
- decreased bowel sounds
- blood in stools
- abnormal color
- cramping/abdominal discomfort
- incontinent of stool
- other

Urinary function: Production and excretion of urine.

Modifiers: Individual/Family/Community *and* Health Promotion/Potential/Actual

SIGNS/SYMPTOMS OF ACTUAL

- burning/painful urination
- incontinent of urine
- urgency/frequency
- difficulty initiating urination

- difficulty emptying bladder
- abnormal amount
- hematuria/abnormal color
- nocturia
- abnormal urinary laboratory results
- other

Reproductive function: Condition of the genital organs and breasts and the ability to reproduce.

Modifiers: Individual/Family/Community *and* Health Promotion/Potential/Actual

SIGNS/SYMPTOMS OF ACTUAL

- abnormal discharge
- abnormal menstrual pattern
- difficulty managing menopause/andropause
- abnormal lumps/swelling/tenderness of genital organs or breasts
- pain during or after sexual intercourse
- infertility
- impotency
- other

Pregnancy: Period from conception to childbirth.

Modifiers: Individual/Family/Community *and* Health Promotion/Potential/Actual

SIGNS/SYMPTOMS OF ACTUAL

- difficulty bonding with unborn baby
- difficulty coping with body changes
- difficulty with prenatal exercise/rest/diet/behaviors
- fears delivery procedure
- prenatal complications/preterm labor
- inadequate social support
- other

Postpartum: Six-week period following childbirth.

Modifiers: Individual/Family/Community *and* Health Promotion/Potential/Actual

SIGNS/SYMPTOMS OF ACTUAL

- difficulty breast-feeding
- difficulty coping with postpartum changes
- difficulty with postpartum exercise/rest/diet/behaviors
- abnormal bleeding/vaginal discharge
- postpartum complications
- abnormal depressed feelings
- other

Communicable/infectious condition: State in which organisms invade/infest and produce superficial or systemic illness with the potential for spreading or transmission.

Modifiers: Individual/Family/Community *and* Health Promotion/Potential/Actual

SIGNS/SYMPTOMS OF ACTUAL

- infection

- infestation
- fever
- biological hazards
- positive screening/culture/laboratory results
- inadequate supplies/equipment/policies to prevent transmission
- does not follow infection control regimen
- inadequate immunity
- other

HEALTH-RELATED BEHAVIORS DOMAIN: Patterns of activity that maintain or promote wellness, promote recovery, and decrease the risk of disease.

Nutrition: Select, consume, and use food and fluids for energy, maintenance, growth, and health.

Modifiers: Individual/Family/Community *and* Health Promotion/Potential/Actual

SIGNS/SYMPTOMS OF ACTUAL

- overweight: adult BMI 25.0 or more; child BMI 95th percentile or more
- underweight: adult BMI 18.5 or less; child BMI 5th percentile or less
- lacks established standards for daily caloric/fluid intake
- exceeds established standards for daily caloric/fluid intake
- unbalanced diet
- improper feeding schedule for age
- does not follow recommended nutrition plan
- unexplained/progressive weight loss
- unable to obtain/prepare food
- hypoglycemia
- hyperglycemia
- other

Sleep and rest patterns: Periods of suspended motor and sensory activity and periods of inactivity, repose, or mental calm.

Modifiers: Individual/Family/Community *and* Health Promotion/Potential/Actual

SIGNS/SYMPTOMS OF ACTUAL

- sleep/rest pattern disrupts family
- frequently wakes during night
- sleepwalking
- insomnia
- nightmares
- insufficient sleep/rest for age/physical condition
- sleep apnea
- snoring
- other

Physical activity: State or quality of body movements during daily living.

Modifiers: Individual/Family/Community *and* Health Promotion/Potential/Actual

SIGNS/SYMPTOMS OF ACTUAL

- sedentary life style

- inadequate/inconsistent exercise routine
- inappropriate type/amount of exercise for age/physical condition
- other

Personal care: Management of personal cleanliness and dressing.

Modifiers: Individual/Family/Community *and* Health Promotion/Potential/Actual

SIGNS/SYMPTOMS OF ACTUAL

- difficulty laundering clothing
- difficulty with bathing
- difficulty with toileting activities
- difficulty dressing lower body
- difficulty dressing upper body
- foul body odor
- difficulty shampooing/combing hair
- difficulty brushing/flossing/mouth care
- unwilling/unable/forgets to complete personal care activities
- other

Substance use: Consumption of medicines, recreational drugs, or other materials likely to cause mood changes and/or psychological/physical dependence, illness, and disease.

Modifiers: Individual/Family/Community *and* Health Promotion/Potential/Actual

SIGNS/SYMPTOMS OF ACTUAL

- abuses over-the-counter/prescription medications
- uses "street"-recreational drugs
- abuses alcohol
- smokes/uses tobacco products
- difficulty performing normal routines
- reflex disturbances
- behavior change
- exposure to cigarette/cigar smoke
- buys/sells illegal substances
- other

Family planning: Practices designed to plan and space pregnancy within the context of values, attitudes, and beliefs.

Modifiers: Individual/Family/Community *and* Health Promotion/Potential/Actual

SIGNS/SYMPTOMS OF ACTUAL

- inappropriate/insufficient knowledge about family planning methods
- inappropriate/insufficient knowledge about preconception health practices
- inaccurate/inconsistent use of family planning methods
- dissatisfied with present family planning method
- fears others' reactions regarding family planning choices
- difficulty obtaining family planning methods
- other

Health care supervision: Management of the health care treatment plan by health care providers.

Modifiers: Individual/Family/Community *and* Health Promotion/Potential/Actual

SIGNS/SYMPTOMS OF ACTUAL

- fails to obtain routine/preventive health care
- fails to seek care for symptoms requiring evaluation/treatment
- fails to return as requested to health care provider
- inability to coordinate multiple appointments/treatment plans
- inconsistent source of health care
- inadequate source of health care
- inadequate treatment plan
- other

Medication regimen: Use or application of over-the-counter and prescribed/recommended medications and infusions to meet guidelines for therapeutic action, safety, and schedule.

Modifiers: Individual/Family/Community *and* Health Promotion/Potential/Actual

SIGNS/SYMPTOMS OF ACTUAL

- does not follow recommended dosage/schedule
- evidence of side effects/adverse reactions
- inadequate system for taking medication
- improper storage of medication
- fails to obtain refills appropriately
- fails to obtain immunizations
- inadequate medication regimen
- unable to take medications without help
- other

Intervention Scheme

CATEGORIES

Teaching, Guidance, and Counseling: Activities designed to provide information and materials, encourage action and responsibility for self-care and coping, and assist the individual, family, or community to make decisions and solve problems.

Treatments and Procedures: Technical activities such as wound care, specimen collection, resistive exercises, and medication prescriptions that are designed to prevent, decrease, or alleviate signs and symptoms for the individual, family, or community.

Case Management: Activities such as coordination, advocacy, and referral that facilitate service delivery, promote assertiveness, guide the individual, family, or community toward use of appropriate resources, and improve communication among health and human service providers.

Surveillance: Activities such as detection, measurement, critical analysis, and monitoring intended to identify the individual, family, or community's status in relation to a given condition or phenomenon.

TARGETS

anatomy/physiology: Structure and function of the human body.

anger management: Activities that decrease or control negative feelings and interactions, including violence.

behavior modification: Activities that change habits, conduct, or patterns of action.

bladder care: Activities that promote urinary bladder function such as bladder retraining, catheter changes, and catheter irrigation.

bonding/attachment: A mutual, positive relationship between two people such as a parent/caregiver and an infant/child.

bowel care: Activities that promote bowel function such as bowel training and enemas.

cardiac care: Activities that promote cardiac or circulatory function such as energy conservation and fluid balance.

caretaking/parenting skills: Activities such as feeding, bathing, discipline, nurturing, and stimulation provided to a dependent child or adult.

cast care: Activities that promote cleanliness, dryness, support, alignment, and relief of pain, pressure, and constriction of an injured body part immobilized by a cast, splint, or other device.

communication: Exchange of verbal or nonverbal information between the individual/family/community and others.

community outreach worker services: Assistance with managing health care, transportation, household, and child/adult care responsibilities provided by qualified employees under the supervision of professional health care providers.

continuity of care: Communication of information among providers/organizations to provide safe and effective care and decrease duplication of efforts/services.

coping skills: Ability to effectively manage challenges and changes such as illness, disability, loss of income, birth of a child, or death of a family member.

day care/respite: Individuals or organizations that provide child/adult supervision while the parent/usual caregiver attends school, works, or has relief from usual responsibilities.

dietary management: Nourishment with balanced food and fluids that sustain life, provide energy, and promote growth and health.

discipline: Nurturing practices that promote appropriate behavior, conduct, and self-control.

dressing change/wound care: Activities that promote wound healing and prevent infection such as observing, measuring, cleansing, irrigating, and/or covering a wound, lesion, or incision.

durable medical equipment: Nondisposable items used while providing care such as special beds, walkers, and apnea monitors.

education: Formal programs that offer general, technical, or individualized studies for students of all ages.

employment: Occupation that provides income.

end-of-life care: Activities that provide physical comfort and emotional calm for those who are dying by involving/including family, friends, spiritual concerns, rituals, pain control, and physical care.

environment: Physical surroundings, conditions, or influences in the residence, neighborhood, and/or community.

exercises: Therapeutic physical activities such as active/passive range of motion, isometrics, stretching, and weight lifting.

family planning care: Activities that support consideration and use of methods to prepare for and space pregnancy.

feeding procedures: Provision of food or fluids using methods such as breast, formula, spoon, tube, and intravenous solutions.

finances: Management of income and expenses.
gait training: Systematic activities that promote walking with or without assistive devices.
genetics: Diagnosis, consultation, and procedures intended to prevent, identify, or treat birth defects, congenital anomalies, or conditions.
growth/development care: Activities that promote progressive maturation in relation to age such as measuring weight, height, and head circumference and stimulating achievement of developmental milestones.
home: Place of residence.
homemaking/housekeeping: Management of activities such as cleaning, laundry, and food preparation in the home or the health care facility.
infection precautions: Activities that decrease the incidence and transmission of contagious disease such as hand washing, isolation, specimen collection, contact follow-up, reporting procedures, and environmental control.
interaction: Reciprocal action or influence among people including parent-child, parent-teacher, and nurse-client.
interpreter/translator services: Assistance with verbal or written communication in other languages provided by qualified employees who are under the supervision of professional health care practitioners.
laboratory findings: Results of fluid and tissue tests such as urine and blood analysis.
legal system: Authority, rules of conduct, or administration of the law.
medical/dental care: Assessment/diagnosis and treatment provided by physicians, dentists, and their staff or assistants.
medication action/side effects: Positive and/or negative consequences of medications.
medication administration: Activities that involve applying or giving medications and that are completed by clients, parents/caregivers, or health care practitioners.
medication coordination/ordering: Communication with those who prescribe and dispense medications and the individual/family/community support systems to ensure that appropriate medications and supplies are obtained in a timely manner.
medication prescription: A formalized pharmaceutical order/official request for medications.
medication set-up: Act of preparing for medication administration by filling/checking an oral medication organizer, prefilling syringes, or inserting intravenous access devices.
mobility/transfers: Body movements that change position or allow participation in activities such as walking.
nursing care: Assessment/diagnosis and treatment provided by nurses and their staff or assistants.
nutritionist care: Assessment/diagnosis and treatment provided by nutritionists/registered dieticians and their staff or assistants.
occupational therapy care: Assessment/diagnosis and treatment provided by occupational therapists and their staff or assistants.
ostomy care: Activities to manage elimination of urine or stool through artificial openings such as a colostomy and ileostomy.
other community resources: Organizations or groups that offer goods or services not specifically identified in other targets such as exercise facilities, food pantries/distribution centers, or faith communities.
paraprofessional/aide care: Assistance provided by qualified aides, home health aides, and nursing assistants under the supervision of professional health care practitioners.
personal hygiene: Individual grooming activities such as bathing, shampooing, and toileting.
physical therapy care: Assessment/diagnosis and treatment provided by physical therapists and their staff or assistants.

positioning: Alignment of the body to promote comfort and function.
recreational therapy care: Assessment/diagnosis and treatment provided by recreational therapists and their staff or assistants.
relaxation/breathing techniques: Activities that relieve muscle tension, induce a quieting body response, and rebuild energy resources such as deep breathing exercises, guided imagery, meditation, and massage.
respiratory care: Activities that promote respiratory or pulmonary function such as suctioning and nebulizer treatments.
respiratory therapy care: Assessment/diagnosis and treatment provided by respiratory therapists and staff or assistants.
rest/sleep: Periodic state of quiet and varying degrees of consciousness.
safety: Freedom from risk, the occurrence of injury, or loss.
screening procedures: Evaluation strategies used to identify risk for conditions, diagnose disease early, and monitor change/progression over time.
sickness/injury care: Activities in response to illness or accidents such as first aid and temperature taking.
signs/symptoms—mental/emotional: Objective or subjective evidence of mental/emotional health problems such as depression, confusion, or agitation.
signs/symptoms—physical: Objective or subjective evidence of physical health problems such as fever, sudden weight loss, or statement of pain.
skin care: Activities that promote skin integrity such as application of lotion and massage.
social work/counseling care: Assessment/diagnosis and treatment provided by social workers, counselors, and their staff or assistants.
specimen collection: Activities designed to obtain samples of human and animal tissue, fluids, secretions, or excreta such as blood, urine, stool, sputum, and drainage.
speech and language pathology care: Assessment/diagnosis and treatment provided by speech and language pathologists and their staff or assistants.
spiritual care: Activities that promote personal serenity and comfort and involve spiritual concerns/practices.
stimulation/nurturance: Activities that promote healthy physical, intellectual, and emotional development.
stress management: Cognitive, emotional, and physical activities that promote healthy functioning during difficult life circumstances.
substance use cessation: Activities that promote discontinuing use of harmful/addicting materials.
supplies: Disposable items used while providing care such as dressings, syringes, tubing, diapers, and baby bottles.
support group: Organized sources of information and assistance such as focused classes and organizations, telephone reassurance, and reliable Internet sites that address a specific topic such as parenting, alcoholism, obesity, and Alzheimer's disease.
support system: Circle of family, friends, and associates that provide love, care, and assistance to promote health and manage illness.
transportation: Methods of travel such as a car, bus, taxi, scooter, or cart.
wellness: Practices that promote physical and mental health such as exercise, nutrition, and immunizations.
other: Persons, places, things, or activities not identified in this list.

Problem Rating Scale For Outcomes

Concepts	1	2	3	4	5
KNOWLEDGE Ability of the client to remember and interpret information	No knowledge	Minimal knowledge	Basic knowledge	Adequate knowledge	Superior knowledge
BEHAVIOR Observable responses, actions, or activities of the client fitting the occasion or purpose	Not appropriate behavior	Rarely appropriate behavior	Inconsistently appropriate behavior	Usually appropriate behavior	Consistently appropriate behavior
STATUS Condition of the client in relation to objective and subjective defining characteristics	Extreme signs/ symptoms	Severe signs/ symptoms	Moderate signs/ symptoms	Minimal signs/ symptoms	No signs/ symptoms

APPENDIX B

Case Studies

Case studies are a valuable strategy to increase accurate and consistent use of the Omaha System. The 18 case studies (stories and answers) in this appendix were submitted by individuals and groups located in the United States, Canada, and Estonia. These case studies are designed to present a rich and diverse set of *realistic but fictitious clients* (individuals, families, and communities) who received equally diverse services from multidisciplinary practitioners in various settings. They are written with the intent to keep the length short, and the content simple and fun. The 18 case studies are copyrighted by Elsevier but may be reproduced for instructional and clinical use without permission.

Typically case studies are used to maximize group interaction and retention of Omaha System concepts. The variation in complexity is evident when the stories and corresponding answers are compared. Most Omaha System terms appear in one or more case studies with each study having an average of three or four problems and several related interventions and outcomes. Therefore, when selecting a case study for a group, evaluate the needs of the participants and the content presented in the case study. For example, novice learners tend to be more comfortable with a story that describes the type of clients they already know. Often, more experienced learners benefit from exposure to less familiar stories and interaction with participants who have varied opinions and professional and life experiences.

Case studies can be used to:

1. Offer practice opportunities for new learners following an introduction of the Omaha System.
2. Provide refresher opportunities for experienced users.
3. Introduce the revised Omaha System. The case studies in this appendix are based on the newly revised problems, modifiers, signs/symptoms, categories, and targets. Review Chapter 2 and Appendix A for information needed to use case studies successfully. Note that several case studies are population-focused and incorporate the *Community* modifier.
4. Examine consistent and accurate use (interrater reliability) among practitioners, students, or researchers regardless of their experience.
5. Offer data from an initial visit, encounter, project, or incident that can be expanded to:
   a. provide a model to develop new case studies that reflect local clients and practice.
   b. create stories about interim visits, visits conducted by other health care professionals, or discharge visits.

c. identify interventions and ratings for additional time intervals than presented in this appendix to provide "before, during, and after" practice opportunities.
6. Promote discussion about particular client groups, holistic practice, expectations about practitioners' and clients' responsibilities, "best practices," trends in medications and treatments, ethical or cultural issues, community resources, documentation standards, the meaning of Omaha System data analysis, and similarities between the Omaha System and other terminologies.
7. Provide opportunities to practice documentation in software programs.
8. Furnish data that practitioner/student actors use to present a role play or prepare a videotape.

Each case study can be used in several ways. The story can be presented by a case study leader to an individual or group, and answers documented using a copy of a worksheet (see Figure 2-5). Participants can complete all Problem Classification Scheme, Intervention Scheme, and Problem Rating Scale for Outcomes answers, and then discuss those answers. A case study can stimulate multiple discussion sessions that focus on client issues and practice, documentation, and information management, as well as Omaha System concepts. The case study can be edited, used incrementally, and/or introduced in segments. Participants can document and discuss details from the Problem Classification Scheme during one session, details from the Intervention Scheme during a second session, and details from the Problem Rating Scale for Outcomes during a third session. Participants can be asked to develop a care plan for the next visit. If an abbreviated story is needed, it is possible to delete details that suggest one or two problems and their related interventions and ratings from both the story and answers. The case studies are presented as software- or form-neutral to increase their usability. However, software screens or manual forms could be used to document answers instead of the Omaha System worksheet.

Case studies have two sections:

1. Information Obtained during a Visit, Encounter, Project, or Incident

The stories are composites that represent real people and situations. The titles of case studies correspond to the first name and first initial of the last name of the clients depicted in the stories; no disrespect was intended by this informal approach. Most stories depict an initial visit or encounter and are identified accordingly. Several are more complex and include answers obtained at different times. The stories include referral details, data that the practitioner or student obtained during the time reflected in the case study, and clues for identification of Omaha System problems, interventions, and ratings. The pertinent information in the stories is designed to be congruent with the answers, which are found in the second section of each case study.

2. Application of the Omaha System

This section provides answers that include Problem Classification Scheme domains, problems, modifiers, signs/symptoms, risk factors, and details; Intervention Scheme categories, targets, and client-specific information; and Problem Rating Scale for Outcomes numeric ratings for *Knowledge*, *Behavior*, and *Status*. Brief comments, usually placed within parentheses, clarify selected answers, including ratings. Often these or similar brief comments are included in client records as free text or narrative generated by practitioners. The answers that are presented have been judged by experts to be accurate and pertinent, and should be considered the standard. However, answers are always viewed through the lens of each unique practice setting, and are meant to be discussed, challenged, and changed if appropriate. Participants should refer to the story for data to support and explain their choices, and have the opportunity to present their opinions.

When reading the answers and using the case studies, remember basic assumptions:

a. Answers reflect care that was actually provided, not a care plan. The time required increases and agreement decreases dramatically if a story is used to develop a care plan.
b. Problems are designated as high priority or low priority, with each having a different amount and style of answers.
c. For each case study, answers such as problems, signs/symptoms, categories, and targets are listed in the same order as they appear in the Omaha System to help readers find information. When using the Omaha System, it is rarely useful to rank or prioritize those terms (i.e., if a client has four high-priority problems, do not prioritize them, but expect to address all four during the period of service).
d. Because "more is not necessarily better," the goal is to list pertinent answers one time and not duplicate answers unnecessarily. Note that answers vary with the context of the stories. In addition, providers may offer health care services to more than one family member. If that occurs, the provider may document specific problems, interventions, and ratings in only one of the client records. The case studies authored by Benavides and Solomon are examples of situations in which another client record might be used.
e. Groups will rarely achieve 100% agreement on all answers. It is more important to achieve agreement at the level of a problem rather than a sign/symptom, or a category rather than client-specific information. The knowledge base and skills of participants vary because of personal attributes, professional perspectives, and life experiences, especially when new learners are involved.
f. Answers and agreement are related to the setting's unique characteristics. Culture, geography, documentation system, data needs, and goals are just some of the factors that influence "best" answers. The documentation system may influence the selection of modifiers, as well as low-priority and high-priority problems. An educator may want undergraduate students to identify and discuss focused sections of a case study for an assignment, and ignore other sections. Provider organizations may develop standard expectations, referred to as practice standards or pathways, for their practitioners to follow for analysis, report generation, accreditation, auditing, or reimbursement (see Chapter 3). For example, a health department manager may want to track the problem *Substance use* among pregnant women. A home care manager may want to track the problem *Pain* and its management among all clients. Practitioners who report to those managers need to understand the purpose of aggregate data collection, the process of outcomes measurement, and their responsibilities as they provide and document care.

Rose Z.: Older Woman Recovering From a Fracture

Lucille Baxter, RN
Nursing Supervisor
Decatur County Public Health and Home Care
Leon, Iowa

Robert Arnold, PT
Physical Therapy Supervisor
Decatur County Public Health and Home Care
Leon, Iowa

JoAnn Dean, RN
Staff Nurse/Home Care Aide Supervisor
Decatur County Public Health and Home Care
Leon, Iowa

Shelley Bickle, BA
Department Supervisor
Decatur County Public Health and Home Care
Leon, Iowa

Information Obtained During the First Visit/Encounter

Rose Z., age 76, fractured her right hip, was hospitalized for 4 days in acute care and was in the rehabilitation unit for 2 weeks. Referral information included toe-touch weight bearing with a walker for 4 weeks; commode and hospital bed with trapeze; home-delivered meals; and nursing, physical therapy, and home health aide services. Medications were to be taken as needed: acetaminophen (extra-strength Tylenol), acetaminophen and hydrocodone (Vicodin), and magnesium hydroxide (Milk of Magnesia). The home care nurse and physical therapist made a shared visit the day after discharge. Rose's daughter, Helen, was staying for several days. The nurse met with Rose and then with Helen; the therapist met with Helen and then with Rose.

The nurse checked Rose's vital signs and blood pressure and noted that they were within normal limits. Her right hip incision was intact and fully granulating. They discussed a few foods that Rose could prepare and the home-delivered meals. The nurse encouraged her to increase her activity as possible, drink six to eight glasses of water each day, and increase her fiber intake. She did not know that pain medications could cause constipation. Rose understood the difference in the two pain medications and the importance of scheduling doses so she was comfortable. Her pain was a 3 on a 0 to 10 pain scale, with 10 being the most severe. Rose had taken pain pills this morning and during the night, but was not certain about the times; the nurse suggested that she start a log to help her remember medication type, dose time, and pain severity. She agreed to take a pill one-half hour before the physical therapist's future visits.

The physical therapist and Helen toured the small, one-story home. The hospital bed was located in Rose's bedroom, with her walker and the commode on left side. The height and condition of the equipment were appropriate. The therapist noted a serious hazard: Rose's house slippers. The physical therapist asked Helen to talk to her mother about the slippers.

The physical therapist asked Rose to remove her slippers and wear supportive shoes. Then Rose used her walker and ambulated more than 100 feet on the carpeted floor. She used the overhead trapeze to get in and out of the bed and demonstrated her exercises. The physical therapist offered suggestions to perform her exercise program more effectively, use the walker while maintaining appropriate weight-bearing status, and properly elevate and position her leg. Rose said that she was anxious to drive again.

The nurse asked Helen how well she thought her mother would manage. Helen was pleased about the sheduled services and meals. Helen had asked several of Rose's friends to establish a schedule to call, stop by, obtain her medication refills, and take her to doctor's appointments. Helen would call her mother daily. Rose, Helen, the nurse, and the therapist reviewed the visit, schedule, and plans and complimented Rose on her progress.

Application of the Omaha System

(Answers reflect care provided by both the nurse and physical therapist.)

DOMAIN: PHYSIOLOGICAL

Problem: Pain (high priority)

Problem Classification Scheme

Modifiers: Individual and Actual

SIGNS/SYMPTOMS OF ACTUAL

- expresses discomfort/pain

Intervention Scheme

Category: Teaching, Guidance, and Counseling

TARGETS AND CLIENT-SPECIFIC INFORMATION

- medication action/side effects (expectations, pain scale, constipation)
- medication administration (schedule, keep log)

Category: Surveillance

TARGETS AND CLIENT-SPECIFIC INFORMATION

- signs/symptoms—physical (pain scale, location, severity, control)

Problem Rating Scale for Outcomes

Knowledge: 3-basic knowledge (understood need for schedule, not aware that pills cause constipation or needed before physical therapy)

Behavior: 3-inconsistently appropriate behavior (took pain medications but unsure about details)

Status: 3-moderate signs/symptoms (pain scale = 3)

Problem: Neuro-musculo-skeletal function (high priority)

Problem Classification Scheme

Modifiers: Individual and Actual

SIGNS/SYMPTOMS OF ACTUAL

- limited range of motion
- decreased muscle strength
- decreased balance
- gait/ambulation disturbance
- difficulty transferring
- fractures

Intervention Scheme

Category: Teaching, Guidance, and Counseling

TARGETS AND CLIENT-SPECIFIC INFORMATION

- communication (Rose's goals of rehabilitation)
- durable medical equipment (use of bed, trapeze, walker)
- exercises (demonstrated)

Category: Treatments and Procedures

TARGETS AND CLIENT-SPECIFIC INFORMATION

- gait training (wear supportive shoes, use walker correctly in home)

Category: Case Management

TARGETS AND CLIENT-SPECIFIC INFORMATION

- continuity of care (shared home visit, met with both Rose and Helen)

Category: Surveillance

TARGETS AND CLIENT-SPECIFIC INFORMATION

- mobility/transfers (techniques, tolerance)
- safety (home check)
- signs/symptoms—physical (vital signs, blood pressure, incision site)

Problem Rating Scale for Outcomes

Knowledge: 3-basic knowledge (knew mobility basics)

Behavior: 3-inconsistently appropriate behavior (demonstrated walker/exercises, but needed suggestions)

Status: 3-moderate signs/symptoms (fracture/pain/restricted activity)

DOMAIN: HEALTH-RELATED BEHAVIORS

Problem: Nutrition (low priority: provide interventions and rate if needed)

Problem Classification Scheme

Modifiers: Individual and Actual

SIGNS/SYMPTOMS OF ACTUAL

- unable to obtain/prepare food

Problem: Personal care (high priority)

Problem Classification Scheme

Modifiers: Individual and Actual

SIGNS/SYMPTOMS OF ACTUAL

- difficulty with bathing
- difficulty with toileting activities
- difficulty dressing lower body
- difficulty shampooing/combing hair

Intervention Scheme

Category: Case Management

TARGETS AND CLIENT-SPECIFIC INFORMATION

- paraprofessional/aide care (scheduled 3 times/week)

Problem Rating Scale for Outcomes

Knowledge: 3-basic knowledge (wants help to regain independence)

Behavior: 4-usually appropriate behavior (will accept home health aide)

Status: 3-moderate signs/symptoms (needs help since surgery)

APPENDIX B

Carmelita S.: Pregnant Teen

Nancy Benavides, RN, BSN
Public Health Nurse
Madison Heights, Michigan

Information Obtained During the First Visit/Encounter

The public health nurse received a referral for Carmelita S., age 15, from the emergency room after she went for abdominal pain and fever. She was approximately 29 weeks' pregnant, and was treated for *Chlamydia* infection.

The nurse visited Carmelita and her mother. The family received governmental medical/financial assistance that they expected to cover Carmelita's expenses and obtained clothing and supplies from other resources. Carmelita and her mother agreed that she needed to start regular prenatal care and obtain supplemental foods; they had transportation. The mother used the phone numbers that the nurse provided and made appointments.

The nurse and Carmelita discussed an appropriate weight gain, a healthy diet, supplemental vitamins, laboratory tests, and exercise. She weighed 130 pounds at the emergency room and was 5′3″ tall. She did not know if she has gained or lost weight since becoming pregnant. However, Carmelita did not take her prenatal vitamin samples because they made her feel nauseated. She usually ate two meals per day and had no appetite until the evening. She did not like milk or meat and ate few vegetables or fruit. She said she would think about exercise.

The nurse and Carmelita agreed on the goal that she would deliver a healthy baby. They discussed her vital signs and blood pressure, which were within normal limits. The nurse described *Chlamydia*, how it is transmitted, and the effect that an untreated infection could have on a baby. The emergency room report indicated that she may not need more treatment, but needed a follow up appointment. Carmelita denied having symptoms. She did not want to discuss labor and delivery or attend expectant parent classes, because "it's too scary." She planned to keep the baby; she had cared for her younger siblings. She and her mother agreed to meet with the nurse next week.

Application of the Omaha System

DOMAIN: ENVIRONMENTAL

Problem: Income (low priority: provide interventions and rate if needed; received maximum medical/governmental assistance, including food, and obtained clothing and supplies)

Problem Classification Scheme

Modifiers: Family and Actual

SIGNS/SYMPTOMS OF ACTUAL

- low/no income

DOMAIN: PHYSIOLOGICAL

Problem: Pregnancy (high priority)

Problem Classification Scheme

Modifiers: Individual and Actual

SIGNS/SYMPTOMS OF ACTUAL

- difficulty with prenatal exercise/rest/diet/behaviors
- fears delivery procedure
- prenatal complications/preterm labor

Intervention Scheme

Category: Teaching, Guidance, and Counseling

TARGETS AND CLIENT-SPECIFIC INFORMATION

- anatomy/physiology (normal changes, exercise/labor/delivery)
- medical/dental care (prenatal care/*Chlamydia*, improve pregnancy outcomes)

Category: Case Management

TARGETS AND CLIENT-SPECIFIC INFORMATION

- medical/dental care (gave information, Carmelita's mother made an appointment)

Category: Surveillance

TARGETS AND CLIENT-SPECIFIC INFORMATION

- signs/symptoms—physical (vital signs, blood pressure)

Problem Rating Scale for Outcomes

Knowledge: 2-minimal knowledge (unware of pregnency/infections; scared of labor)
Behavior: 2-rarely appropriate behavior (did not recognize/admit pregnancy, seek care)
Status: 2-severe signs/symptoms (29 weeks' pregnant with no prenatal care)

Problem: Communicable/infectious condition (low priority: provide interventions and rate if evidence of another infection)

Problem Classification Scheme

Modifiers: Individual and Potential

RISK FACTORS (*Chlamydia* treated in emergency room; no more symptoms)

DOMAIN: HEALTH-RELATED BEHAVIORS

Problem: Nutrition (high priority)

Problem Classification Scheme

Modifiers: Individual and Actual

SIGNS/SYMPTOMS OF ACTUAL

- lacks established standards for daily caloric/fluid intake
- unbalanced diet

Intervention Scheme

Category: Teaching, Guidance, and Counseling

TARGETS AND CLIENT-SPECIFIC INFORMATION

- dietary management (monitor weight, take vitamins, improve diet, laboratory tests)

APPENDIX B

Category: Case Management

TARGETS AND CLIENT-SPECIFIC INFORMATION

- other community resources (mother made appointment for supplemental foods)

Category: Surveillance

TARGETS AND CLIENT-SPECIFIC INFORMATION

- dietary management (food history/needed changes)

Problem Rating Scale for Outcomes

Knowledge: 2-minimal knowledge (not aware of balanced nutrition, effect on fetus, or weight gain)

Behavior: 2-rarely appropriate behavior (did not eat nutritious diet, take vitamins, or monitor weight)

Status: 3-moderate signs/symptoms (appeared healthy based on color and self-report)

Sally D.: Woman With Hepatitis B

Stephanie C. Bryant, RN, MSN, PHN
Senior Public Health Nurse
County of Riverside Department of Public Health
Riverside, California

Shawna R. Johnson, RN, BA, PHN
Public Health Nurse
County of Riverside Department of Public Health,
Riverside, California

Information Obtained During the First Visit/Encounter

The public health nurse made a home visit for communicable disease investigation to Sally D., a 45-year-old female, who tested positive for hepatitis B. She was employed part time but did not work for the last 2 weeks due to persistent fatigue, nausea, and vomiting. She noticed that her urine was dark brown. She did not seek care because she did not have medical insurance or a car. A friend noticed that Sally's skin and eyes were yellow and took her to the emergency room.

She did not know how she contracted hepatitis B. She stated that she had not used drugs for 3 months and was attending a local substance abuse program.

The nurse told Sally about hepatitis B, including sources of infection, treatment, and ways to prevent transmission. Sally knew that she needed to get another blood test in 6 months but did not understand why or what it meant if she continued to test positive for hepatitis B. The nurse described what options were available, encouraged Sally to seek the help of friends, urged her to keep well hydrated and nourished during the acute phase of the disease, and listed foods that might be easy to tolerate. They discussed her finances and lack of medical insurance. The nurse referred Sally to the local health department clinic for follow-up care and to the social services office to apply for indigent medical insurance and income assistance. She referred Sally to a hepatitis B support group in her area and gave her a bus schedule with vouchers and the phone number for a local, free medical van service. She scheduled a follow-up visit with Sally in 2 weeks.

Application of the Omaha System

DOMAIN: ENVIRONMENTAL

Problem: Income (high priority)

Problem Classification Scheme

Modifiers: Individual and Actual

SIGNS/SYMPTOMS OF ACTUAL

- low/no income
- uninsured medical expenses
- difficulty buying necessities

Intervention Scheme

Category: Teaching, Guidance, and Counseling

TARGETS AND CLIENT-SPECIFIC INFORMATION

- finances (Sally's income and expenses, lack of insurance)

Category: Case Management

TARGETS AND CLIENT-SPECIFIC INFORMATION

- social work/counseling care (referred for indigent insurance/income assistance)

Category: Surveillance

APPENDIX B

TARGETS AND CLIENT-SPECIFIC INFORMATION
- finances (status, follow up with referral)

Problem Rating Scale for Outcomes
Knowledge: 2-minimal knowledge (did not know how to obtain care)
Behavior: 2-rarely appropriate behavior (unemployed, insurance)
Status: 2-severe signs/symptoms (ill; needed income, care, transportation)

DOMAIN: PHYSIOLOGICAL

Problem: Communicable/infectious condition (high priority)

Problem Classification Scheme
Modifiers: Individual and Actual
SIGNS/SYMPTOMS OF ACTUAL
- infection
- positive screening/culture/laboratory results
- does not follow infection control regimen

Intervention Scheme
Category: Teaching, Guidance, and Counseling
TARGETS AND CLIENT-SPECIFIC INFORMATION
- anatomy/physiology (disease process, source/transmission)
- dietary management (need for food that Sally can tolerate, high fluid intake)
- laboratory findings (interpretation of tests)
- signs/symptoms—physical (current status and possible progression, employment)
- support system (need for friends and others to help and encourage)

Category: Case Management
TARGETS AND CLIENT-SPECIFIC INFORMATION
- medical/dental care (referred to health department clinic for follow-up)
- support group (referred to hepatitis B support group)
- transportation (provided bus vouchers and van information)

Category: Surveillance
TARGETS AND CLIENT-SPECIFIC INFORMATION
- medical/dental care (follow up with appointments and laboratory tests)
- signs/symptoms—physical (changes)

Problem Rating Scale for Outcomes
Knowledge: 2-minimal knowledge (did not know about disease, transmission)
Behavior: 2-rarely appropriate behavior (did not seek care)
Status: 2-severe signs/symptoms (acute phase of disease, few resources)

DOMAIN: HEALTH-RELATED BEHAVIORS

Problem: Substance use (low priority: provide interventions and rate if evidence of drug use)

Problem Classification Scheme
Modifiers: Individual and Potential
RISK FACTORS (reports previous drug use; attends substance abuse program)

Jerry H.: Man With a Chronic Respiratory Condition

Ida Clark, RN, BSN
Clinical Director
Health Systems Research Center
Carle Foundation Hospital
Urbana, Illinois

Donna Dworak, RN, MS
Outcomes Analyst
Health Systems Research Center
Carle Foundation Hospital
Urbana, Illinois

Information Obtained During the First Visit/Encounter

Jerry H., a 68-year-old man, lived with his wife of 46 years in a small, rural community. He was a self-employed farmer until he retired 2 years ago; his son managed the farm. Every morning, Jerry drove to the coffee shop, where he drank several cups of coffee with his friends and smoked three to four cigarettes. He said if his wife ever caught him smoking, she would be "VERY upset." He also "snuck" cigarettes on other occasions. He did not plan to quit smoking.

Jerry came to the clinic for a routine 3-month evaluation of his chronic obstructive pulmonary disease (COPD). He had been hospitalized several times during the last year for exacerbations. During the clinic visit, he complained of increased shortness of breath and a chronic cough, especially in the morning. His temperature was 98.3° F, his pulse was 106, his blood pressure was 102/52, and oxygen saturation was 92% on room air. He had bibasilar crackles.

Jerry's medication regimen included furosemide (Lasix) 20 mg daily, potassium 10 mEq daily, enalapril (Vasotec) 5 mg daily, ipratropium (Atrovent MDI) 2 inhalations three times a day, salmeterol (Serevent MDI) 2 inhalations three times a day, and albuterol (Ventolin) 2 inhalations as needed. His last potassium level was 4.6 mEq/L. Jerry's medication costs were increasing each month. He did not use his inhalers consistently; insurance did not cover them, "they cost a 'pretty penny,' and they do not help anyway." Last month, when Jerry had to choose between buying his inhalers and paying his electric bill, he knew he must pay the electric bill. The nurse explained the relationship between his diagnosis, his symptoms, and his medications. When the nurse described some financial options and offered to help with a referral for assistance, he said he would participate. The nurse sent an e-mail to the low-income drug program and gave Jerry the necessary form to present. Jerry took his other medications under the watchful eye of his wife. He admitted that if something happened to her, he would be in trouble because he did not know what medications he took or why he took them. Although the nurse reviewed Jerry's medication profile with him and demonstrated correct inhaler use, the nurse questioned if he benefited. Jerry did not like to go to the doctor. He said he would return when he was sick and may return for his follow-up appointments. He had previously refused influenza and pneumonia immunizations.

Application of the Omaha System

DOMAIN: ENVIRONMENTAL

Problem: Income (high priority)

Problem Classification Scheme

Modifiers: Family and Actual

SIGNS/SYMPTOMS OF ACTUAL

- low/no income
- uninsured medical expenses
- difficulty buying necessities

Intervention Scheme

Category: Teaching, Guidance, and Counseling

TARGETS AND CLIENT-SPECIFIC INFORMATION

- finances (options, how to contact and obtain assistance)
- other community resources (how to obtain drugs from low-income drug program)

Category: Case Management

TARGETS AND CLIENT-SPECIFIC INFORMATION

- other community resources (referred to low-income drug program)

Problem Rating Scale for Outcomes

Knowledge: 2-minimal knowledge (did not know how to obtain medications or help with power bill)

Behavior: 4-usually appropriate behavior (consistently paid his bills)

Status: 2-severe signs/symptoms (did not buy inhalers because of other expenses)

DOMAIN: PHYSIOLOGICAL

Problem: Respiration (high priority)

Problem Classification Scheme

Modifiers: Individual and Actual

SIGNS/SYMPTOMS OF ACTUAL

- abnormal breath patterns
- cough
- abnormal breath sounds

Intervention Scheme

Category: Teaching, Guidance, and Counseling

TARGETS AND CLIENT-SPECIFIC INFORMATION

- anatomy/physiology (disease process)
- respiratory care (treatment regimen that could help)
- signs/symptoms—physical (shortness of breath, cough)

Category: Surveillance

TARGETS AND CLIENT-SPECIFIC INFORMATION

- signs/symptoms—physical (vital signs, bibasilar crackles, changes)

Problem Rating Scale for Outcomes

Knowledge: 2-minimal knowledge (did/would not understand relationship between diagnosis, symptoms, and medications; not interested in preventive care)
Behavior: 2-rarely appropriate behavior (came to clinic for symptoms/usually for follow up, smoked, used inhalers inconsistently)
Status: 2-severe signs/symptoms (chronic cough, shortness of breath, bibasilar crackles, rapid pulse)

DOMAIN: HEALTH-RELATED BEHAVIORS

Problem: Substance use (low priority: provide interventions and rate if Jerry is willing)

Problem Classification Scheme

Modifiers: Individual and Actual

SIGNS/SYMPTOMS OF ACTUAL

- smokes/uses tobacco products

Problem: Medication regimen (high priority)

Problem Classification Scheme

Modifiers: Individual and Actual

SIGNS/SYMPTOMS OF ACTUAL

- does not follow recommended dosage/schedule
- fails to obtain refills appropriately
- unable to take medications without help

Intervention Scheme

Category: Teaching, Guidance, and Counseling

TARGETS AND CLIENT-SPECIFIC INFORMATION

- medication action/side effects (all medications including inhalers)
- medication administration (proper method of using inhalers, need for refills)

Category: Surveillance

TARGETS AND CLIENT-SPECIFIC INFORMATION

- signs/symptoms—physical (effects of medications)

Problem Rating Scale for Outcomes

Knowledge: 1-no knowledge (did not know what/why about medications)
Behavior: 3-inconsistently appropriate behavior (did not use inhalers/get refills, took oral medications because of his wife)
Status: 2-severe signs/symptoms (hospitalizations, bibasilar crackles, rapid pulse, did not use inhalers)

Pete F.: Boy With a Recent Asthma Exacerbation

Loretta Conner, RN, BSN
Public Health Nurse
Marion County Health Department
Indianapolis, Indiana

Lisa Norquest, RN, BSN, MSN
Public Health Nurse
Marion County Health Department
Indianapolis, Indiana

Information Obtained During the First Visit/Encounter

The public health nurse, Lisa Lobe, visited the home of 9-year-old Pete Flow. He was diagnosed with asthma 4 months ago and had been released from the hospital recently following an asthma exacerbation. His physician, Dr. Al Buterol, requested a home visit because he was concerned about the home environment and medication management. Pete's mother, Sarah Vent, explained that he was feeling much better and was at school. She said he still had a cough and runny nose.

During the visit, the nurse observed aerosol cans and dust on the furniture and carpet; there was a roach trap on the floor, and a cat asleep on the couch. The nurse and Sarah talked about asthma triggers. Sarah had received much asthma material at the hospital and remembered hearing about triggers, but could not explain what they were. They discussed asthma, the need for timely and consistent health care, the relationship between asthma and growth, and Sarah's need to monitor his symptoms and treatment.

The nurse asked about Pete's medications. Sarah showed the nurse Pete's inhaler and the decongestant that he took regularly. He was discharged from the hospital with a prescription for prednisone, but Sarah was unclear about the tapered schedule and purpose. They reviewed details. Although Pete would like to be responsible for taking his own medicines, Sarah recognized that he was too young. "I think this is why he had problems and had to go to the hospital; I want him to be healthy and grow, not go to the hospital again. I guess I need to be around at the right times." Sarah left for work before Pete went to school and she was not home after school. Nurse Lobe offered to call Dr. Al Buterol during the visit to alter Pete's medication schedule so Sarah could be more involved. Sarah was pleased and said she appreciated the nurse's help.

Application of the Omaha System

DOMAIN: ENVIRONMENTAL

Problem: Sanitation (high priority)

Problem Classification Scheme

Modifiers: Family and Actual

SIGN/SYMPTOMS OF ACTUAL

- allergens
- infectious/contaminating agents

Intervention Scheme

Category: Teaching, Guidance, and Counseling

TARGETS AND CLIENT-SPECIFIC INFORMATION

- anatomy/physiology (potential impact of allergens on Pete)
- coping skills (needed to make difficult changes)

- environment (change to decrease Pete's symptoms and risk)

Category: Surveillance

TARGETS AND CLIENT-SPECIFIC INFORMATION

- environment (changes that Sarah makes)

Problem Rating Scale for Outcomes

Knowledge (Sarah): 2-minimal knowledge (received much information but limited understanding)

Behavior (Sarah): 2-rarely appropriate behavior (has not altered home or habits; indicated willingness)

Status: 2-severe signs/symptoms (multiple allergens present)

DOMAIN: PHYSIOLOGICAL

Problem: Respiration (high priority)

Problem Classification Scheme

Modifiers: Individual (Pete) and Actual

SIGNS/SYMPTOMS OF ACTUAL

- cough
- rhinorrhea/nasal congestion

Intervention Scheme

Category: Teaching, Guidance, and Counseling

TARGETS AND CLIENT-SPECIFIC INFORMATION

- anatomy/physiology (disease process)
- caretaking/parenting skills (Sarah's responsibilities)
- signs/symptoms—physical (triggers that alter breathing/coughing patterns)

Category: Surveillance

TARGETS AND CLIENT-SPECIFIC INFORMATION

- growth/development care (physical-mental activity/weight/height)
- signs/symptoms—physical (Sarah's observations and recall about Pete's status)

Problem Rating Scale for Outcomes

Knowledge (Sarah): 3-basic knowledge (accurate and inaccurate information)

Behavior: 3-inconsistently appropriate behavior (Pete told Sarah that he has been breathing regularly; she cannot confirm)

Status: 3-moderate signs/symptoms (Pete improved; only cough and runny nose)

DOMAIN: HEALTH-RELATED BEHAVIORS

Problem: Medication regimen (high priority)

Problem Classification Scheme

Modifiers: Individual (Pete) and Actual

SIGNS/SYMPTOMS OF ACTUAL

- does not follow recommended dosage/schedule
- inadequate system for taking medication
- unable to take medications without help

Intervention Scheme

Category: Teaching, Guidance, and Counseling

TARGETS AND CLIENT-SPECIFIC INFORMATION

- behavior modification (improve administration technique and regularity)
- caretaking/parenting skills (Sarah needed to supervise and encourage Pete)
- medical/dental care (importance of timely, consistent care)

Category: Case Management

TARGETS AND CLIENT-SPECIFIC INFORMATION

- medical/dental care (nurse and Sarah communicate with physician)

Category: Surveillance

TARGETS AND CLIENT-SPECIFIC INFORMATION

- coping skills (how Sarah and Pete are managing)
- medication action/side effects (observe and discuss)

Problem Rating Scale for Outcomes

Knowledge (Sarah): 2-minimal knowledge (has materials but needs to focus on the basics)

Behavior: 3-inconsistently appropriate behavior (questionable self administration technique and frequency)

Status: 3-moderate signs/symptoms (ineffective medication therapy resulted in hospitalization)

Sadiya M.: Woman With Active Tuberculosis

Luanne S. Crinion, RN, MS
Supervisor
Public Health Nursing, State of Maine
Augusta, Maine

Beth B. Patterson, RN, MN
Director
Public Health Nursing, State of Maine
Augusta, Maine

Information Obtained During the First Visit/Encounter

Sadiya M. was a 55-year-old woman who emigrated from Somalia 1 year ago with her daughter and other relatives. She was recently diagnosed with active pulmonary tuberculosis; she had a history of hypertension and congestive heart failure. The referral indicated that she was not taking her cardiac medications as prescribed.

The public health nurse wore a protective particulate air respirator to give Sadiya her first dose of oral medications as part of directly observed therapy (DOT). DOT is recommended as the standard protocol for active tuberculosis, and includes administration of isoniazid (INH), rifampin, pyrazinamide, and ethambutol. For at least the first 8 weeks, public health nurses visit clients 5 days a week and set up their four medications in a reminder box for the weekends.

Sadiya did not speak or understand English. In order for Sadiya and the nurse to converse, an interpreter joined the conversation by telephone. Sadiya had a productive cough during the visit; the nurse complimented her for appropriate tissue disposal and washing her hands. The nurse took Sadiya's vital signs and blood pressure, and listened to her lung sounds and recorded that they were within normal limits. They reviewed infection precaution guidelines, the risk to her family and close contacts, and why the nurse wore a respirator. The nurse described the sputum specimen that would be part of the next visit. Previously, Sadiya had received translated written information; she and the nurse reviewed this with the interpreter's assistance. The information described the disease, transmission, DOT treatment, potential toxic effects of the medications, medical care, and when to contact providers. The nurse also described the need to avoid alcohol and restrict social activity temporarily. Based on Sadiya's comments, the nurse questioned if she understood tuberculosis and the health care system in this country.

APPENDIX B

Sadiya showed the public health nurse the three medications prescribed for her congestive heart failure and hypertension. She shrugged her shoulders when asked about the pill schedule but agreed to take them as prescribed. She said she did not want to return to the primary care clinic but did not say why not. When the visit began, Sadiya had given the nurse a note from her daughter, indicating that the nurse could call her at work. The nurse called the daughter; they decided to meet during the next DOT appointment to review Sadiya's treatment plan. The nurse also wanted to determine if Sadiya took her cardiac medications as prescribed and if she could read.

Application of the Omaha System

DOMAIN: PSYCHOSOCIAL

Problem: Communication with community resources (high priority)

Problem Classification Scheme

Modifiers: Individual and Actual

SIGNS/SYMPTOMS OF ACTUAL

- difficulty understanding roles/regulation of services providers
- language barrier
- cultural barrier

Intervention Scheme

Category: Case Management

TARGETS AND CLIENT-SPECIFIC INFORMATION

- communication (scheduled appointment with daughter to check on Sadiya's coping with treatment regimen, and ability to read/understand materials)
- interpreter/translator services (scheduled/used interpreter by telephone)

Category: Surveillance

TARGETS AND CLIENT-SPECIFIC INFORMATION

- continuity of care (facilitate communication between Sadiya, family, interpreter, providers)

Problem Rating Scale for Outcomes

Knowledge: 3-basic knowledge (may not understand/be overwhelmed by health care system)

Behavior: 3-inconsistently appropriate behavior (needed nurse to arrange interpreter; does not want to return to primary care clinic)

Status: 3-moderate signs/symptoms (barriers for communication and obtaining services)

DOMAIN: PHYSIOLOGICAL

Problem: Communicable/infectious condition (high priority)

Problem Classification Scheme

Modifiers: Individual and Actual

SIGNS/SYMPTOMS OF ACTUAL

- infection
- positive screening/culture/laboratory results

Intervention Scheme

Category: Teaching, Guidance, and Counseling

TARGETS AND CLIENT-SPECIFIC INFORMATION

- anatomy/physiology (may not understanding although materials were in her language)
- infection precautions (disposal of tissues, hand washing; risk to family and others; nurse wore respirator)

- signs/symptoms—physical (cough/other symptoms of tuberculosis, when to contact providers)
- specimen collection (scheduled sputum specimen during next visit)

Category: Surveillance

TARGETS AND CLIENT-SPECIFIC INFORMATION

- signs/symptoms—physical (monitor cough, vital signs, blood pressure)

Problem Rating Scale for Outcomes

Knowledge: 2-minimal knowledge (seemed to know little about tuberculosis)
Behavior: 4-usually appropriate behavior (following respiratory precautions and beginning DOT)
Status: 2-severe signs/symptoms (productive cough)

DOMAIN: HEALTH-RELATED BEHAVIORS

Problem: Medication regimen (high priority)

Problem Classification Scheme

Modifiers: Individual and Actual

SIGNS/SYMPTOMS OF ACTUAL

- inadequate system for taking medication
- unable to take medications without help

Intervention Scheme

Category: Teaching, Guidance, and Counseling

TARGETS AND CLIENT-SPECIFIC INFORMATION

- medication actions/side effects (information about cardiac medication and DOT standard protocol, need to avoid alcohol)

Category: Treatment and Procedures

TARGETS AND CLIENT-SPECIFIC INFORMATION

- medication administration (DOT standard protocol)

Category: Case Management

TARGETS AND CLIENT-SPECIFIC INFORMATION

- interpreter/translator services (materials about disease, medications, DOT)

Category: Surveillance

TARGETS AND CLIENT-SPECIFIC INFORMATION

- medication administration (schedule, Sadiya's knowledge about cardiac medications)

Problem Rating Scale for Outcomes

Knowledge: 2-minimal knowledge (questionable understanding of medication management)
Behavior: 3-inconsistently appropriate behavior (home for visit and says she will be tomorrow, and willing to take medications)
Status: 3-moderate signs/symptoms (questionable cardiac medication therapy; needs DOT standard protocol)

APPENDIX B

Irma L.: Older Woman Needing Help With Bathing and Nutrition

Helin J. Eelsalu, RN, MD, MPH
Senior Lecturer
Tartu Medical School
Tartu, Estonia

Birgit K. Uiga, RN, BScN
Senior Lecturer
Tartu Medical School
Tartu, Estonia

Information Obtained During the First Visit/Encounter

Irma L., 78 years old, lived alone in a one-bedroom apartment. The home care nurse scheduled a visit because Irma asked to have a social care worker assist her with bathing and shampooing. Irma told the nurse that she did not have any relatives who could help. Recently, she stopped using the bathtub because she was afraid of falling. When they looked at the tub, the nurse agreed that the tub was high. They decided that the nurse would make arrangements for the nurse and social care worker to return together later in the week. They would determine if it was safe for Irma to use the tub and, if so, what type of assistance she needed. Irma was pleased with the plan.

The nurse weighed and measured Irma and noted that her weight was 160 pounds, her height was 5′4″, and her BMI was 27.0. Irma admitted that her mealtimes were irregular and that she loved candy. When Irma described her eating patterns, the nurse asked if she was willing to change the schedule and type of food she ate, and suggested that losing weight might help her step in and out of her bathtub. Irma said that she was willing, especially if she could use the tub. They identified gradual dietary changes that Irma agreed to make during the next 2 weeks. The nurse and Irma developed a calendar with a summary of her nutrition plan. When they discussed Irma's need to eat more vegetables and drink more water, Irma reported that she had occasional problems with constipation and took laxative tablets. Irma described more details and showed the bottle of tablets. The nurse told Irma that changing her diet should decrease her constipation and need for laxatives. They discussed the possibility of having a nutritionist visit, but decided to talk about that option during a later visit.

Application of the Omaha System

DOMAIN: PHYSIOLOGICAL

Problem: Bowel function (low priority: provide interventions and rate if needed; if Irma changed her diet, she should be less constipated)

Problem Classification Scheme

Modifiers: Individual and Actual

SIGNS/SYMPTOMS OF ACTUAL

- abnormal frequency/consistency of stool

DOMAIN: HEALTH-RELATED BEHAVIORS

Problem: Nutrition (high priority)

Problem Classification Scheme

Modifiers: Individual and Actual

SIGNS/SYMPTOMS OF ACTUAL

- overweight: adult BMI 25.0 or more; child BMI 95th percentile or more
- exceeds established standards for daily caloric/fluid intake
- unbalanced diet

Intervention Scheme

Category: Teaching, Guidance, and Counseling

TARGETS AND CLIENT-SPECIFIC INFORMATION

- dietary management (increase vegetables and water, decrease candy, and change schedule to improve nutrition and decrease weight)

Category: Surveillance

TARGETS AND CLIENT-SPECIFIC INFORMATION

- signs/symptoms—physical (weight, height, BMI)

Problem Rating Scale for Outcomes

Knowledge: 3-basic knowledge (acknowledged need to change habits)
Behavior: 3-inconsistently appropriate behavior (some nutritious foods, many others)
Status: 3-moderate signs/symptoms (weight, height, BMI)

Problem: Personal care (high priority)

Problem Classification Scheme

Modifiers: Individual and Actual

SIGNS/SYMPTOMS OF ACTUAL

- difficulty with bathing
- difficulty shampooing/combing hair

Intervention Scheme

Category: Teaching, Guidance, and Counseling

TARGETS AND CLIENT-SPECIFIC INFORMATION

- personal hygiene (requested help with bathing and shampooing)

Category: Case Management

TARGETS AND CLIENT-SPECIFIC INFORMATION

- paraprofessional/aide care (schedule social care worker)

Category: Surveillance

TARGETS AND CLIENT-SPECIFIC INFORMATION

- mobility/transfers (height of bathtub in comparison to Irma's agility)

Problem Rating Scale for Outcomes

Knowledge: 4-adequate knowledge (requested help)
Behavior: 4-usually appropriate behavior (stopped trying to use tub for safety reasons)
Status: 3-moderate signs/symptoms (bathing without using bathtub)

APPENDIX B

Compliance Checks: Strategies To Decrease Tobacco Sales to Teens in the Community

Patricia Galligher, RD, MPH, LN
Senior Community Health Specialist
Washington County Department of Public Health and Environment
Stillwater, Minnesota

Minnesota Omaha System Users Group

Information Obtained During a Project/Incident

Studies have shown that if teens do not smoke by the time they are 18 years old, they are much less likely to begin. Legislation and ordinances have been passed to support a population-focused approach to such research. It is illegal for teens who are less than 18 years of age to possess or use tobacco products in Minnesota or buy tobacco or tobacco products in Washington County. It is the responsibility of the health department to educate businesses about the county ordinance and enforce it; the businesses are the client for this case study.

The health department provided an educational program for businesses and law enforcement officers. The department also sent letters to 24 businesses explaining the new procedures, and enclosed a copy of the county ordinance and a notice about a public hearing. A community health specialist inspected the businesses for compliance. Some objected to sections of the ordinance. The ordinance was amended and officially adopted following the public hearing. A license renewal form was sent to the businesses. The health department began to perform compliance checks every 6 months.

- An underage teen trained to purchase tobacco was sent into a business.
- A community health specialist accompanied the underage teen and waited outside during the attempt.
- If a purchase was not made, the community health specialist entered the store immediately with a commendation letter to the business and spoke with the clerk.
- If a purchase was made, the community health specialist entered the store immediately with a notice of violation to the business and the clerk.

APPENDIX B

The problem *Substance use* was modified as *Individual* when data were collected about each business, and as *Community* when data were aggregated to analyze the community impact of the program. *Substance use* was also modified as *Potential* for businesses that passed compliance checks, and as *Actual* when businesses did not pass. The following case study describes a typical failed compliance check. That example and the results of the data analysis are described below.

A teen entered a business and attempted to purchase cigarettes. The clerk, who was also the store owner, thought the teen looked old enough to buy cigarettes and asked the teen's age, but did not check identification. When the teen exited the store with cigarettes, the community health specialist immediately entered and gave the clerk and business a notice of failure. This was the business's third violation within 24 months. The owner of the business appeared before the county's appeal board to explain his case and appeal his fine and suspension. He stated that he supported the youth access ordinance and did not think underage teens should be able to buy tobacco products.

He was not denying that he made an illegal sale, but that the fine was too high for his small business. He promised to check identification in the future. The fine was reduced.

Data for the 24 businesses that each had two consecutive compliance checks in 6 months were analyzed. Paired samples *t*-test of *Knowledge, Behavior,* and *Status* ratings showed significant improvement in mean *Knowledge* (3.0 before to 3.79 after, p = 0.036), improvements in mean *Behavior* (3.67 before to 4.67 after, p = 0.056), and mean *Status* (4.67 before to 4.92 after, p = 0.056) approached significance.

Application of the Omaha System

(Problem Classification and Intervention Scheme answers reflect a business that failed a compliance check; Problem Rating Scale for Outcomes answers reflect aggregate county data.)

DOMAIN: HEALTH-RELATED BEHAVIORS

Problem: Substance use (high priority)

Problem Classification Scheme

Modifiers: Community and Actual

SIGNS/SYMPTOMS OF ACTUAL

- buys/sells illegal substances

Intervention Scheme

Category: Teaching, Guidance, and Counseling

TARGETS AND CLIENT-SPECIFIC INFORMATION

- legal system (about ordinance and enforcement)
- substance use cessation (about youth access and addiction to tobacco)

Category: Case Management

TARGETS AND CLIENT-SPECIFIC INFORMATION

- continuity of care (collaboration with law enforcement groups to establish a compliance plan)
- legal system (collaboration with businesses, county attorneys, and the county board to create and approve the ordinance)

Category: Surveillance

TARGETS AND CLIENT-SPECIFIC INFORMATION

- substance use cessation (compliance checks to see if businesses are selling tobacco)

Problem Rating Scale for Outcomes

Knowledge: 3-basic knowledge (*t*-test was 3.0 before to 3.79 after, p = 0.036; many knew about the ordinance and that they would be fined if they sold to a minor; most supported the ordinance, even some who were fined in the past)

Behavior: 3-inconsistently appropriate behavior (*t*-test was 3.67 before to 4.67 after, p = 0.056; some sold to minors, some asked age, but not identification)

Status: 4-minimal signs/symptoms (*t*-test was 4.67 before to 4.92 after, p = 0.056; few were out of compliance, especially by the second check)

APPENDIX B

Rocky S.: Older Man With Diabetes

Nancy A. Gamache, RN
Staff Nurse
LakeWood Nursing Service
Baudette, Minnesota

Information Obtained during the First Visit/Encounter

Rocky S., age 78, was referred to home care following a 24-hour hospital stay for hypoglycemia. He returned from a day of fishing with his friends, was tired, and took a nap. When his wife, age 75, was unable to rouse him, she called the ambulance, and he was transported to the hospital. The ambulance crew reported that his blood sugar was 36 mg/dL. He responded to glucose quickly. The home care referral listed Rocky's diagnosis as non–insulin dependent diabetes, his medications as glipizide (Glucotrol) 10 mg twice a day 30 minutes before meals and pioglitazone hydrochloride (Actos) 15 mg daily, and a request to organize the medications. During the visit, the nurse concluded that Mrs. S. understood her husband's disease and medications, even though she had macular degeneration and rheumatoid arthritis. The couple continually "picked" at each other. Mrs. S. said that she would not think of touching her husband's medications, and Rocky made it clear that he did not want her to touch them either.

Rocky was willing to let the nurse see his bag of medications. Rocky could read the labels, but knew little else. He did not know why or when he should take medications, and told the nurse that he "never took his diabetes very seriously, but got 'a good scare' recently." Rocky admitted that it was time to learn more about his diabetes and pills. He grudgingly agreed that the nurse could take those pill bottles that were long outdated and no longer prescribed. They used an egg carton to arrange his pills until the next visit, when the nurse would bring a pill organizer. The nurse provided basic information about diabetes and oral hypoglycemics, and asked if he would read materials. He laughed and said he would; previously he threw it away.

The nurse documented Rocky's current physical findings: height, 5′ 7″; weight, 190 pounds; blood pressure, 140/86; pulse, 84 and regular; respirations, 20; and lungs, clear. The nurse used the agency's glucometer, noted that his blood sugar was 260 mg/dL, and expressed concern. When Rocky said he had not taken any medications yet today, they decided which medications he would take now and which later, and which diabetic symptoms to note. Rocky said he did not have a glucometer; Mrs. S. confirmed that report. The nurse agreed to order one to use during the next visit.

The nurse explained that while medications were very important, Rocky also needed to manage and monitor his diet, exercise, blood sugar, and other aspects of his life. His typical daily schedule was to drive to the restaurant for coffee and two donuts, return home about noon, watch television while snacking on nuts and sweets, and doze in his recliner. Their evening meal usually consisted of fried or roasted meat, boiled or fried potatoes, and sometimes a vegetable or a dessert. In the evening, he and Mrs. S. watched television, or he drank a beer with his friends. During pleasant weather, he mowed their lawn with a riding lawn mower and fished. The nurse asked Rocky what he was willing to change to decrease his risk of more trips to the hospital and other serious problems. He said he would start on food because he was already spending time outdoors. The nurse said that their evening meal was quite healthy and asked if he could replace the donuts at the restaurant. Rocky agreed to try eating a scrambled egg and a piece of white toast with a small amount of butter. The nurse suggested that they continue their discussion about food and his glucometer next week and ask Mrs. S. to help, knowing that Mrs. S had listened to the entire conversation. For the second time, he grudgingly agreed.

Application of the Omaha System

DOMAIN: HEALTH-RELATED BEHAVIORS

Problem: Nutrition (high priority)

Problem Classification Scheme

Modifiers: Individual and Actual

SIGNS/SYMPTOMS OF ACTUAL

- overweight: adult BMI 25.0 or more; child BMI 95th percentile or more
- exceeds established standards for daily caloric/fluid intake
- unbalanced diet
- does not follow recommended nutrition plan
- hypoglycemia
- hyperglycemia

Intervention Scheme

Category: Teaching, Guidance, and Counseling

TARGETS AND CLIENT-SPECIFIC INFORMATION

- behavior modification (start dietary changes with breakfast)
- dietary management (diet guidelines for diabetes; control versus likely future events)
- laboratory findings (interpretation of today's and previous blood sugars)

Category: Treatments and Procedures

TARGETS AND CLIENT-SPECIFIC INFORMATION

- specimen collection (glucose test)

Category: Case Management

TARGETS AND CLIENT-SPECIFIC INFORMATION

- durable medical equipment (ordered glucometer)

Category: Surveillance

TARGETS AND CLIENT-SPECIFIC INFORMATION

- dietary management (diet history completed)
- signs/symptoms—physical (blood sugar, weight [Rocky's BMI=30.0], height, vital signs, blood pressure, lung sounds)

Problem Rating Scale for Outcomes

Knowledge: 1-no knowledge (no recall of previous diet instructions; threw away materials)

Behavior: 2-rarely appropriate behavior (poor eating habits, except for evening meal; not testing blood sugar)

Status: 2-severe signs/symptoms (low blood sugar prompted hospitalization, high today)

Problem: Physical activity (low priority: provide interventions and rate as soon as Rocky is willing)

Problem Classification Scheme

Modifiers: Individual and Actual

SIGNS/SYMPTOMS OF ACTUAL

- sedentary life style
- inadequate/inconsistent exercise routine
- inappropriate type/amount of exercise for age/physical condition

Problem: Medication regimen (high priority)

Modifiers: Individual and Actual

SIGNS/SYMPTOMS OF ACTUAL

- does not follow recommended dosage/schedule
- evidence of side effects/adverse reactions
- inadequate system for taking medication

Intervention Scheme

Category: Teaching, Guidance, and Counseling

TARGETS AND CLIENT-SPECIFIC INFORMATION

- medication action/side effects (initiated instruction and gave materials)
- medication administration (take pills accurately and consistently)

Category: Treatments and Procedures

TARGETS AND CLIENT-SPECIFIC INFORMATION

- medication set-up (used egg carton to set up pills)

Category: Case Management

TARGETS AND CLIENT-SPECIFIC INFORMATION

- durable medical equipment (ordered pill organizer)

Category: Surveillance

TARGETS AND CLIENT-SPECIFIC INFORMATION

- medication action/side effects (Rocky poorly informed; Mrs. S. well informed but does not participate)
- medication set-up (Rocky-determined to be independent in past; sorted through bag of medications and disposed as needed)

Problem Rating Scale for Outcomes

Knowledge: 2-minimal knowledge (knew schedule but not what medications or when)

Behavior: 2-rarely appropriate behavior (no medication system/schedule)

Status: 2-severe signs/symptoms (very low blood glucose required hospitalization, elevated results today)

Michael O.: Teen With Diabetes

Andrea E. Johnson, RN, BSN, MA
Licensed School Nurse
New Spirit Schools
St. Paul, Minnesota

Information Obtained During the School Year

Michael O., age 16, was diagnosed with insulin-dependent diabetes mellitus a year ago. This case study reflects his progress during that year. Michael's mother, a single parent, worked full time as a nurse's aide.

Michael often skipped eating breakfast at home and then walked about a mile to school. Sometimes, he purchased breakfast in the school cafeteria where he also ate lunch. Although he tried to eat well, he admitted to eating some sweets and junk food. Michael wore an insulin pump. His glucometer, insulin, snacks, and glucagon were stored in the school health office. Every day before lunch, he went to the school health office to check his blood sugar, and gave himself a bolus of insulin, based on an established sliding scale. Several times a week but with decreasing frequency and severity, Michael needed to leave class because he felt shaky or dizzy. He went to the health office, checked his blood sugar, ate a snack, rested, and returned to class. Often the school nurse was not in the office. On other occasions, the nurse checked his vital signs, blood pressure, weight, height, and skin.

Michael and the school nurse talked frequently about diabetes, the effect of dietary and medication management on his concentration and school work, participation in exercise and sports, and his future. The school nurse and Michael's mother communicated by telephone or e-mail weekly or several times a month about the same topics, and met several times during the school year. The nurse sent reports to Michael's diabetes specialist physician, who he visited quarterly, and to the neighborhood family practice doctor, who knew his family well. The nurse received reports from both offices. Michael did not miss the appointments with either physician.

APPENDIX B

One of the meetings occurred when Michael, his mother, and the nurse updated his health plan. His mother and the nurse congratulated Michael for his progress and the responsibility he had assumed for managing his diabetes. They discussed the *Nutrition* and *Medication regimen* problems, interventions, and ratings on the care plan. Specifically, they reviewed the initial *Knowledge, Behavior,* and *Status* ratings and established new, interim ratings. Based on the new ratings, they considered ways that they could work together. First, Michael agreed to change his breakfast habits by selecting some breakfast food the night before, set the alarm to ring 10 minutes earlier, and not get upset if his mother left notes or called to remind him to eat before leaving for school. Second, because Michael admitted that he did not always administer the bolus of insulin correctly, they developed a 1-month plan. Michael would try to be more accurate, and record the glucometer reading and the amount of the bolus on a log. The school nurse and Michael planned to meet briefly each Thursday in the health office and review his blood sugar reading before he added the insulin; his mother agreed to do the same on either Saturday or Sunday. At the end of the month, they would determine if the number of times he became shaky or dizzy had decreased. After the meeting, the nurse visited Michael's teachers and coaches to discuss the revised plan, and remind them about Michael's supplies in the health office, and his diabetes emergency care plan. A team meeting was scheduled for a future date.

Application of the Omaha System

(Answers reflect current rather than initial problems and interventions; both initial and current ratings are listed.)

DOMAIN: HEALTH-RELATED BEHAVIORS

Problem: Nutrition (high priority)

Problem Classification Scheme

Modifiers: Individual and Actual

SIGNS/SYMPTOMS OF ACTUAL

- does not follow recommended nutrition plan
- hypoglycemia
- hyperglycemia

Intervention Scheme

Category: Teaching, Guidance, and Counseling

TARGETS AND CLIENT-SPECIFIC INFORMATION

- anatomy/physiology (disease process)
- behavior modification (change certain habits, especially breakfast)
- dietary management (reviewed foods patterns that created symptoms/interfered with learning)
- signs/symptoms—physical (responses to hypo/hyperglycemia, vital signs, weight, height, skin)

Category: Case Management

TARGETS AND CLIENT-SPECIFIC INFORMATION

- continuity of care (met with Michael and his mother to update the health and emergency plans and with his teachers and coaches; communicated regularly with 2 doctors)

Category: Surveillance

TARGETS AND CLIENT-SPECIFIC INFORMATION

- continuity of care (communicate with Michael, mother, doctors, school personnel)
- dietary management (improve choices/patterns, especially breakfast)
- signs/symptoms—physical (frequency of hypo/hyperglycemia, vital signs, weight, height, skin)

Problem Rating Scale for Outcomes

***Initial* Knowledge:** 1-no knowledge (not informed about relationship of diet to blood sugar and ability to concentrate)

***Initial* Behavior:** 2-rarely appropriate behavior (did not select correct foods or schedule; mother purchases/prepares healthy foods)

APPENDIX B

***Initial* Status:** 1-extreme signs/symptoms (blood sugar levels were outside the normal range almost daily)
***Current* Knowledge:** 4-adequate knowledge (understood medication management and relationship of diet to blood sugar and ability to concentrate)
***Current* Behavior:** 3-inconsistently appropriate behavior (reasonable diet at home, did not select correct foods or schedule consistently, especially at school)
***Current* Status:** 3-moderate signs/symptoms (blood sugars were outside the normal range less often, now averaging once a week)

Problem: Medication regimen (high priority)

Problem Classification Scheme

Modifiers: Individual and Actual

SIGNS/SYMPTOMS OF ACTUAL

- does not follow recommended dosage/schedule
- evidence of side effects/adverse reactions

Intervention Scheme

Category: Teaching, Guidance, and Counseling

TARGETS AND CLIENT-SPECIFIC INFORMATION

- medication administration (use pump and add insulin accurately based on blood sugar)

Category: Surveillance

TARGETS AND CLIENT-SPECIFIC INFORMATION

- medication administration (accurate and consistent use of pump and insulin)

Problem Rating Scale for Outcomes

***Initial* Knowledge:** 1-no knowledge (new diagnosis that required detailed information to use pump correctly)
***Initial* Behavior:** 1-rarely appropriate behavior (struggled to use pump accurately/consistently)
***Initial* Status:** 1-extreme signs/symptoms (blood sugars were outside the normal range almost daily)
***Current* Knowledge:** 4-adequate knowledge (understood medication management and pump)
***Current* Behavior:** 3-inconsistently appropriate behavior (made progress but not using pump accurately/consistently)
***Current* Status:** 3-moderate signs/symptoms (decreasing severity of hypo/hyperglycemia)

West Nile Virus Outbreak: Reduce Disease Transmission in a Community

Linda Olson Keller, RN, CS, MS
Coordinator, Center for Public Health Nursing
Minnesota Department of Public Health
St. Paul, Minnesota

Minnesota Omaha System Users Group

Information Obtained During a Project/Incident

West Nile Virus is transmitted to people through the bite of an infected mosquito. Because there is no treatment, prevention is essential. Bloom County, population 120,000, became the client of this case study. The county's environmental engineers, public health nurses, and other epidemiology staff worked diligently with state health department officials. The health department launched an aggressive community education campaign with the help of the media, pharmacists, physicians, health care facilities, stores, churches, and other community groups. Fliers and announcements described the urgency of residents using personal protection measures, such as the use of mosquito repellents, avoiding outdoor exposure at dusk and dawn, and wearing long-sleeved shirts and long pants.

A door-to-door campaign was conducted to identify and eradicate potential breeding sites and to notify homeowners about the spraying schedule. Residents were urged to remove water-holding containers such as buckets, tires, and swimming pool covers and to clean gutters. Horse owners and veterinarians were encouraged to vaccinate horses. The public was asked to follow specific steps to report and deliver dead blue jays and crows to the local health department so the virus could be diagnosed and mosquito-infected areas sprayed. Despite the aggressive efforts, many residents did not heed warnings; they believed that they and their families would not contract the virus. When the first person who developed encephalitis died, the public began to panic. Worried residents with real and imagined symptoms began to crowd local clinics and emergency departments. Bloom County experienced 113 cases of West Nile Virus and 6 deaths. One third of the horses that developed the virus died or had to be killed.

Application of the Omaha System

(Answers reflect information at the beginning of the incident.)

DOMAIN: ENVIRONMENTAL

Problem: Neighborhood/workplace safety (high priority)

Problem Classification Scheme

Modifiers: Community and Actual

SIGNS/SYMPTOMS OF ACTUAL

- uncontrolled/dangerous/infected animals

Intervention Scheme

Category: Teaching, Guidance, and Counseling

Targets and Client-specific Information

- environment (distributed guidelines to reduce mosquito population)

Category: Case Management

Targets and Client-specific Information

- communication (health department organized widely supported media campaign)
- infection precautions (areas sprayed, residents asked to deliver dead birds)
- medical/dental care (shared information with physicians about diagnosis and treatment of human cases and horse owners and veterinarians about vaccinating horses)

Category: Surveillance

Targets and Client-specific Information

- environment (conducted public and door-to-door efforts)
- specimen collection (asked public to deliver dead birds)

Problem Rating Scale for Outcomes

Knowledge: 3-basic knowledge (most knew about risks and needed modifications but viewed risks impersonally)

Behavior: 3-inconsistently appropriate behavior (did not follow needed modifications)

Status: 2-severe signs/symptoms (increasing number of infected people/animals)

DOMAIN: PHYSIOLOGICAL

Problem: Communicable/infectious condition (high priority)

Problem Classification Scheme

Modifiers: Community and Actual

Signs/Symptoms of Actual

- infection
- fever
- positive screening/culture/laboratory results
- does not follow infection control regimen

APPENDIX B

Intervention Scheme

Category: Teaching, Guidance, and Counseling

Targets and Client-specific Information

- behavior modification (needed changes)
- communication (publicized prevention information repeatedly)
- infection precautions (effective preventive measures and actions)

Category: Surveillance

Targets and Client-specific Information

- infection precautions (monitor adherence, track reports of cases and deaths)

Problem Rating Scale for Outcomes

Knowledge: 3-basic knowledge (most residents were aware of risk and needed actions; some did not personalize risk while others were overly concerned)

Behavior: 3-inconsistently appropriate behavior (many residents did not follow warnings initially and later crowded emergency health care facilities)

Status: 2-severe signs/symptoms (many infections/deaths; monitored statistics)

Adam C.: Older Man Admitted to Long-term Care Facility Because of a Stroke

Beverly M. King, RN, BScN, MS
Clinical Nurse Educator
Baycrest Centre for Geriatric Care
Toronto, Ontario, Canada

Gilda Waltman, BScOT, OT Reg (Ont)
Clinical Occupational Therapist
Baycrest Centre for Geriatric Care
Toronto, Ontario, Canada

Information Obtained During the First Visit/Encounter

Adam C., age 72, was admitted to the continuing complex care unit a week ago. His wife visited when she could. Three years ago, Adam had a left-sided stroke followed by right hemiplegia and aphasia; he had no further strokes.The clinical team scheduled a meeting to review Adam's care and consider strategies to ease his transition. The unit staff reported that he was oriented but became easily agitated and depressed when his environment changed or he experienced disruptions in his routine and threw objects. His behavior was described as disruptive and erratic. About a year ago, Adam was evaluated by a psychologist; the report indicated that he was able to learn, but was very impulsive and mildly perseverative in that he repeated familiar words or phrases. The team identified ways unit staff could minimize changes in Adam's environment, help increase his comfort level, and alert staff to protect themselves from injury. A nurse who was a team member had developed the most rapport with Adam and volunteered to serve as his primary care provider and work on strategies with him and his wife. The team initiated the referral process for another psychological evaluation and planned to revise their strategies.

Adam communicated effectively using single words or short phrases and a communication board. Unit staff reported that his vital signs were stable and that he had no physical changes since admission. He required care for toileting, bathing/skin care, and dressing; was transferred in and out of his wheelchair with a mechanical lifter; and spent most of his time in the wheelchair. He used a closed-cell cushion in his wheelchair for pressure relief, and a tray to support his right arm. He had no history of pressure ulcers. Adam wore splints on his right wrist and ankle to reduce deformities. His care and range-of-motion exercises progressed safely as long as staff provided adequate reminders to him. The team suggested that the primary nurse observe others when they provided care and identify any needed changes, especially if those changes could reduce his disruptive behavior.

Application of the Omaha System

(Answers reflect multidisciplinary care and information available during the first team meeting.)

DOMAIN: PSYCHOSOCIAL

Problem: Mental health (high priority)

Problem Classification Scheme

Modifiers: Individual and Actual

SIGNS/SYMPTOMS OF ACTUAL

- irritable/agitated/aggressive
- purposeless/compulsive activity
- difficulty managing stress
- mood swings

Intervention Scheme

Category: Teaching, Guidance, and Counseling

TARGETS AND CLIENT-SPECIFIC INFORMATION

- anger management (decrease triggers, use control techniques, involve wife)
- coping skills (increase Adam's comfort in his new residence)

Category: Case Management

TARGETS AND CLIENT-SPECIFIC INFORMATION

- medical/dental care (referred to psychologist)
- nursing care (primary nurse to work on behavior, supervise rest of care)

Category: Surveillance

TARGETS AND CLIENT-SPECIFIC INFORMATION

- signs/symptoms—mental/emotional (frequency/severity of behavior, throws objects)

Problem Rating Scale for Outcomes

Knowledge: 2-minimal knowledge (did not acknowledge need to change behavior)
Behavior: 2-rarely appropriate behavior (became agitated, disruptive; threw objects)
Status: 2-severe signs/symptoms (many incidents during past week)

DOMAIN: PHYSIOLOGICAL

Problem: Speech and language (low priority: provide interventions and rate if Adam needs additional assistance with communication)

Problem Classification Scheme

Modifiers: Individual and Actual

SIGNS/SYMPTOMS OF ACTUAL

- absent/abnormal ability to speak/vocalize
- limited enunciation/clarity
- inappropriate word usage

Problem: Neuro-musculo-skeletal function (high priority)

Problem Classification Scheme

Modifiers: Individual and Actual

SIGNS/SYMPTOMS OF ACTUAL

- limited range of motion
- decreased muscle strength
- decreased muscle tone
- gait/ambulation disturbance
- difficulty transferring

Intervention Scheme

Category: Teaching, Guidance, and Counseling

Targets and Client-specific Information

- exercises (regular reminders to do active range of motion)
- positioning (regular reminders to change positions, use cushion, tray, splints)
- safety (with care, transfers)

Category: Surveillance

Targets and Client-specific Information

- safety (use of lift, wheelchair, on premises and when leaves premises)
- signs/symptoms—physical (vital signs, blood pressure, pain, skin)

Problem Rating Scale for Outcomes

Knowledge: 3-basic knowledge (usually knew correct steps to transfer/use wheelchair, needed reminders for position changes/range of motion)

Behavior: 3-inconsistently appropriate behavior (usually cooperated but did not initiate position changes or active range of motion)

Status: 3-moderate signs/symptoms (residual from stroke, skin intact, transferred safely)

Problem: Circulation (low priority: provide interventions and rate problem if status changes)

Problem Classification Scheme

Modifiers: Individual and Potential

Risk Factors (left-sided stroke 3 years ago; blood pressure stable since then)

DOMAIN: HEALTH-RELATED BEHAVIORS

Problem: Personal care (high priority)

Problem Classification Scheme

Modifiers: Individual and Actual

Signs/Symptoms of Actual

- difficulty with bathing
- difficulty with toileting activities
- difficulty dressing lower body
- difficulty dressing upper body
- difficulty shampooing/combing hair

Intervention Scheme

Category: Treatments and Procedures

Targets and Client-specific Information

- paraprofessional/aide care (health care aides provide daily care)

Category: Surveillance

Targets and Client-specific Information

- paraprofessional/aide care (minimize risks from thrown objects)
- signs/symptoms—mental/emotional (agitation/behavior changes)
- signs/symptoms—physical (evidence of good health/illness/injury)

Problem Rating Scale for Outcomes

Knowledge: 3-basic knowledge (aware of need for assistance if routine consistent)
Behavior: 3-inconsistently appropriate behavior (cooperated unless routine changed)
Status: 3-moderate signs/symptoms (hemiplegia; required consistent assistance)

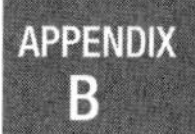

Mabel G.: Older Woman With a Chronic Cardiac Condition

Maureen E. Leonardo, RN, CRNP, BC, MN
Associate Professor, School of Nursing
Duquesne University
Pittsburgh, Pennsylvania

Lenore K. Resick, RN, CRNP, BC, MSN
Associate Professor, School of Nursing
Duquesne University
Pittsburgh, Pennsylvania

Information Obtained During an Interim Visit/Encounter

Mabel G. was a 73-year-old widow who routinely visited the nurse-managed wellness center to monitor her blood pressure, manage her severe degenerative joint disease of the knees, and discuss her 1200-calorie, low-sodium diet. Mabel was 4′9″ tall and weighed 168 pounds. She participated in the wellness center's weight loss program and lost approximately 40 pounds during the last 18 months. She had chronic venous insufficiency, which she managed by restricting her sodium intake, using compression, and administering consistent skin care. Mabel ambulated approximately 40 feet with her walker in her apartment. Otherwise she used a scooter.

During a recent visit, Mabel complained of extreme fatigue and trouble sleeping the last 2 nights because of "coughing and some shortness of breath." She could not put on her antiembolism (TED) hose that she wore "except when it is hot outside." Vital signs revealed a weight gain of 5 pounds, an increase in systolic blood pressure of 20 mm Hg, and tachycardia. Her skin was warm and clammy. She had dyspnea, coarse crackles to one-half of posterior lung fields, an S_3, and bilateral 2+ pitting edema to mid-calf.

Mabel reported that she saw her primary care provider for a "cough and cold" about 2 weeks ago and was given fexofenadine (Allegra) and omeprazole (Prilosec) for allergic rhinitis and gastroesophageal reflux. She visited friends and ate a bag of potato chips, two pieces of pizza, and diet soda—foods that she usually avoided. The nurse practitioner and Mabel discussed her signs and symptoms and decided she needed to see by her primary care provider that day. The nurse helped apply her TED hose, reviewed ways to relieve edema, including leg elevation, and reiterated the importance of a low sodium diet and rest. The nurse assisted her to contact her family and physician and arranged immediate transportation.

Application of the Omaha System

DOMAIN: PHYSIOLOGICAL

Problem: Circulation (high priority)

Problem Classification Scheme

Modifiers: Individual and Actual

SIGNS/SYMPTOMS OF ACTUAL

- edema
- abnormal blood pressure reading
- excessively rapid heart rate
- abnormal heart sounds/murmurs

Intervention Scheme

Category: Teaching, Guidance, and Counseling

Targets and Client-specific Information

- cardiac care (relief of edema, pacing rest/activity)
- signs/symptoms—physical (about condition, vital signs, when to notify physician; see Nutrition for weight)

Category: Treatments and Procedures

Targets and Client-specific Information

- cardiac care (applied TED hose)

Category: Case Management

Targets and Client-specific Information

- medical/dental care (helped make an appointment)
- transportation (arranged immediate transportation)

Category: Surveillance

Targets and Client-specific Information

- signs/symptoms—physical (status, edema, shortness of breath; see Nutrition for weight)

Problem Rating Scale for Outcomes

Knowledge: 3-basic knowledge (knew effect of sodium intake on fluid retention, recognized worsening condition)
Behavior: 3-inconsistently appropriate behavior (did not wear TED hose consistently)
Status: 1-extreme signs/symptoms (pitting edema of feet, ankles, and lower extremities, elevated blood pressure, crackles, S_3, tachycardia, and dyspnea)

DOMAIN: HEALTH-RELATED BEHAVIORS

Problem: Nutrition (high priority)

Problem Classification Scheme

Modifiers: Individual and Actual

Signs/Symptoms of Actual

- overweight: adult BMI 25.0 or more; child BMI 95th percentile or more
- exceeds established standards for daily caloric/fluid intake
- does not follow recommended nutrition plan

Intervention Scheme

Category: Teaching, Guidance, and Counseling

Targets and Client-specific Information

- dietary management (repeated sodium restriction details; praised continuing weight loss)

Category: Surveillance

Targets and Client-specific Information

- signs/symptoms—physical (weight)

Problem Rating Scale for Outcomes

Knowledge: 3-basic knowledge (knew effect of sodium intake on fluid retention)
Behavior: 4-usually appropriate behavior (only followed diet plan when home)
Status: 3-moderate signs/symptoms (significant fluid retention; lost 40 pounds in last 18 months but still overweight)

APPENDIX B

Maria G.: Older Woman Injured in an Auto Accident

Kathi Nelson, RN, BSN
Administrator
Hancock County Public Health Services
Garner, Iowa

Information Obtained During the First Visit/Encounter

Maria G., a 78-year-old woman, recently moved to a small rural town with her daughter and her daughter's family. Beginning this week, Maria was alone in the home from 5:00 AM until 4:00 PM while the family members were at work about 30 miles away.

Maria's grandson met with Maria and the home care nurse during the first visit. The grandson was fluent in Spanish and English. The nurse spoke and read English and had minimal Spanish skills. Maria spoke Spanish and did not understand or speak English. The grandson explained that Maria's mobility was limited and she had contractures as a result of injures sustained in an auto accident about 5 years ago. She required assistance with bathing, dressing, transferring, and toileting. Maria wore supportive walking shoes, and could ambulate about 20 feet with her walker, which was in good condition. She did not have a history of falls. She fed herself if a meal was placed before her.

Before the family moved, Maria's daughter stayed home and cared for her; now she was employed. The grandson smiled and told the nurse that Maria said she did not know why her daughter started working, rather than stay home with her, and she could not understand many things in this country. The family was happy to have Maria living with them, but was overwhelmed by her needs, fearful for her safety during their daily absence, and uninformed about available services.

The nurse and grandson toured the home. The nurse complimented the grandson that the doorways and walkways accommodated Maria's walker, a commode was located beside her bed, a bathroom adjoined her bedroom, and no throw rugs were on the floor. He said his mother would appreciate the compliment. The nurse suggested that a toilet riser, toilet bars, and bathroom grab bars would increase bathroom safety, and provided details about obtaining them. The nurse asked if Maria used the telephone. He replied that she would not initiate calls and would not answer the phone when it rang. They discussed a personal alert/alarm system; he thought she would be willing to use it.

The nurse took Maria's vital signs and blood pressure, and listened to her lung sounds; all were within normal limits. The nurse also completed a limited physical assessment, noting evidence of healed fractures and contractures, and provided various suggestions. For Maria to maintain her current mobility and intact skin, she needed to change position regularly, complete active range of motion exercises, and have family members perform other exercises. Options were available for daytime care including several day care/respite programs, one of which had a staff member who spoke Spanish. Home health aide services could be scheduled several times a week for personal care. The grandson said his mother had to participate in the plans; he called her at work and they scheduled another visit with the nurse for the next day.

Application of the Omaha System

DOMAIN: PSYCHOSOCIAL

Problem: Communication with community resources (high priority)

Problem Classification Scheme

Modifiers: Family and Actual

SIGNS/SYMPTOMS OF ACTUAL

- unfamiliar with options/procedures for obtaining services
- difficulty understanding roles/regulations of service providers
- language barrier
- cultural barrier
- unable to use/has inadequate communication devices/equipment

Intervention Scheme

Category: Teaching, Guidance, and Counseling

TARGETS AND CLIENT-SPECIFIC INFORMATION

- day care/respite (several options; one has a Spanish-speaking staff member)
- durable medical equipment (may use personal alert/alarm system; will not use phone)

Problem Rating Scale for Outcomes

Knowledge: 2-minimal knowledge (knew little about local services)
Behavior: 4-usually appropriate behavior (called public health; indicated intent to use services)
Status: 3-moderate signs/symptoms (needs are complex, difficult to obtain appropriate services)

Problem: Caretaking/parenting (high priority)

Problem Classification Scheme

Modifiers: Family and Actual

SIGNS/SYMPTOMS OF ACTUAL

- difficulty providing physical care/safety
- difficulty providing preventive and therapeutic health care

Intervention Scheme

Category: Teaching, Guidance, and Counseling

TARGETS AND CLIENT-SPECIFIC INFORMATION

- paraprofessional/aide care (provide personal care several times a week)

Problem Rating Scale for Outcomes

Knowledge: 3-basic knowledge (understands physical/social care needs)
Behavior: 2-rarely appropriate behavior (adequate care when home, but Maria alone during day)
Status: 3-moderate signs/symptoms (overwhelmed with the responsibilities)

APPENDIX B

DOMAIN: PHYSIOLOGICAL

Problem: Neuro-musculo-skeletal function (high priority)

Problem Classification Scheme

Modifiers: Individual and Actual

Signs/Symptoms of Actual

- limited range of motion
- decreased muscle strength
- decreased muscle tone
- decreased balance
- gait/ambulation disturbance
- difficulty transferring

Intervention Scheme

Category: Teaching, Guidance, and Counseling

Targets and Client-specific Information

- exercises (need range of motion and others)
- positioning (frequent change to prevent skin breakdown)

Category: Case Management

Targets and Client-specific Information

- durable medical equipment (toilet riser/toilet bars; grab bars in bathroom)

Category: Surveillance

- safety (checked home)
- signs/symptoms—physical (vital signs, blood pressure, skin)

Problem Rating Scale for Outcomes

Knowledge (Family): 3-basic knowledge (few safety hazards in home; not aware that exercises needed)

Behavior: 2-rarely appropriate behavior (Maria performed minimal exercises; walks little)

Status: 2-severe signs/symptoms (activity restricted due to fractures and contractures)

Garbage Odors: Resolving a Problem at a Senior Apartment Building in the Community

Barbara B. Ottinger, RN, MS, PHN
Public Health Nurse
Scott County Public Health Department
Shakopee, Minnesota

Information Obtained During a Project/Incident

In July the public health nurse started spending Wednesday afternoons at a senior apartment building, the client for this case study. A resident stopped to discuss her health problems and reported that the first floor "smelled just awful—like rotten fish" during the previous weekend. The resident asked if the nurse could resolve the problem. A second resident described the same building odor. He said that some residents frequently go fishing on pleasant summer days and had observed one of the non–English speaking residents emptying paper bags containing fish scraps into the trash chute. This resident stated that the odor was most offensive before the scheduled Monday and Thursday garbage days. The nurse asked the resident to keep notes about when he smelled the odor and speak to the building manager.

The nurse returned to the office the following week and smelled a foul odor near the elevator next to the trash chute. The nurse talked to the manager, who acknowledged that the odor had been a problem for a number of weeks. The manager stated that all residents were informed about the trash removal policy when they moved in, and that she had posted signs about the policy on each floor beside the trash chute. No food was to be disposed in the trash chute unless it was placed in plastic bags and tied, and fish remains were to be disposed only in the outside dumpster. The building manager and the nurse took a tour of the building and saw the posted signs. When the nurse asked the manager if all residents could read the English signs, the manager responded that a number of residents spoke other languages, but she assumed that they could read English. She could not translate the information. The nurse provided the manager with contact information for a county department that had translation services. Within a week, the manager had the signs translated into the languages spoken by residents and posted new signs beside the trash chutes. They did not receive trash odor complaints during the past 6 months.

Application of the Omaha System

(Answers reflect information at the beginning of the incident.)

DOMAIN: ENVIRONMENTAL

Problem: Sanitation (high priority)

Problem Classification Scheme

Modifiers: Community and Actual
SIGNS/SYMPTOMS OF ACTUAL
- inadequate food storage/disposal
- foul odor

Intervention Scheme
Category: Teaching, Guidance, and Counseling
TARGETS AND CLIENT-SPECIFIC INFORMATION
- behavior modification (residents needed to change disposal patterns)

Category: Surveillance
TARGETS AND CLIENT-SPECIFIC INFORMATION
- environment (residents and manager continued to monitor for foul odors)

Problem Rating Scale for Outcomes
Knowledge: 2-minimal knowledge (only residents who read English signs knew the disposal policy)
Behavior: 2-rarely appropriate behavior (residents who knew the policy disposed of trash properly but others did not)
Status: 2-severe signs/symptoms (offensive odor strongest on weekends)

Problem: Communication with community resources (high priority)

Problem Classification Scheme
Modifiers: Community and Actual
SIGNS/SYMPTOMS OF ACTUAL
- unfamiliar with options/procedures for obtaining services
- difficulty understanding roles/regulations of service providers
- language barrier

Intervention Scheme
Category: Teaching, Guidance, and Counseling
TARGETS AND CLIENT-SPECIFIC INFORMATION
- communication (shared trash disposal policy in a language all could understand)

Category: Case Management
TARGETS AND CLIENT-SPECIFIC INFORMATION
- interpreter/translator services (provided contact capable of translating signs)

Category: Surveillance
TARGETS AND CLIENT-SPECIFIC INFORMATION
- communication (toured building to check for appropriate signs)

Problem Rating Scale for Outcomes
Knowledge: 2-minimal knowledge (residents who did not read English did not know disposal policy)
Behavior: 2-rarely appropriate behavior (residents who did not know policy did not dispose of trash properly)
Status: 2-severe signs/symptoms (those who did not follow the policy produced odor problems for all residents)

James N.: Man Who Received Total Parenteral Nutrition

Julie Pahlen, RN, BS, PHN
Director
Roseau County Home Health Care
Roseau, Minnesota

Information Obtained During the First Visit/Encounter

James N., a 47-year-old man, was referred to a home care agency following a 2-week hospital stay. The referral listed current diagnoses as malnutrition, electrolyte imbalance, weakness, anorexia, indigestion, and cardiomegaly, and previous diagnoses as ischemic heart disease and myocardial infarction. A porta-catheter was inserted to instill daily total parenteral nutrition (TPN) with lipids and multi-vitamins during a 12-hour period for 8 weeks. James said he would not learn about or assume responsibility for self-administration. Fortunately, his wife and daughter, Jan, were willing. Mrs. N. received written TPN instructions at the hospital, but only a brief explanation.

During the first visit, the home care nurse started the TPN and reviewed the detailed instructions with Mrs. N. and Jan. They discussed storing, protecting, and preparing the TPN bags; hand washing; clean and sterile technique; starting and discontinuing TPN; flushing the line; observing the site; providing catheter care; and troubleshooting problems including the alarm. Although Mrs. N. said she felt overwhelmed, she took notes and observed the nurse closely. The nurse scheduled two return visits to discontinue the TPN and for Mrs. N. to begin participating in the TPN procedure.

The home care nurse gave Mrs. N. a form to use as a diary, and instructed her to record TPN instillations and side effects such as fever, pain, nausea, or taste sensation. They recorded the following: temperature, 98.8° F.; pulse, 104 and slightly irregular; respirations, 30; blood pressure, 90/62; comfortable; and pale, cool skin. They compared the previous measurements to the hospital discharge form. The nurse described reasons to call providers. The nurse and Mrs. N. discussed how to measure and record intake and output. Mrs. N. mentioned James' long cardiac history and that she had requested the recent admission. They discussed his weight recorded in the hospital; Mrs. N. will weigh him and document the information twice a week. Mrs. N. understands that James should have small amounts of soft foods as tolerated and at least one healthy shake daily. She will record what he eats and when his appetite improves. The nurse will check James' blood sugar every third day, draw blood weekly for a complete blood count and liver enzyme/complete metabolic panel, and note these procedures in the diary.

The medications, pump, and pole were delivered before the nurse arrived. The nurse described the steps for obtaining more supplies, and called the infusion and equipment companies to confirm the plans. Mrs. N. and Jan thanked the nurse, indicating that the plan for James and their responsibilities were much clearer.

Application of the Omaha System

DOMAIN: PHYSIOLOGICAL

Problem: Digestion-hydration (low priority: provide interventions and rate if current needs are not met by Nutrition and Medication regimen)

Problem Classification Scheme

Modifiers: Individual and Actual

SIGNS/SYMPTOMS OF ACTUAL

- nausea/vomiting
- difficulty/inability to chew/swallow/digest
- indigestion
- anorexia
- electrolyte imbalance

Problem: Circulation (high priority)

Problem Classification Scheme

Modifiers: Individual and Actual

SIGNS/SYMPTOMS OF ACTUAL

- discoloration of skin/cyanosis
- temperature change in affected area
- abnormal blood pressure reading
- irregular heart rate
- excessively rapid heart rate

Intervention Scheme

Category: Teaching, Guidance, and Counseling

TARGETS AND CLIENT-SPECIFIC INFORMATION

- signs/symptoms—physical (compared vital signs, blood pressure, skin color, and temperature to hospital notes and history; use diary)

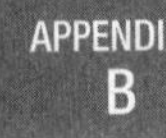

Category: Surveillance

TARGETS AND CLIENT-SPECIFIC INFORMATION

- signs/symptoms—physical (vital signs/blood pressure, skin color, temperature)

Problem Rating Scale for Outcomes

Knowledge (Family): 4-adequate knowledge (aware of extent of disease)
Behavior (Family): 4-usually appropriate (provided care at home, requested hospitalization)
Status: 2-severe symptoms (assessment confirmed disease status)

DOMAIN: HEALTH-RELATED BEHAVIORS

Problem: Nutrition (high priority)

Problem Classification Scheme

Modifiers: Individual and Actual

SIGNS/SYMPTOMS OF ACTUAL

- underweight: adult BMI 18.5 or less; child BMI 5th percentile or less
- lacks established standards for daily caloric/fluid intake

Intervention Scheme

Category: Teaching, Guidance, and Counseling

Targets and Client-specific Information

- dietary management (follow recommended diet, record intake)
- signs/symptoms—physical (record weight)

Category: Surveillance

Targets and Client-specific Information

- dietary management (status of food intake)

Problem Rating Scale for Outcomes

Knowledge (Family): 2-minimal knowledge (did not understand nutrition plan)
Behavior (Family): 2-rarely appropriate behavior (did not begin recommended plan)
Status: 2-severe signs/symptoms (James improved since hospital admission, still malnourished)

Problem: Medication regimen (high priority)

Problem Classification Scheme

Modifiers: Individual and Actual

Signs/Symptoms of Actual

- unable to take medications without help

Intervention Scheme

Category: Teaching, Guidance, and Counseling

Targets and Client-specific Information

- feeding procedures (steps of TPN procedure)
- infection precautions (hand washing, good technique, protect supplies)
- laboratory findings (expect blood sugar, CBC, and metabolic panel regularly)
- medication action/side effects (what to observe/report to providers)
- signs/symptoms—physical (evidence of infection at site, intake and output)

Category: Treatments and Procedures

Targets and Client-specific Information

- medication administration (started TPN instillation)

Category: Case Management

Targets and Client-specific Information

- durable medical equipment (confirmed pump/pole arrangements with company)
- supplies (confirmed solution arrangements with infusion company)

Category: Surveillance

Targets and Client-specific Information

- signs/symptoms—physical (no evidence of infection at site, intake and output)

Problem Rating Scale for Outcomes

Knowledge (Family): 2-minimal knowledge (received instructions at hospital; did not understand)
Behavior (Family): 2-rarely appropriate behavior (had not participated in TPN procedure)
Status: 2-severe signs/symptoms (compromised health, improvement will be slow)

Mary E.: Woman With a Wound

Gretchen M. Sampson, RN, MPH
Director/Health Officer
Polk County Health Department
Balsam Lake, Wisconsin

Information Obtained During the First Visit/Encounter

Mary E., age 34, lived with her husband in a trailer home in a rural area of the county. She had insulin-dependent diabetes for 10 years. One week ago, Mary had a total abdominal hysterectomy and a right salpingo-oophorectomy. After returning home, dehiscence occurred. When the home care nurse arrived, Mary was lying on the couch, propped up with pillows. She confirmed the referral information by indicating that she could not care for her incision. Her oral temperature was 99.6° F, radial pulse was 76 and apical pulse was 80, respirations were 18, lung sounds were clear, and blood pressure was 106/70. Mary's weight was listed as 310 pounds, and her height as 5′3″ on the referral information.

The nurse asked Mary about her eating and exercise patterns. Mary complained of nausea, especially after eating, although she had not vomited. She showed the nurse her diabetic diet, but said, especially since her surgery, she was not following it or drinking extra fluids. She was not using her blood glucose monitor 3 times a day; they discussed her log and some elevated entries. Mary reported having considerable pain when she tried to walk or do daily activities; she was not trying to do her other exercises now.

Mary could not see the wound area due to the size of her abdomen. Her mother was present during the visit, but was not willing to learn to change the dressing. Mary's husband changed it yesterday and agreed to help regularly. They decided to schedule the next and most future visits when he was home to participate in wound care and discuss related symptoms. Using appropriate clean technique, the nurse removed the dressing and observed an inflamed incision and copious amounts of red, serosanguinous drainage. The wound measured 16 cm long, 7.5 cm wide, and 8 cm deep. The nurse cleansed and covered the wound, following the recommended protocol. Mary was diaphoretic and grimacing during the procedure. Based on a pain scale of 0 to 10 with 10 being most severe, Mary said that her level pain was often an 8. When she took her pain medication, propoxyphene napsylate and acetaminophen (Darvocet N), the level decreased to a 2, and she could turn in bed and walk from her bed to the bathroom and back. She placed pillows tightly around her in bed, and used them to brace her abdomen when she walked. Mary and the nurse discussed the need to change positions every 1 to 2 hours, increase activity, and schedule pain medication administration regularly to coincide with movement and dressing changes. The nurse gave Mary a form to use as a diary and record her pain, wound care, temperature, activities, and intake. Mary agreed to call the nurse or physician if her entries were above or below the values the nurse listed.

Application of the Omaha System

DOMAIN: PHYSIOLOGICAL

Problem: Pain (high priority)

Problem Classification Scheme

Modifiers: Individual and Actual

SIGNS/SYMPTOMS OF ACTUAL

- expresses discomfort/pain
- compensated movement/guarding
- facial grimaces
- pallor/perspiration

Intervention Scheme

Category: Teaching, Guidance, and Counseling

TARGETS AND CLIENT-SPECIFIC INFORMATION

- positioning (change positions regularly, support abdomen with pillows when lying down)
- signs/symptoms—physical (establish a schedule for Darvocet, considering activity and dressing changes)

Category: Surveillance

TARGETS AND CLIENT-SPECIFIC INFORMATION

- exercises (limited until pain controlled)
- signs/symptoms—physical: (pain status, effectiveness of control measures)

Problem Rating Scale for Outcomes

Knowledge: 3-basic knowledge (knew which medication relieves pain)
Behavior: 3-inconsistently appropriate behavior (did not schedule medications effectively, uses other pain control techniques sometimes)
Status: 2-severe signs/symptoms (reported/exhibited frequent severe pain)

Problem: Skin (high priority)

Problem Classification Scheme

Modifiers: Individual and Actual

SIGNS/SYMPTOMS OF ACTUAL

- lesion/pressure ulcer
- inflammation
- drainage
- delayed incisional healing

Intervention Scheme

Category: Teaching, Guidance, and Counseling

TARGETS AND CLIENT-SPECIFIC INFORMATION

- signs/symptoms—physical (needed observations, when to report to providers)
- support system (include Mary's husband in next/other visits)

Category: Treatments and Procedures

TARGETS AND CLIENT-SPECIFIC INFORMATION

- dressing change/wound care (used clean technique, measured wound, and followed protocol)

Category: Surveillance

TARGETS AND CLIENT-SPECIFIC INFORMATION

- signs/symptoms—physical (vital signs, measurements, evidence of healing, signs of infection)

Problem Rating Scale for Outcomes

Knowledge: 3-basic knowledge (recognized severity and treatment of lesion but not cause or stages of healing)

Behavior: 3-inconsistently appropriate behavior (tried to care for surgical incision, but cannot)

Status: 2-severe signs/symptoms (stage III lesion with minimal healing)

DOMAIN: HEALTH-RELATED BEHAVIORS

Problem: Nutrition (high priority)

Problem Classification Scheme

Modifiers: Individual and Actual

SIGNS/SYMPTOMS OF ACTUAL

- overweight: adult BMI 25.0 or more; child BMI 95th percentile or more
- does not follow recommended nutrition plan
- hyperglycemia

Intervention Scheme

Category: Teaching, Guidance, and Counseling

TARGETS AND CLIENT-SPECIFIC INFORMATION

- dietary management (recommended plan, extra fluids)
- durable medical equipment (needed to use glucose monitor regularly)

Category: Surveillance

TARGETS AND CLIENT-SPECIFIC INFORMATION

- dietary management (status, weight)
- laboratory findings (blood glucose trends)

Problem Rating Scale for Outcomes

Knowledge: 3-basic knowledge (understood relationship of diet to blood sugar)

Behavior: 2-rarely appropriate behavior (not following diet plan or monitoring glucose)

Status: 2-severe signs/symptoms (blood sugar within normal limits occasionally)

Lydia Y.: Woman With a Pressure Ulcer and Cancer

Debra A. Solomon, RN, FNP, MSN
Clinical Coordinator
HomeCaring and Hospice, Fairview Lakes Regional Health Care
Chisago City, Minnesota

Information Obtained During the First Visit/Encounter

Lydia Y., a 52-year-old woman, was referred to the home care agency for daily wound care. About 2 months ago, she had surgery, was told that her diagnosis was cancer of the liver, and was admitted to a long-term care facility. During the nurse's first visit, the niece reported that she and her husband offered to take Lydia into their home and care for her. Lydia was pleased to be with them, knew her diagnosis was terminal and that she would need more services in the future, and planned to request admission to the home care agency's hospice program or to a hospice facility.

Lydia's vital signs and blood pressure were within normal limits; her weight was 120 pounds and her height was 5′5″. The nurse did not see evidence of jaundice. Lydia ambulated slowly with a four-prong cane. She said she tired easily. Lydia had a stage 2 pressure ulcer on her right heel measuring 1.5 × 1.5 × 0.3 cm. The nurse used clean technique and removed the dressing, noted a small amount of serous drainage, and demonstrated the steps of the wound care procedure: she rinsed with normal saline, cleansed and dried surrounding skin, applied collagenase (Collagenase Santyl Ointment) to the wound bed, filled it loosely with saline moistened gauze, covered it with ABD pad to absorb drainage, and secured the dressing with kerlix wrap and a cotton stocking.

The niece asked the nurse if there was anything more they could do for Lydia. They discussed how wounds heal, ways to keep the area free from injury, signs of infection, and when to notify providers. They developed a plan for showering; the nurse will order a shower chair. Lydia knew she needed to elevate her leg several times a day and limit weight bearing on her right leg. The nurse demonstrated proper positioning and asked Lydia to change her position frequently and to be as active as she could, but to use various energy conservation techniques. Lydia denied having pain. The nurse indicated that a diet high in protein, iron, and vitamin C and a high fluid intake would stimulate wound healing. The nurse suggested that Lydia drink high protein supplements. The nurse planned to return tomorrow to continue teaching wound care and bring more supplies.

Application of the Omaha System

DOMAIN: PHYSIOLOGICAL

Problem: Skin (high priority)

Problem Classification Scheme

Modifiers: Individual and Actual

SIGNS/SYMPTOMS OF ACTUAL

- lesion/pressure ulcer
- drainage

Intervention Scheme

Category: Teaching, Guidance, and Counseling

TARGETS AND CLIENT-SPECIFIC INFORMATION

- anatomy/physiology (skin, healing process)
- dietary management (high protein/iron/vitamin C diet, high fluid intake)
- dressing change/wound care (protocol, keep dry/free from injury/infection)
- mobility/transfers (limit weight bearing on right leg)
- personal hygiene (plan for showering)
- positioning (frequent change, proper elevation)
- rest/sleep (rest/activity balance, energy conservation techniques)
- signs/symptoms—physical (wound changes, when to notify providers)

Category: Treatments and Procedures

TARGETS AND CLIENT-SPECIFIC INFORMATION

- dressing change/wound care (followed wound care protocol)

Category: Case Management

TARGETS AND CLIENT-SPECIFIC INFORMATION

- durable medical equipment (shower chair)
- supplies (dressing supplies)

Category: Surveillance

TARGETS AND CLIENT-SPECIFIC INFORMATION

- dressing change/wound care (skin status, wound size, signs of healing)
- mobility/transfers (use of four-prong cane, denied pain, tires easily)
- signs/symptoms—physical (vital signs, blood pressure, color/jaundice)

Problem Rating Scale for Outcomes

Knowledge (Niece): 2-minimal knowledge (does not know wound care, other aspects of care)

Behavior (Niece): 4-usually appropriate behavior (willing to learn wound care, seems motivated)

Status: 3-moderate signs/symptoms (stage 2 pressure ulcer)

DOMAIN: HEALTH-RELATED BEHAVIORS

Problem: Nutrition (low priority: provide interventions and rate if situation changes; current needs may be met with Skin interventions)

Problem Classification Scheme

Modifiers: Individual and Potential

RISK FACTORS: (pressure ulcer; needs high protein/iron/vitamin C diet and high fluid intake)

Problem: Personal care (low priority: provide interventions and rate problem if situation changes; current needs may be met with Skin interventions)

Problem Classification Scheme:

Modifiers: Individual and Potential

RISK FACTORS (pressure ulcer; niece seems willing to provide assistance)

APPENDIX

C

Client Problems Frequently Associated With Selected Conditions, Medical Diagnoses, and Treatments

This appendix is a list of selected conditions, medical diagnoses, and treatments associated with a nonexhaustive list of problems. It is designed to help new users compare the Omaha System's Problem Classification Scheme to their previous assessment and documentation methods, and to offer suggestions for experienced users who are working with new types of clients. This appendix is a guide, not a set of rules. Users should review the following lists, refer to the corresponding sections in the User's Guide, and choose the one or several problems that are the focus of their individual, family, or community client's concerns as they provide and document health-related services. It is possible that the most appropriate choice does not appear on the list in this appendix. Also, all problems in these lists will not apply to every client, especially when selected conditions, medical diagnoses, and treatments have been combined to create one list. Users should *not* select and document all problems in a list for a client.

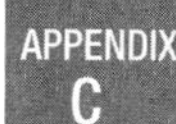

Addiction

Income
Residence
Neighborhood/workplace safety
Communication with community resources
Role change
Interpersonal relationship
Mental health
Neglect
Abuse
Pain
Physical activity
Personal care
Substance use
Health care supervision
Medication regimen

Alzheimer's Disease/Dementia

Residence
Communication with community resources
Social contact
Role change
Interpersonal relationship
Grief
Caretaking/parenting
Cognition
Sleep and rest patterns
Personal care
Medication regimen

Arthritis/Chronic Back Pain

Residence
Role change
Grief
Pain
Neuro-musculo-skeletal function
Physical activity
Personal care
Medication regimen

Asthma/Allergies

Sanitation
Role change
Respiration
Communicable/infectious condition
Sleep and rest patterns
Physical activity
Medication regimen

Cancer/Chemotherapy

Income
Communication with community resources
Spirituality
Grief
Mental health
Caretaking/parenting
Cognition
Pain
Consciousness
Neuro-musculo-skeletal function
Bowel function
Urinary function
Reproductive function
Communicable/infectious condition
Nutrition
Personal care
Health care supervision
Medication regimen

Cerebral Palsy/Multiple Sclerosis/Muscular Dystrophy/Spinal Cord Injury

Income
Residence
Neighborhood/workplace safety
Communication with community resources
Grief
Caretaking/parenting
Neglect
Abuse
Growth and development
Speech and language
Pain
Skin
Neuro-musculo-skeletal function
Respiration
Circulation
Digestion-hydration
Bowel function
Urinary function
Communicable/infectious condition
Nutrition
Sleep and rest patterns
Health care supervision
Medication regimen

Chronic Obstructive Pulmonary Disease (COPD)/Emphysema

Sanitation
Neighborhood/workplace safety
Role change
Sexuality
Neuro-musculo-skeletal function
Respiration
Circulation
Communicable/infectious condition
Sleep and rest patterns
Physical activity
Personal care
Substance use
Health care supervision
Medication regimen

Cirrhosis/Liver Disease

Pain
Skin
Circulation
Digestion-hydration
Nutrition
Substance use
Medication regimen

Congestive Heart Failure

Residence
Pain
Respiration
Circulation
Digestion-hydration
Communicable/infectious condition
Nutrition
Sleep and rest patterns
Physical activity
Substance use
Health care supervision
Medication regimen

Depression

Income
Sanitation
Communication with community resources
Social contact
Role change
Interpersonal relationship
Mental health
Sexuality
Caretaking/parenting
Nutrition
Sleep and rest patterns
Physical activity
Personal care
Substance use
Health care supervision
Medication regimen

Diabetes

Grief
Skin
Circulation
Reproductive function
Pregnancy
Nutrition
Physical activity
Health care supervision
Medication regimen

Domestic Violence

Income
Communication with community resources
Social contact
Interpersonal relationship
Mental health
Sexuality
Caretaking/parenting
Neglect
Abuse
Pregnancy
Postpartum
Communicable/infectious condition
Nutrition
Sleep and rest patterns
Substance use
Family planning

Gastric/Peptic Ulcer

Mental health
Pain
Digestion-hydration
Bowel function
Nutrition
Substance use
Medication regimen

Gastrostomy/Nasogastric Feedings

Role change
Skin
Digestion-hydration
Bowel function
Nutrition
Medication regimen

Head Lice

Sanitation
Communication with community resources
Caretaking/parenting
Neglect
Abuse
Growth and development
Communicable/infectious condition
Personal care
Medication regimen

HIV/AIDS

Income
Sanitation
Communication with community resources
Social contact
Role change
Grief
Mental health
Sexuality
Caretaking/parenting
Pain
Consciousness
Skin
Neuro-musculo-skeletal function
Respiration
Circulation
Digestion-hydration
Personal care
Substance use
Health care supervision
Medication regimen

Hypertension

Role change
Respiration
Circulation
Nutrition
Physical activity
Health care supervision
Medication regimen

Infusion Therapy

Role change
Spirituality
Grief
Mental health
Sexuality
Pain
Skin
Digestion-hydration
Bowel function
Urinary function
Communicable/infectious condition
Nutrition
Physical activity
Health care supervision
Medication regimen

Lead Poisoning

Sanitation
Residence
Neighborhood/workplace safety
Communication with community resources
Pain
Neuro-musculo-skeletal condition
Digestion-hydration
Urinary function
Nutrition
Medication regimen

Mental Illness

Communication with community resources
Social contact
Interpersonal relationship
Mental health
Sexuality
Caretaking/parenting
Neglect
Abuse
Cognition
Nutrition
Sleep and rest patterns
Personal care
Health care supervision
Medication regimen

Myocardial Infarction

Residence
Communication with community resources
Role change
Mental health
Sexuality
Pain
Circulation
Bowel function
Nutrition
Physical activity
Health care supervision
Medication regimen

Obesity

Residence
Communication with community resources
Interpersonal relationship
Mental health
Growth and development
Neuro-musculo-skeletal function
Respiration
Circulation
Digestion-hydration
Reproductive function
Nutrition
Sleep and rest patterns
Physical activity
Personal care
Medication regimen

Osteoporosis/Parkinson's Disease

Residence
Communication with community resources
Role change
Caretaking/parenting
Cognition
Pain
Neuro-musculo-skeletal function
Digestion-hydration
Bowel function
Nutrition
Physical activity
Personal care
Health care supervision
Medication regimen

Pregnancy/Complications of Pregnancy

Role change
Caretaking/parenting
Circulation
Digestion-hydration
Bowel function
Urinary function
Pregnancy
Postpartum
Nutrition
Sleep and rest patterns
Physical activity
Family planning
Health care supervision
Medication regimen

Prematurity/Failure to Thrive

Communication with community resources
Caretaking/parenting
Neglect
Abuse
Growth and development
Skin
Digestion-hydration
Communicable/infectious condition
Nutrition
Health care supervision
Medication regimen

Pressure Ulcer

Sanitation
Pain
Skin
Neuro-musculo-skeletal function
Circulation
Communicable/infectious condition
Nutrition
Personal care
Medication regimen

Renal Disease

Communication with community resources
Role change
Skin
Circulation
Urinary function
Nutrition
Medication regimen

Stroke

Residence
Communication with community resources
Role change
Mental health
Vision
Speech and language
Cognition
Skin
Neuro-musculo-skeletal function
Circulation
Bowel function
Urinary function
Nutrition
Physical activity
Personal care
Health care supervision
Medication regimen

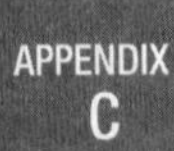

Terminal Illness/Palliative Care

Income
Communication with community resources
Spirituality
Grief
Mental health
Caretaking/parenting
Pain
Consciousness
Skin
Neuro-musculo-skeletal function
Respiration
Circulation
Digestion-hydration
Bowel function
Urinary function
Reproductive function
Nutrition
Sleep and rest patterns
Personal care
Health care supervision
Medication regimen

Tracheostomy

Role change
Caretaking/parenting
Speech and language
Skin
Respiration
Medication regimen

Tuberculosis

Sanitation
Communication with community resources
Social contact
Caretaking/parenting
Respiration
Communicable/infectious condition
Nutrition
Sleep and rest patterns
Physical activity
Substance use
Health care supervision
Medication regimen

Violence

Income
Neighborhood/workplace safety
Communication with community resources
Interpersonal relationship
Mental health
Sexuality
Abuse
Growth and development
Pain
Substance use

APPENDIX D

Omaha System Revision Process

Revising the Omaha System has been an ongoing process since its initial development began in 1975. The last revision was published in 1992 in two books: *The Omaha System: Applications for Community Health Nursing* and *The Omaha System: A Pocket Guide for Community Health Nursing*. The need to revise the System has been tempered by the reality that change poses serious challenges, especially as the number and the type of users with automated and manual client records increase globally. From the onset, the goals have been that the vocabulary and structure be stable, follow taxonomic principles, be as simple and easy to use as possible, and that the same, current version be used consistently across sites (Box D-1). It is not possible to aggregate or compare data when multiple versions of a terminology are included in clinical information software systems and manual forms, or included in electronic forms such as the National Library of Medicine's Metathesaurus and SNOMED CT® and printed literature.

STEPS OF THE ONGOING PROCESS

Omaha System user surveys have been collected since 1993 (Appendix F contains the current user survey). New organizations are asked to submit a survey so they are counted as users; experienced users are asked to submit periodic surveys or other written communication about their Omaha System experiences and suggestions for improvement. Table 1-3 in Chapter 1 provides a summary of the number and type of organizations that submitted surveys from 2001-2003.

Criteria for revising the Omaha System were developed and used throughout the initial 1975-1993 research; those criteria have been updated for this book and are listed in Box D-1. Steps for submitting recommendations for future revisions and the review process are described in Box D-2. In 2001, a 12-member advisory board, Consortium for the Omaha System International, was formed; it is comprised of representatives from diverse service and educational settings nationally and globally (Box D-3). Board members are involved in diverse Omaha System activities, which are summarized in Chapter 1. They and their organizations participated in essential revision steps including terminology review, field testing, pocket guide section review, and coding review that resulted in the 2005 version of the Omaha System (Chapter 2 and Appendixes A and E). They are also authors of many sections of this book.

PROCESS THAT RESULTED IN THE 2005 REVISION

Suggestions for revisions came from many sources in addition to the surveys. The Minnesota Users Group has met regularly since 2001 to discuss their use of the Omaha System and suggestions (see Chapter 1). Record audits have been conducted in many user organizations, sometimes annually. Two international conferences have been held that provided reports from practitioners, managers, educators, students, and researchers (see Chapter 1). Software developers and experts such as the National Library of Medicine staff discussed coding options (Appendix E). The Board met in person in 2001 and 2003, and communicated by telephone and e-mail numerous times. One Board member conducted an extensive review of research literature and identified strengths and possible areas for improvement (see Chapter 5).

Based on recommendations, a pilot test was conducted in late 2002 and early 2003 to consider incorporating the concept of communicable disease into the Omaha System. Two agencies in California, one in Maine, and three in Minnesota completed more than 30 data collection forms developed for the pilot test. Each form represented a summary of a prac-

OMAHA SYSTEM BOX D-1
Criteria for Revising the Omaha System

For inclusion in the Omaha System, terms and definitions need to be:

1. Client focused.
2. Congruent with the concepts of the problem-solving process, critical thinking, and the Omaha System model.
3. Designed to enhance practice, documentation, and information management.
4. Congruent with the following taxonomic principles:
   a. Hierarchical (i.e., flows from general to specific; domains, problems, modifiers, and signs/symptoms are linked, as are categories, targets, and client-specific information).
   b. Comparable levels of specificity (i.e., all problems should represent a similar level of abstraction).
   c. Limited repetition or redundancy; mutual exclusivity (i.e., a sign/symptom should not appear with more than one problem).
   d. Clearly defined and easy to use terms.
   e. Allows for expansion.
5. Simple
6. Brief.
7. Reflective of both objective and subjective data.
8. Capable of use by multidisciplinary practitioners who provide health-related care to individuals, families, and communities in diverse settings globally.
9. Reflective of the most current health care organizational practices.
10. Representative of new or changed information, not repeating existing information.
11. Compatible with but not attempting to replace other data sets or models (e.g., ICD, OASIS, CPT Codes, Healthy People 2010, Core Functions of Public Health, SNOMED CT®, Read Codes).
12. Suitable for use in automated or manual client record systems.

titioner's experiences working with clients who had diagnoses of tuberculosis, varicella, hepatitis A and B, and *Salmonella* and *Shigella* infections. The six agencies also conducted focus groups. The consensus of the participating practitioners and managers was that a communicable disease problem and target would be useful additions to the Omaha System, but that new terms should avoid duplicating other terms. Agencies agreed to review and respond to future rounds of information gathering.

During 2003, Board members reviewed and discussed the results of the communicable disease pilot test and numerous other recommendations. The Board agreed that the pilot test should serve as the model for conducting a field test of the proposed additions to the Omaha System. A list of terms and definitions was completed and prepared for use with field test forms. The field test was conducted during 2003 and 2004. Thirty experienced service agencies and educational programs located in the United States and Wales participated and completed 431 forms. In addition, many field test sites conducted focus groups with fellow practitioners or educators before submitting detailed suggestions. While the field test was in progress, two or more user groups from the United States, Canada, and New Zealand representing a total of 91 organizations were recruited to review each problem, intervention, and outcome section in the 1992 pocket guide.

Results were considered by many key stakeholders, including members of the Consortium for the Omaha System International Board and users. The finalized Omaha System (2005) that appears in Appendixes A and E represents a limited, but necessary, number of revisions that address changes in practice and coding requirements globally.

OMAHA SYSTEM BOX D-2
The Omaha System Review Process

1. Steps for Submitting Recommendations
   a. Comments about the Omaha System in general, as well as suggestions for additions or changes, are welcome. Review the criteria for revising the Omaha System and the current terms and definitions.
   b. Complete the Omaha System survey found in Appendix F or on the Omaha System Web site (www.omahasystem.org), or submit a typed statement. Include a brief rationale for suggested changes; the practice, education, and/or research experiences of the user; and references when appropriate.
   c. Submit recommendations to a member of the Consortium for the Omaha System International, follow the submission directions on the Web site, or send them to Karen Martin via e-mail at martinks@tconl.com.
2. Validation and testing
   a. Board members serve as validation experts and discuss suggested revisions every two years at their meetings. If a change is essential, steps will be taken to incorporate that change into the Omaha System quickly. Most revisions will be completed during a 5-year review cycle.
   b. Validation by expert practitioners and field testing is an integral part of the review process for revisions. Groups who are using the Omaha System will continue to be asked to compare the proposed revision to actual client data and indicate if the revision improves practice, documentation, and information management.

OMAHA SYSTEM BOX D-3
Board Members of the Consortium for the Omaha System International

Linda K. Ament, RN, BSN
Director
Beatrice Community Home Care
Beatrice, Nebraska

Mary Jo Baisch, RN, MS
Clinical Assistant Professor
College of Nursing
University of Wisconsin-Milwaukee
Milwaukee, Wisconsin

Amy J. Barton, RN, PhD
Associate Dean for Clinical Affairs
School of Nursing
University of Colorado Health Sciences Center
Denver, Colorado

Kathryn H. Bowles, RN, PhD
Associate Professor
School of Nursing
University of Pennsylvania
Philadelphia, Pennsylvania

Christine M. Broeker, RN, BSN
Home Care/Hospice Manager
St. Joseph's Area Health Services
Park Rapids, Minnesota

Jean R. Christensen, RN, RHV, BSc (Hons)
Project Manager
Welsh Assembly Government
Cardiff, Wales, United Kingdom

Victoria L. Elfrink, RNBC, PhD
Senior Associate
iTelehealth, Inc.
Frederick, Maryland;
Adjunct Professor
UNITEC Polytechnic Institute
Auckland, New Zealand

Karen S. Martin, RN, MSN, FAAN
Health Care Consultant
Martin Associates
Omaha, Nebraska

Karen A. Monsen, RN, MS
Program Manager
Washington County Department of Public Health and Environment
Stillwater, Minnesota

Gretchen M. Sampson, RN, MPH
Director/Health Officer
Polk County Health Department
Balsam Lake, Wisconsin

Nancy J. Scheet, RN, MSN
Quality Management Director
Magellan Behavioral Health
Lincoln, Nebraska

Bonnie L. Westra, RN, PhD
Vice President, Planning
CareFacts Information Systems, Inc.
St. Paul, Minnesota

APPENDIX E

Omaha System Codes

The Omaha System now appears in diverse private and commercially available clinical information system software, the UMLS Metathesaurus (a collection of health care terminology), SNOMED CT® (a reference terminology), LOINC (a clinical vocabulary), and HL7 (a messaging standard). Because the number and type of software applications that include the Omaha System are expected to continue expanding rapidly, this book represents a significant change from the books published in 1992. The new terms and codes presented in Appendix E are necessary for Omaha System software to operate compatibly with diverse systems nationally and globally. As described in Appendix D, the taxonomic structure and hierarchical order are maintained, but certain terms (concepts) were retired, added, or edited, and the codes were removed from the domains, problems, signs/symptoms, categories, and targets.

National and global organizations, including the National Library of Medicine, provided recommendations regarding the Omaha System coding revision decisions. In order to meet current criteria and standards for terminologies, each discrete term needs a unique identifier. The identifier or code is a numeric representation that does not have an inherent meaning. This appendix presents the Problem Classification Scheme and Intervention Scheme changes in the following way:

- Obsolete or retired terms and codes are represented by a ~~strikethrough.~~ Obsolete terms and their corresponding codes must be permanently retired and not used again.
- New terms and codes are represented by an underline. Newly added terms or those that were significantly revised by changing, separating, or combining terms must have new codes.
- Edited terms and codes are represented by *italics.* If the term's meaning does not change, the term's code remains the same even if the name of the term was edited.

Appendixes A and E present the terms and codes of the 2005 revision of the Omaha System. As such, this information is public domain and available for unrestricted use. The appendixes are designed for two different purposes and groups. Appendix A is the complete Problem Classification Scheme, Intervention Scheme, and Problem Rating Scale for Outcomes, the three components of the Omaha System. It is intended primarily for practitioners, managers, educators, and students. These individuals and organizations provide and document client care using the Omaha System, review others' documentation, and aggregate and analyze client data. Numerous practice, education, and research

Health Connections Press does not claim ownership of the terms, definitions, and codes embodied in the Omaha System.

applications that illustrate how to increase the usability, accuracy, and consistency of Omaha System data, documentation, reports, and software are described in Chapters 3 to 6. Note that the codes were removed from Appendix A and the User's Guide. Practitioners view the Omaha System in logical order rather than out of sequence and do not need to learn a significantly different coding system.

In contrast, Appendix E presents both the 1992 and the 2005 versions of the Omaha System. *Terms* continue to be displayed in order. However, *codes* are displayed out of order to reflect how the Problem Classification and Intervention Schemes were revised to meet terminology criteria and standards. Signs/symptoms were added at the end of a problem cluster, except when the flow suggested changing the order of the list. A retired sign/symptom is listed with its unique code before its corresponding new sign/symptom with its new code. The same pattern was used for targets. Appendix E is designed primarily for:

- Manual users need to update their forms to include the revised Omaha System, and recognize the similarities and differences between the two versions to conduct their own statistical analysis and compare data with other users.
- Experienced users, especially those who have teaching, quality improvement, or data analysis responsibilities in practice and educational settings, need to become familiar with the revisions. This group includes automated and manual users.
- Private and commercial software developers and vendors who incorporated the 1992 version of the Omaha System need to replace it with the 2005 version. Such changes require significant effort. The changes require developing new tables and fields and updating databases. Developers need to examine the options for presenting both old and new information. They should evaluate the alternatives to manage existing client records that are open for service, represent retrospective data, and compare data abstracted from client records between sites *or* software systems. One option is to present old records in the old format and new records in the new format. Another option is to convert old records into the new format.

To understand this appendix, consider Mental health, a problem that has a number of signs/symptoms italicized and underlined. In the 1992 version the same problem, Emotional stability, had a total of 12 signs/symptoms: 11 that were unique and one that was "other." Initially it may appear that the problem changed significantly because the name was edited to Mental health and 23 signs/symptoms appear in the problem cluster in this appendix. However, when the 1992 and 2005 versions are compared, the revisions are not dramatic: 7 of the original 11 signs/symptoms remain the same, with 2 of those marked with italics for limited editing; 5 are marked as obsolete ~~(strikethrough)~~, and 11 are marked as new <u>(underlined)</u> for a total of 18 signs/symptoms in the 2005 version. Note the dramatic difference in the way the Omaha System is displayed for users in Appendix A compared to this appendix.

Coding changes in the Intervention Scheme follow the same pattern of markings. Health is omitted from the first category to signify that it was removed. The italics indicate that *Teaching, Guidance, and Counseling* is the new name of the category, and that its definition continues to have the same meaning. *~~Bronchial hygiene~~* is marked as an obsolete (strikethrough) target, and *<u>respiratory care</u>* as new (underlined), because the definition reflects a change that exceeds limited editing and italics. Again, practitioners do not see the marks or revisions in Appendix A.

Many principles, characteristics, terms, definitions, and rules of the Omaha System remain the same in this book. Rules for expansion and customization appear in Chapter 2. Reliability, validity, and usability of the Omaha System increase when content, order, and the relationships between terms are presented consistently and reflected in software and manual forms. Problem Classification Scheme domains, problems, modifiers, and sign/symptoms continue to be linked. Likewise, Intervention Scheme categories, targets, and client-specific information continue to be linked as are Problem Rating Scale for Outcome concepts and numeric ratings. For example, in the Problem Classification Scheme, each unique sign/symptom is associated with one and only one unique problem. The exception is the sign/symptom "other," which appears at the end of each sign/symptom cluster. For the Intervention Scheme, one or more unique targets can be linked to one unique category. Any one target from the alphabetized target list may be linked to any of the four categories if practitioners indicate that the linkage represents services appropriately. Because some combinations of categories and targets are possible according to the rules, but are not logical, the User's Guide includes suggested linkages. The target "other" appears at the end of the target list.

In order to link client data from a software application to a reference terminology or exchange data between two software systems via HL7 messaging, recognized coding conventions are needed. The sequence of characters representing terms need to be the same or capable of translation. To facilitate translation, the Roman numerals for the domains and categories were replaced with Arabic numbers. Although this appendix does not illustrate linkages between Problem Classification or Intervention Scheme codes, it is possible to create those linkages. The coding schema recommended for Omaha System use is as follows:

- Problem Classification Scheme: 12.01 *Mental health* (problem=12.) and *sadness/hopelessness/decreased self-esteem* (first sign/symptom=.01). These are the codes for a problem and one of its signs/symptoms, using the principle of concatenating the problem and a sign/symptom with a decimal as a separator.
- Intervention Scheme: 01.80 *Teaching, Guidance, and Counseling* (category=01.) and *respiratory care* (target=.80). These are the codes for a category and a target with a decimal as a separator.

Problem Classification Scheme

Modifiers (select one):
Individual
Family
Community

Modifiers (select one):
Health Promotion
Potential
Actual

01. ENVIRONMENTAL DOMAIN

01. Income

APPENDIX E

SIGNS/SYMPTOMS OF ACTUAL:

01. low/no income
02. uninsured medical expenses
03. *difficulty with* money management
04. able to buy only necessities
05. difficulty buying necessities
06. other

02. Sanitation

Signs/Symptoms of Actual:

01. soiled living area
02. inadequate food storage/disposal
03. insects/rodents
04. foul odor
05. inadequate water supply
06. inadequate sewage disposal
07. inadequate laundry facilities
08. allergens
09. infectious/contaminating agents
11. presence of mold
12. excessive pets
10. other

03. Residence

Signs/Symptoms of Actual:

01. structurally unsound
02. inadequate heating/cooling
03. steep/*unsafe* stairs
04. inadequate/obstructed exits/entries
05. cluttered living space
06. unsafe storage of dangerous objects/substances
07. unsafe mats/throw rugs
08. inadequate safety devices
09. presence of lead-based paint
10. unsafe *appliances/equipment*
11. inadequate/crowded living space
14. exposed wiring
15. structural barriers
12. homeless
13. other

04. Neighborhood/workplace safety

Signs/Symptoms of Actual:

01. high crime rate
02. high pollution level
03. uncontrolled/*dangerous/infected* animals
05. *inadequate/*unsafe play/*exercise* areas
07. inadequate space/resources to foster health
08. threats/reports of violence
04. physical hazards
09. vehicle/traffic hazards
10. chemical hazards
11. radiological hazards
06. other

~~05. Other~~

~~01. other~~

02. PSYCHOSOCIAL DOMAIN

06. Communication with community resources

SIGNS/SYMPTOMS OF ACTUAL:

01. unfamiliar with options/procedures for obtaining services
02. difficulty understanding roles/regulations of service providers
03. unable to communicate concerns *to provider*
04. dissatisfaction with services
06. inadequate/unavailable resources
05. language barrier
08. cultural barrier
09. educational barrier
10. transportation barrier
11. limited access to care/services/goods
12. unable to use/has inadequate communication devices/equipment
07. other

07. Social contact

SIGNS/SYMPTOMS OF ACTUAL:

01. limited social contact
02. uses health care provider for social contact
03. minimal outside stimulation/leisure time activities
04. other

08. Role change

SIGNS/SYMPTOMS OF ACTUAL:

~~01. involuntary reversal of traditional male/female roles~~
~~02. involuntary reversal of dependent/independent roles~~
06. involuntary role reversal
03. assumes new role
04. loses previous role
05. other

09. Interpersonal relationship

SIGNS/SYMPTOMS OF ACTUAL:

01. difficulty establishing/maintaining relationships
02. minimal shared activities
03. incongruent values/goals/*expectations/schedules*
04. inadequate interpersonal communication skills
05. prolonged, unrelieved tension
~~06. inappropriate suspicion/manipulation/compulsion/aggression~~
08. inappropriate suspicion/manipulation/control
09. physically/emotionally abusive to partner
10. difficulty problem solving without conflict
07. other

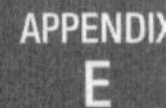

10. *Spirituality*

Signs/Symptoms of Actual:

01. expresses spiritual concerns
02. disrupted spiritual rituals
03. disrupted spiritual trust
04. conflicting spiritual beliefs and medical/*health care* regimen
05. other

11. Grief

Signs/Symptoms of Actual:

01. fails to recognize *stages of grief/process of healing*
02. difficulty coping with grief responses
03. difficulty expressing grief responses
04. conflicting stages of grief among *individuals/families*
05. other

12. *Mental health*

Signs/Symptoms of Actual:

01. sadness/hopelessness/*decreased self-esteem*
02. apprehension/undefined fear
03. loss of interest/involvement in activities/self-care
~~04. narrowed perceptual focus~~
~~05. scattering of attention~~
<u>13. narrowed to scattered attention/focus</u>
06. flat affect
~~07. irritable/agitated~~
<u>14. irritable/agitated/aggressive</u>
~~08. purposeless activity~~
<u>15. purposeless/compulsive activity</u>
09. difficulty managing stress
<u>16. difficulty managing anger</u>
10. somatic complaints/*fatigue*
<u>17. delusions</u>
<u>18. hallucinations/illusions</u>
~~11. expresses wish to die/attempts suicide~~
<u>19. expresses suicidal/homicidal thoughts</u>
<u>20. attempts suicide/homicide</u>
<u>21. self-mutilation</u>
<u>22. mood swings</u>
<u>23. flash-backs</u>
12. other

13. *Sexuality*

Signs/Symptoms of Actual:

01. difficulty recognizing consequences of sexual behavior
02. difficulty expressing intimacy
03. sexual identity confusion

04. sexual value confusion
05. dissatisfied with sexual relationships
07. unsafe sexual practices
08. sexual acting out/provocative behaviors/harassment
09. sexual perpetration/assault
06. other

14. Caretaking/parenting

Signs/Symptoms of Actual:

01. difficulty providing physical care/safety
02. difficulty providing emotional nurturance
03. difficulty providing cognitive learning experiences and activities
04. difficulty providing preventive and therapeutic health care
05. expectations incongruent with stage of growth and development
06. dissatisfaction/difficulty with responsibilities
10. difficulty interpreting or responding to verbal/nonverbal communication
07. neglectful
08. abusive
09. other

15. *Neglect*

Signs/Symptoms of Actual:

01. lacks adequate physical care
02. lacks emotional nurturance/support
03. lacks appropriate stimulation/cognitive experiences
04. inappropriately left alone
05. lacks necessary supervision
06. inadequate/delayed medical care
07. other

16. *Abuse*

Signs/Symptoms of Actual:

01. harsh/excessive discipline
02. welts/burns/*other injuries*
03. questionable explanation of injury
04. attacked verbally
05. fearful/hypervigilant behavior
06. violent environment
07. consistent negative messages
08. assaulted sexually
09. other

17. Growth and development

Signs/Symptoms of Actual:

01. abnormal results of developmental screening tests
02. abnormal weight/height/head circumference in relation to growth/*age standards*

03. age-inappropriate behavior
04. inadequate achievement/maintenance of developmental tasks
05. other

~~18. Other~~

~~01. other~~

03. PHYSIOLOGICAL DOMAIN

19. Hearing

SIGNS/SYMPTOMS OF ACTUAL:

01. difficulty hearing normal speech tones
05. difficulty hearing speech in large group settings
06. difficulty hearing high frequency sounds
02. absent/abnormal response to sound
03. abnormal results of hearing screening test
04. other

20. Vision

SIGNS/SYMPTOMS OF ACTUAL:

01. difficulty seeing small print/calibrations
02. difficulty seeing distant objects
03. difficulty seeing close objects
04. absent/abnormal response to visual stimuli
05. abnormal results of vision screening test
06. squinting/blinking/tearing/blurring
09. floaters/flashes
07. difficulty differentiating colors
08. other

21. Speech and language

SIGNS/SYMPTOMS OF ACTUAL:

01. absent/abnormal ability to speak*/vocalize*
02. absent/abnormal ability to understand
03. lacks alternative communication skills*/gestures*
04. inappropriate sentence structure
05. limited enunciation/clarity
06. inappropriate word usage
07. other

~~22. Dentition~~

SIGNS/SYMPTOMS OF ACTUAL:

~~01. abnormalities of teeth~~
~~02. sore/swollen/bleeding gums~~
~~03. ill-fitting dentures~~
~~04. malocclusion~~
~~05. other~~

APPENDIX E

45. Oral health

SIGNS/SYMPTOMS OF ACTUAL:

01. missing/broken/malformed teeth
02. caries
03. excess tartar
04. sore/swollen/bleeding gums
05. malocclusion
06. ill-fitting/missing dentures
07. sensitivity to hot or cold
08. other

23. Cognition

SIGNS/SYMPTOMS OF ACTUAL:

01. diminished judgment
02. disoriented to time/place/person
03. limited recall of recent events
04. limited recall of long past events
05. limited calculating/sequencing skills
06. limited concentration
07. limited reasoning/abstract thinking ability
08. impulsiveness
09. repetitious language/behavior
11. wanders
10. other

24. Pain

SIGNS/SYMPTOMS OF ACTUAL:

01. expresses discomfort/pain
02. elevated pulse/respirations/blood pressure
03. compensated movement/guarding
04. restless behavior
05. facial grimaces
06. pallor/perspiration
07. other

25. Consciousness

SIGNS/SYMPTOMS OF ACTUAL:

01. lethargic
02. stuporous
03. unresponsive
04. comatose
05. other

APPENDIX E

26. *Skin*

SIGNS/SYMPTOMS OF ACTUAL:

01. lesion/*pressure ulcer*
02. rash

03. excessively dry
04. excessively oily
05. inflammation
06. pruritus
07. drainage
08. *bruising*
09. hypertrophy of nails
11. delayed incisional healing
10. other

27. Neuro-musculo-skeletal function

SIGNS/SYMPTOMS OF ACTUAL:

01. limited range of motion
02. decreased muscle strength
03. decreased coordination
04. decreased muscle tone
05. increased muscle tone
06. decreased sensation
07. increased sensation
08. decreased balance
09. gait/ambulation disturbance
~~10. difficulty managing activities of daily living~~
13. difficulty transferring
14. fractures
11. tremors/seizures
15. difficulty with thermoregulation
12. other

28. Respiration

SIGNS/SYMPTOMS OF ACTUAL:

01. abnormal breath patterns
02. unable to breathe independently
03. cough
04. unable to cough/expectorate independently
05. cyanosis
06. abnormal sputum
07. noisy respirations
08. rhinorrhea/*nasal congestion*
09. abnormal breath sounds
11. abnormal respiratory laboratory results
10. other

29. Circulation

SIGNS/SYMPTOMS OF ACTUAL:

01. edema
02. cramping/pain of extremities
03. decreased pulses

04. discoloration of skin
05. temperature change in affected area
06. varicosities
07. syncopal episodes *(fainting)/dizziness*
08. abnormal blood pressure reading
09. pulse deficit
10. irregular heart rate
11. excessively rapid heart rate
12. excessively slow heart rate
13. anginal pain
14. abnormal heart sounds/murmurs
16. abnormal clotting
17. abnormal cardiac laboratory results
15. other

30. Digestion-hydration

SIGNS/SYMPTOMS OF ACTUAL:

01. nausea/vomiting
02. difficulty/inability to chew/swallow/digest
03. indigestion
04. reflux
05. anorexia
06. anemia
07. ascites
08. jaundice/liver enlargement
09. decreased skin turgor
10. cracked lips/dry mouth
11. electrolyte imbalance
12. other

31. Bowel function

SIGNS/SYMPTOMS OF ACTUAL:

01. abnormal frequency/consistency of stool
02. painful defecation
03. decreased bowel sounds
04. blood in stools
05. abnormal color
06. cramping/abdominal discomfort
07. incontinent of stool
08. other

~~32. Genito-urinary function~~

SIGNS/SYMPTOMS OF ACTUAL:

~~01. incontinent of urine~~
~~02. urgency/frequency~~
~~03. burning/painful urination~~
~~04. difficulty emptying bladder~~

~~05. abnormal urinary frequency/amount~~
~~06. hematuria~~
~~07. abnormal discharge~~
~~08. abnormal menstrual pattern~~
~~09. abnormal lumps/swelling/tenderness of male/female reproductive organs~~
~~10. dyspareunia~~
~~11. other~~

46. Urinary function

Signs/Symptoms of Actual:

01. burning/painful urination
02. incontinent of urine
03. urgency/frequency
04. difficulty initiating urination
05. difficulty emptying bladder
06. abnormal amount
07. hematuria/abnormal color
08. nocturia
09. abnormal urinary laboratory results
10. other

47. Reproductive function

Signs/Symptoms of Actual:

01. abnormal discharge
02. abnormal menstrual pattern
03. difficulty managing menopause/andropause
04. abnormal lumps/swelling/tenderness of genital organs or breasts
05. pain during or after sexual intercourse
06. infertility
07. impotency
08. other

~~33. Antepartum/postpartum~~

Signs/Symptoms of Actual:

~~01. difficulty coping with pregnancy/body changes~~
~~02. inappropriate exercise/rest/diet/behaviors~~
~~03. discomfort~~
~~04. complications~~
~~05. fears delivery procedure~~
~~06. difficulty breast feeding~~
~~07. other~~

48. Pregnancy

Signs/Symptoms of Actual:

01. difficulty bonding with unborn baby
02. difficulty coping with body changes
03. difficulty with prenatal exercise/rest/diet/behaviors
04. fears delivery procedure

05. prenatal complications/preterm labor
06. inadequate social support
07. other

49. Postpartum

Signs/Symptoms of Actual:

01. difficulty breast-feeding
02. difficulty coping with postpartum changes
03. difficulty with postpartum exercise/rest/diet/behaviors
04. abnormal bleeding/vaginal discharge
05. postpartum complications
06. abnormal depressed feelings
07. other

50. Communicable/infectious condition

Signs/Symptoms of Actual:

01. infection
02. infestation
03. fever
04. biological hazards
05. positive screening/culture/laboratory results
06. inadequate supplies/equipment/policies to prevent transmission
07. does not follow infection control regimen
08. inadequate immunity
09. other

~~34. Other~~

~~01. other~~

04. HEALTH-RELATED BEHAVIORS DOMAIN

35. Nutrition

Signs/Symptoms of Actual:

~~01. weighs 10% more than average~~
12. overweight: adult BMI 25.0 or more; child BMI 95th percentile or more
~~02. weighs 10% less than average~~
13. underweight: adult BMI 18.5 or less; child BMI 5th percentile or less
03. lacks established standards for daily caloric/fluid intake
04. exceeds established standards for daily caloric/fluid intake
05. unbalanced diet
06. improper feeding schedule for age
07. *does not follow recommended nutrition plan*
08. unexplained/progressive weight loss
14. unable to obtain/prepare food
09. hypoglycemia
10. hyperglycemia
11. other

APPENDIX E

36. Sleep and rest patterns

Signs/Symptoms of Actual:

01. sleep/rest pattern disrupts family
02. frequently wakes during night
03. *sleepwalking*
04. insomnia
05. nightmares
06. insufficient sleep/rest for age/physical condition
08. sleep apnea
09. snoring
07. other

37. Physical activity

Signs/Symptoms of Actual:

01. sedentary life style
02. inadequate/inconsistent exercise routine
03. inappropriate type/amount of exercise for age/physical condition
04. other

38. Personal *care*

Signs/Symptoms of Actual:

01. *difficulty* laundering clothing
02. *difficulty with* bathing
07. difficulty with toileting activities
08. difficulty dressing lower body
09. difficulty dressing upper body
03. *foul* body odor
04. *difficulty* shampooing/combing hair
05. *difficulty* brushing/flossing/mouth care
10. unwilling/unable/forgets to complete personal care activities
06. other

39. Substance use

Signs/Symptoms of Actual:

~~01. abuses over-the-counter/street drugs~~
08. abuses over-the-counter/prescription medications
09. uses "street"-recreational drugs
02. abuses alcohol
03. smokes/*uses tobacco products*
04. difficulty performing normal routines
05. reflex disturbances
06. behavior change
10. exposure to cigarette/cigar smoke
11. buys/sells illegal substances
07. other

APPENDIX E

40. Family planning

SIGNS/SYMPTOMS OF ACTUAL:

01. inappropriate/insufficient knowledge *about* family planning methods
05. inappropriate/insufficient knowledge about preconception health practices
02. inaccurate/inconsistent use of family planning methods
03. dissatisfied with present family planning method
06. fears others' reactions regarding family planning choices
07. difficulty obtaining family planning methods
04. other

41. Health care supervision

SIGNS/SYMPTOMS OF ACTUAL:

01. fails to obtain routine/*preventive health care*
02. fails to seek care for symptoms requiring *evaluation/treatment*
03. fails to return as requested to *health care provider*
04. inability to coordinate multiple appointments/*treatment plans*
05. inconsistent source of *health* care
08. inadequate source of health care
06. inadequate *treatment plan*
07. other

42. Medication regimen

SIGNS/SYMPTOMS OF ACTUAL:

01. *does not follow recommended* dosage/schedule
02. *evidence of* side effects/*adverse reactions*
03. inadequate system for taking medication
04. improper storage of medication
05. fails to obtain refills appropriately
06. fails to obtain immunizations
08. inadequate medication regimen
09. unable to take medications without help
07. other

~~43. Technical procedure~~

SIGNS/SYMPTOMS OF ACTUAL:

~~01. unable to demonstrate/relate procedure accurately~~
~~02. does not follow/demonstrate principles of safe/aseptic techniques~~
~~03. procedure requires nursing skill~~
~~04. unable/unwilling to perform procedures without assistance~~
~~05. unable/unwilling to operate special equipment~~
~~06. other person(s) unable/unavailable to assist~~
~~07. other~~

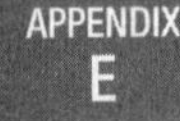

~~44. Other~~

~~01. other~~

INTERVENTION SCHEME

CATEGORIES

01. Teaching, Guidance, and Counseling
02. Treatments and Procedures
03. Case Management
04. Surveillance

TARGETS

01. anatomy/physiology
64. anger management
02. behavior modification
03. bladder care
04. bonding/*attachment*
05. bowel care
~~06. bronchial hygiene~~
07. cardiac care
08. caretaking/parenting skills
09. cast care
10. communication
65. community outreach worker services
66. continuity of care
11. coping skills
12. day care/respite
67. dietary management
13. discipline
14. dressing change/wound care
15. durable medical equipment
16. education
17. employment
68. end-of-life care
18. environment
19. exercises
20. family planning *care*
21. feeding procedures
22. finances
~~23. food~~
24. gait training
69. genetics
25. growth/development *care*
27. *home*
~~26. homemaking~~
70. homemaking/housekeeping
71. infection precautions
28. interaction

72. interpreter/translator services
29. *laboratory* findings
30. legal system
31. medical/dental care
32. medication action/side effects
33. medication administration
73. medication coordination/ordering
74. medication prescription
34. medication set-up
35. mobility/transfers
~~36. nursing care, supplementary~~
75. nursing care
~~37. nutrition~~
38. nutritionist *care*
76. occupational therapy care
39. ostomy care
40. other community resource*s*
77. paraprofessional/aide care
41. personal *hygiene*
78. physical therapy care
42. positioning
79. recreational therapy care
~~43. rehabilitation~~
44. relaxation/breathing techniques
80. respiratory care
81. respiratory therapy care
45. rest/sleep
46. safety
47. screening *procedures*
48. sickness/injury care
49. signs/symptoms-mental/emotional
50. signs/symptoms-physical
51. skin care
52. social work/counseling *care*
53. specimen collection
82. speech and language pathology care
54. spiritual care
55. stimulation/nurturance
56. stress management
~~57. substance use~~
83. substance use cessation
58. supplies
59. support group
60. support system
61. transportation
62. wellness
63. other

Problem Rating Scale For Outcomes

Concepts	1	2	3	4	5
KNOWLEDGE (K) Ability of the client to remember and interpret information	No knowledge	Minimal knowledge	Basic knowledge	Adequate knowledge	Superior knowledge
BEHAVIOR (B) Observable responses, actions, or activities of the client fitting the occasion or purpose	Not appropriate behavior	Rarely appropriate behavior	Inconsistently appropriate behavior	Usually appropriate behavior	Consistently appropriate behavior
STATUS (S) Condition of the client in relation to objective and subjective defining characteristics	Extreme signs/ symptoms	Severe signs/ symptoms	Moderate signs/ symptoms	Minimal signs/ symptoms	No signs/ symptoms

APPENDIX

F

Omaha System Survey

Survey

Please complete this survey! Your response will provide current information about the use of the Omaha System and suggestions for revision. Copy and share this form with other Omaha System users you know, and/or share their names with us. Individual data will remain confidential; summary data will be shared in publications and presentations. You may use the back of this survey to elaborate on your answers.

Your Name____________________ Title____________________

Organization____________________ Phone (____) ____________________

Address____________________ Email____________________

1. How did you learn about the Omaha System?____________________

2. Do you currently use the Omaha System? ❑ Yes ❑ No

a. If yes, when did you start?____________ Check which parts* you use: ❑ PCS ❑ IS ❑ PRSO
Check how you use it: ❑ Document services ❑ Orient/teach ❑ Reimbursement ❑ Quality improvement ❑ Case management ❑ Reports ❑ Research ❑ Develop software ❑ Other____________

b. If no, do you plan to use it? ❑ Yes ❑ No When?________ Which parts?* ❑ PCS ❑ IS ❑ PRSO

3. If you are employed by an organization that provides services:

a. Services offered: ❑ Home Health ❑ Public Health ❑ Clinics/Centers ❑ Acute ❑ Schools ❑ Long-term care ❑ Case management ❑ Other (specify)____________

b. Approx. no. of practitioner users:† RNs____ PTs____ OTs____ SW/Cs____ MDs____ DDSs____ SLPs____ N/RDs____ RTs____ RPhs____ P/A/T/OWs____ Other____________

c. Is your organization's client record: ❑ Automated ❑ Handwritten

❑ Other (describe)____________________

4. If you are employed by an education program:

a. Programs using: RNs____ PTs____ OTs____ SW/Cs____ MDs____ DDSs____ SLPs____ N/RDs____ RTs____ RPhs____ P/A/T/OWs____

b. Degrees offered: ❑ AD ❑ Dip ❑ BS/BA ❑ MS/MSN ❑ PhD/DNS ❑ Continuing ed.

c. Approximate annual no. of student users (count students using during classes and at clinical sites):
AD____ Dip____ BS/BA____ MS/MSN____ PhD/DNS____ Cont. ed.____ ❑ Other____________

d. Approximate annual no. of faculty users (count faculty using during classes and at clinical sites):________

5. From your experiences as a user, can you offer suggestions and/or revisions? Describe your experience and

publications:____________________

____

6. Other comments:____________________

____

* *PCS*, Problem Classification Scheme; *IS*, Intervention Scheme; *PRSO*, Problem Rating Scale for Outcomes.

† *RN*, registered nurse; *PT*, physical therapist; *OT*, occupational therapist; *SW/C*, social worker/counselor; *MD*, physician; *DDS*, dentist; *SLP*, speech and language pathologist; *N/RD*, nutritionist/registered dietician; *RT*, recreational therapist; *RPh*, pharmacist; *P/A/T/OW*, paraprofessional/aide/outreach worker/translator.

Thanks for your time! Please return this survey to:
Karen S. Martin, 2115 South 130th Street, Omaha, NE 68144

Glossary

General Glossary

Acute Care Health care and social services provided at hospitals, emergency rooms, or health care inpatient systems.

Advanced Beginner Second stage in the Dreyfus model of skill acquisition, in which the practitioner has enough background experience to recognize recurring, meaningful aspects of a situation and can demonstrate marginally acceptable performance (Benner, 1984).

Caregiver Family member, friend, or private employee who provides care to a dependent adult or child.

Case Mix System that classifies clients into homogeneous groups according to their acuity of their illness, amount of care they require, and/or their use of resources.

Client Individual, family, or community that receives health care and social services. Synonyms include resident, patient, customer, consumer, and constituency.

Client Record Official document completed by practitioners that typically includes client identification and demographic data, assessment data, care planning data, reports of services provided, and evidence of client progress. May include health history, laboratory data, screening reports, and other pertinent information.

Competent Third stage in the Dreyfus model of skill acquisition, in which the practitioner has considerable conscious, deliberate planning, predictable accomplishments, and an increased level of efficiency (Benner, 1984).

Data Pertinent specifics that are collected and reported, but are not organized, analyzed, or interpreted. Examples include weight, height, blood pressure reading, and the number of fluid ounces of milk that a baby drank.

Documentation Automated or manual record system used by practitioners to report and store client data.

eHealth Convenient, readily accessible health-related information and communication available by using e-mail, the World Wide Web, and rapidly developing technology devices.

Electronic Health Record Longitudinal collection of clinical and demographic client-specific data that are stored in a computer readable format. Used instead of electronic medical record or computerized patient record.

Etiology Causal factors.

Expert Fifth stage in the Dreyfus model of skill acquisition, in which the practitioner has an intuitive grasp of a problem because of extensive background experience, and accurately identifies the problem without considering a large number of alternatives (Benner, 1984).

Hardware Physical components of a computer system.

Health State of complete physical, mental, and social well-being and not merely the absence of disease or infirmity (World Health Organization, 2004).

Home Care Health care and social services provided by freestanding and facility-based community agencies at the client's residence, work site, or other location. Synonyms include community health, visiting nurse, and district nursing services.

Hospice Care Health care and social services provided to the terminally ill. Services focus on physical, emotional, and spiritual needs rather than on cure.

Information Collection of related data that has been organized and has meaning.

Informatics Study of the structure/properties of information and the process of communication.

Information Management Integration of clinical, demographic, financial, administrative, and staffing data; manipulation or processing of these data; and production of various reports that transform data into meaningful information for decision making.

Information Technology Development and use of diverse hardware, software, networks, and procedures to process and communicate data.

Interoperability Ability to exchange coded data between and among computerized documentation systems after comparability and compatibility are established.

Knowledge Information that has been organized, analyzed, and synthesized.

Long-Term Care Health care and social services provided by home care agencies, residential facilities, or rehabilitation centers that are designed for dependent clients.

Novice First stage in the Dreyfus model of skill acquisition, in which the practitioner has no background understanding of the situation requiring that performance is based on rules (Benner, 1984).

Nurse-Managed Center Health care site that primarily offers outpatient nursing clinic services designed for a target population.

Nurse Practitioner Registered nurse with a master's degree or certificate who is licensed to diagnose, treat, and prescribe medications to a specific group of clients.

Objective Data Client observations and measurements obtained by practitioners.

Other Community Care Health care and social services provided at ambulatory care centers, occupational health offices, and other sites not included in the other definitions.

Point-of-Care Technology Automated information system that is designed to receive data where client care is provided and send those data to multiple locations.

Practice Use of knowledge and skill by a practitioner to provide health care and social services that improve and maintain health and prevent, assess, and treat illness.

Practitioner Professional who provides health care and/or social services to clients.

Primary Prevention Measures designed to promote clients' optimal health and provide specific protection against illness, injuries, and disabilities; implemented before a problem develops.

Proficient Fourth stage in the Dreyfus model of skill acquisition, in which the practitioner perceives a situation as a whole; performance is guided by an intuitive grasp based on a background understanding (Benner, 1984).

Provider Organization whose employees offer formalized health care and social services.

Public Health Care Health care and social services provided by local, county, and state health departments at the client's residence or work site or at schools or clinics. Synonyms include community health and health visitor services.

Quality Improvement Process of continuously evaluating and enhancing the level of excellence, effectiveness, and efficiency of services.

Record Audit Review and critique of client records intended to provide positive feedback to practitioners for accurate and consistent documentation, identify missing or incorrect entries, and stimulate improved documentation in the future.

Reliability Degree of consistency an instrument/classification provides when measuring the attribute for which it was designed.

Secondary Prevention Measures designed to reduce the duration and severity of illness or injury by identifying problems early and providing effective interventions; implemented soon after a problem develops.

Software Computer program providing the instructions to enable computer hardware to operate.

Standards Statements that describe acceptable levels of achievement. Includes practice standards (quality improvement programs, guidelines, policies, and regulations), professional standards (educational requirements, scope of practice, and licensure), and technical standards (interchange, integration, storage, and retrieval among diverse data systems).
Subjective Data Pertinent specifics obtained from the client or another person that reflect the client's viewpoint.
Tertiary Prevention Measures designed to reduce residual defects and disabilities that follow illness, primarily by providing rehabilitation to maximize the remaining capacities; implemented after a problem has developed.
Validity Degree to which an instrument/classification measures what it is designed to measure.
Wisdom Knowledge that is understood and applied with sound judgment.

Omaha System Glossary

GENERAL TERMS

Aggregate Data Problem, intervention, and/or outcome data that are grouped together.
Assessment Collection of pertinent objective and subjective client data; first step or concept of the problem solving process. Use of the Problem Classification Scheme enables the practitioner to operationalize assessment before completing problem identification.
Classification Process of arranging similar terms into groups according to a specific model.
Concepts Ideas that represent a merger of specific, familiar, concrete terms or objects into more general levels of abstraction; building blocks of a classification or taxonomy.
Critical Thinking Careful analysis using facts, intuition, and experience intended to result in sound judgment.
Decision Making Selection of a course of action after considering the advantages and disadvantages of alternatives.
Evaluation Process designed to measure outcomes and compare results of care to designated standards; fourth step or concept of the problem solving process. Use of the Problem Rating Scale for Outcomes enables the practitioner to operationalize evaluation.
Evidenced-Based Practice Selection of interventions based on accurate client data and current research. The practitioner combines critical thinking and the problem solving process, and often refers to best practices, guidelines, standards, protocols, or clinical pathways.
Planning and Intervention Proposed and completed care actions and activities for diverse clients; third step or concept of the problem solving process. Use of the Intervention Scheme enables the practitioner to operationalize planning and intervention.
Omaha System Research-based approach to practice, documentation, and information management that incorporates the Problem Classification Scheme, Intervention Scheme, and Problem Rating Scale for Outcomes.
Omaha System Model Circular, dynamic, epidemiological, interactive conceptual model that represents the standardized instruments of the Omaha System and is based on the problem solving process, client-practitioner relationship/partnership, and concepts of critical thinking, clinical decision making, and quality improvement.
Problem Identification Clinical judgment based on assessment data; identification or diagnosis of client interests, potential risks, signs, or symptoms; second step or concept of the problem solving process. Use of the Problem Classification enables the practitioner to operationalize problem identification after completing assessment.

Problem-Solving Process Assessment, problem identification, planning and intervention, and evaluation steps or concepts that guide multidisciplinary health care practice and provide feedback loops to practitioners. Nurses often use the synonym *nursing process* whereas physicians use *medical diagnostic process.*

Relationship Development Art of establishing a therapeutic partnership between practitioners and clients by combining health care services, understanding, self-respect, motivation, professionalism, and a genuine concern for others; a partnership arrangement. The existence of this partnership provides a context for interactions within the Omaha System model.

Taxonomy Science of classification and arrangement of terms and concepts at levels from general to specific, according to established principles and rules.

Terminology Study of symbols or terms used by one or more disciplines in health care and social services. The American Nurses Association developed a recognition process for diverse terminologies.

Theory Coherent set of concepts; the relationships among the concepts can be described.

PROBLEM CLASSIFICATION SCHEME TERMS

Actual Client problem status characterized by the existence of one or more signs and symptoms. Used as a problem modifier that appears at the third level of the Problem Classification Scheme.

Community Groups, schools, clinics, neighborhoods, or other larger geographic areas that share a common physical environment and ownership of a health-related problem. Used as a problem modifier that appears at the third level of the Problem Classification Scheme.

Details Descriptive data that explain client interest in or concern about a specific problem. The practitioner identifies, describes, and documents details when selecting the modifier Health Promotion.

Domains Four general areas that represent health care practice and provide organizational groupings for client problems. Appear at the first level of the Problem Classification Scheme.

Environmental Domain Material resources and physical surroundings both inside and outside the living area, neighborhood, and broader community. Appears at the first level of the Problem Classification Scheme.

Family Social unit or related group of individuals who live together and share ownership of a health-related problem. Used as a problem modifier that appears at the third level of the Problem Classification Scheme.

Health Promotion Client status characterized by interest in increasing knowledge, behavior, and health expectations, as well as developing strengths and resources to enhance well-being in the absence of risk factors, signs, or symptoms. Used as a problem modifier that appears at the third level of the Problem Classification Scheme.

Health-Related Behaviors Domain Patterns of activities that maintain or promote wellness, promote recovery, and decrease the risk of disease. Appears at the first level of the Problem Classification Scheme.

High Priority Practitioner's judgment that a problem should be addressed promptly, based on recommendations from clients, referral sources, and others. When a problem is considered high priority, the practitioner documents the problem, provides interventions, and completes ratings.

Individual Person who experiences a health-related problem. Used as a problem modifier that appears at the third level of the Problem Classification Scheme.

Low Priority Practitioner's judgment that a problem is of secondary concern as compared to other problems, based on recommendations from clients, referral sources, and others. When a problem is considered low priority, the practitioner documents the problem, but does not provide interventions or complete ratings until the client's needs change or increase.

Modifiers Two sets of terms (Individual, Family, Community and Health Promotion, Potential, Actual) used in conjunction with problems, which allow practitioners to identify to whom the problem pertains and the degree of severity in relation to client strengths, concerns, risk factors, signs, and symptoms.

Physiological Domain Functions and processes that maintain life. Appears at the first level of the Problem Classification Scheme.

Potential Client status characterized by the absence of signs and symptoms and the presence of patterns, practices, behaviors, or risk factors that may preclude optimal health. Used as a problem modifier that appears at the third level of the Problem Classification Scheme.

Problem Classification Scheme Comprehensive, orderly, nonexhaustive, mutually exclusive taxonomy designed to identify clients' health-related concerns. One of the three components or standardized instruments of the Omaha System.

Problems Unique client concerns, needs, strengths, issues, foci, or conditions that affect any aspect of the client's well-being; nursing diagnoses stated from the client's perspective. There are 42 problems at the second level of the Problem Classification Scheme.

Psychosocial Domain Patterns of behavior, emotion, communication, relationships, and development. Appears at the first level of the Problem Classification Scheme.

Risk Factors Circumstances that increase the client's vulnerability to the development of a health problem. The practitioner identifies, describes, and documents risk factors when selecting the modifier Potential.

Signs Objective evidence about a client's problem. The practitioner identifies, describes, and documents signs and/or symptoms when selecting the modifier Actual. Appear at the fourth level of the Problem Classification Scheme.

Symptoms Subjective evidence about a client's problem. The practitioner identifies, describes, and documents symptoms and/or signs when selecting the modifier Actual. Appear at the fourth level of the Problem Classification Scheme.

INTERVENTION SCHEME TERMS

Case Management Activities such as coordination, advocacy, and referral that facilitate service delivery; promote assertiveness; guide the individual, family, or community toward use of appropriate resources; and improve communication among health and human service providers. Applicable to a specific problem. Appears at the first level of the Intervention Scheme.

Categories Four broad areas that provide a structure for describing practitioner actions or activities. Appear at the first level of the Intervention Scheme.

Client-Specific Information Detailed portion of a plan or intervention statement that is developed and documented by the practitioner. The User's Guide includes suggested client-specific information for all problems. Appears at the third level of the Intervention Scheme.

Interventions Actions or activities implemented to address a specific client problem and to improve, maintain, or restore health or prevent illness. An intervention statement consists of a category, one or more targets, and client-specific information.

Intervention Scheme Comprehensive, orderly, nonexhaustive, mutually exclusive taxonomy used to describe practitioners' actions and activities. One of the three components or standardized instruments of the Omaha System.

Plans Proposed actions or activities designed to establish a course of care for a particular client problem. A plan statement consists of a category, one or more targets, and client-specific information.

Surveillance Activities such as detection, measurement, critical analysis, and monitoring intended to identify the individual, family, or community's status in relation to a given condition or phenomenon. Applicable to a specific problem. Appears at the first level of the Intervention Scheme.

Targets Unique objects of practitioner actions or activities that serve to further describe interventions. There are 75 targets at the second level of the Intervention Scheme.

Teaching, Guidance, and Counseling Activities designed to provide information and materials, encourage action and responsibility for self-care and coping, and assist the individual, family, or community to make decisions and solve problems. Applicable to a specific problem. Appear at the first level of the Intervention Scheme.

Treatments and Procedures Technical activities such as wound care, specimen collection, resistive exercises, and medication prescriptions that are designed to prevent, decrease, or alleviate signs and symptoms for the individual, family, or community. Applicable to a specific problem. Appear at the first level of the Intervention Scheme.

PROBLEM RATING SCALE FOR OUTCOMES TERMS

Admission Ratings Problem-specific numeric ratings for Knowledge, Behavior, and Status completed the first time the problem is identified as high priority for the client.

Behavior Observable responses, actions, or activities of the client fitting the occasion or purpose. Describes what a client "does." One of the three separate scales of the Problem Rating Scale for Outcomes.

Discharge Ratings Problem-specific numeric ratings for Knowledge, Behavior, and Status completed at the time the problem is resolved, is changed to low priority, or when the client is discharged.

Interim Ratings Problem-specific numeric ratings for Knowledge, Behavior, and Status completed at periodic intervals during the course of service delivery to the client and while the problem is identified as high priority.

Knowledge Ability of the client to remember and interpret information. Describes what a client "knows." One of the three separate scales of the Problem Rating Scale for Outcomes.

Outcomes Management Systematic process of aggregating, analyzing, and interpreting data graphically followed by the dissemination of information.

Problem Rating Scale for Outcomes Comprehensive, systematic, recurring/evaluation framework designed to measure client progress in relation to specific health-related problems. One of the three components or standardized instruments of the Omaha System.

Ratings Five numeric choices that comprise three Likert-type scales; the numeric choices and scales depict the most negative to the most positive state of a problem area in relation to the client's Knowledge, Behavior, and Status. Practitioners need to determine ratings based on the client's data, not their values or biases.

Status Condition of the client in relation to objective and subjective characteristics. Describes how a client "is." One of the three separate scales of the Problem Rating Scale for Outcomes.

REFERENCES

Benner, P. (1984). *From Novice to Expert: Excellence and Power in Clinical Nursing Practice.* Menlo Park, California, Addison-Wesley.

World Health Organization. (2004). *Constitution of the World Health Organization.* Retrieved February 20, 2004 from the Internet: *http://www.policy.who.int/cgi-bin/om-isapi.*

INDEX

B

C

INDEX

I

INDEX

O

P

Q

INDEX

INDEX

INDEX